ACE→

Coaching Senior Fitness

Empowering Older Adults Through a Client-centered Approach

AMERICAN COUNCIL ON EXERCISE®

EDITORS

SABRENA JO, MS

CHRIS GAGLIARDI, MS

CEDRIC X. BRYANT, PHD, FACSM

DANIEL J. GREEN

Library of Congress Control Number: 2020920284

ISBN 978-890720-81-0

Distributed by:
American Council on Exercise
4851 Paramount Drive
San Diego, CA 92123
(858) 576-6500
(858) 576-6564 FAX
ACEfitness.org

Project Editor: Daniel J. Green
Technical Editors: Sabrena Jo, MS, Chris Gagliardi, MS, Cedric X. Bryant, PhD, Dianne McCaughey, PhD, and Jan Schroeder, PhD
Art Direction: Devon Browning
Creative Design and Cover Design: Rick Gray
Production: Nancy Garcia
Photography: Rob Andrew, Matt Gossman, Vertex Photography
Anatomical Illustration: James Staunton
Stock Images: Getty.com, AdobeStock.com
Index: Kathi Unger
Cover and Exercise Models: Courtney Brickner, Jermaine Castaneda, Mary Cherwink, Jacque Crockford, Sabrena Jo, Chris Kiepfer, Kelli Lessie, Martha Ranson, Jessica Talbi, Tiffany Tate, Nicole Thompson, Don Thibedeau

Production Services provided by Westchester Education Services of Dayton, Ohio — A U.S. Employee-owned Company

Acknowledgments:
Thanks to the entire American Council on Exercise staff for their support and guidance through the process of creating this textbook. Thank you to Hoist Fitness for hosting photo shoots for this publication.

NOTICE
The field of health and wellness is ever-changing. As new research and clinical experience broaden our knowledge, changes in programming and standards are required. The authors and the publisher of this work have checked with sources believed to be reliable in their efforts to provide information that is complete and generally in accord with the standards accepted at the time of publication. However, in view of the possibility of human error or changes in industry standards, neither the authors nor the publisher nor any other party who has been involved in the preparation or publication of this work warrants that the information contained herein is in every respect accurate or complete, and they are not responsible for any errors or omissions or the results obtained from the use of such information. Readers are encouraged to confirm the information contained herein with other sources.

DISCLAIMERS
Moving forward, ACE will use "they" and "their" in place of "he/she" and "his/her." This change eliminates gender biases associated with these pronouns and is more inclusive of all individuals across the gender spectrum. Note that all ACE content moving forward will reflect this update, and previous content will be updated as needed. It is ACE's goal to share our mission to Get People Moving with all people, regardless of race, gender, sexual orientation, physical or intellectual abilities, religious beliefs, ethnic background, or socioeconomic status.

Due to restrictions related to COVID-19, we were not able to conduct photoshoots during the production of this text. For this reason, some assessments and exercises are depicted using non-senior models.

ACE's Mission Is to Get People Moving.
Job # P21-001

Table of Contents

Contributors and Reviewers

SABRENA JO, MS, is the Director of Science and Research for the American Council on Exercise and ACE Liaison to the Scientific Advisory Panel. Jo has been actively involved in the fitness industry since 1987. As an ACE Certified Group Fitness Instructor, Personal Trainer, and Health Coach, she has taught group exercise and owned her own personal-training and health-coaching businesses and is a relentless pursuer of finding ways to help people start and stick with physical activity. Jo is a former full-time faculty member in the Kinesiology and Physical Education Department at California State University, Long Beach. She has a bachelor's degree in exercise science, a master's degree in physical education/biomechanics, and is pursuing a PhD in exercise psychology from the University of Kansas.

CHRISTOPHER GAGLIARDI, MS, is the Scientific Education Content Manager of the American Council on Exercise, where he creates, reviews, edits, and updates educational resources and serves as a key contributor to the development and revision of written, audio, and video content. He also serves as a subject matter expert for video and photoshoots and for media requests. Gagliardi is an ACE Certified Personal Trainer, Health Coach, Group Fitness Instructor, and Medical Exercise Specialist, NSCA Certified Strength and Conditioning Specialist, National Board Certified Health and Wellness Coach (NBC-HWC), and NASM Certified Personal Trainer who loves to share his enthusiasm for fitness with others and is committed to lifelong learning. He holds a bachelor's degree in kinesiology from San Diego State University, a master's degree in kinesiology from A.T. Still University, and a certificate in orthotics from Northwestern University Fienberg School of Medicine.

CEDRIC X. BRYANT, PHD, FACSM, is the President and Chief Science Officer of the American Council on Exercise, where he stewards ACE's development of strategies to deliver exercise-science and behavior-change education. He's responsible for driving innovation in the area of behavior-change programming, overseeing the development of programs that ACE Certified Professionals can utilize to help people adopt and sustain healthier lifestyles. Furthermore, he leads ACE's exploration of how science-based programs and interventions appropriately integrate into healthcare and public health. Bryant has authored, co-authored or edited more than 35 books and written over 300 articles and columns in fitness trade magazines and peer-reviewed exercise science journals. He represents ACE as a national and international presenter, writer and subject-matter expert (SME), and highly sought-after media spokesperson. Finally, Dr. Bryant shares his expertise as a member of the National Academy of Medicine's Obesity Solutions Roundtable, the National Board for Health & Wellness Coaching's Council of Advisors, the Arthritis Foundation's Expert Panel – Exercise Science and Fitness

SME, the Physical Activity Alliance, Exercise Is Medicine's Credentialing Committee, the Centers for Disease Control and Prevention's *Active People, Healthy Nation* Partner Committee, and the World Health Organization's *Global Action Plan on Physical Activity*. He earned both his doctorate in physiology and master's degree in exercise science from Pennsylvania State University, where he received the Penn State Alumni Fellow Award, the school's highest alumni honor that is given to select alumni who are considered leaders in their professional fields.

DIANNE McCAUGHEY, PHD, is an award-winning fitness specialist with 35-plus years of experience in personal training, group exercise, coaching, and post-rehabilitation. Dr. McCaughey is an international speaker, author, and presenter who has traveled the world touching lives and emphasizing optimal wellness of the mind, body, and spirit. She has been a master trainer for ACE since 2000. As a gerontologist, her expertise is successful aging in all domains. The two books she has authored are designed to coach individuals on mental and emotional wellness, as well as physical health, to help them age with grace and vigor. In addition, Dr. McCaughey is an international corporate and private seminar facilitator for personal growth, empowerment, and team building; some of her previous clients included Hewlett-Packard and the United Nations.

NATALIE DIGATE MUTH, MD, MPH, RDN, CSSD, FAAP, FACSM, is a board-certified pediatrician, obesity medicine specialist, and registered dietitian. She directs a healthy weight clinic in Carlsbad, California, and is an Adjunct Assistant Professor at UCLA Fielding School of Public Health. She is a member of the Motivational Interviewing Network of Trainers. Dr. Muth has published over 100 articles, books, and book chapters, including *Coaching Behavior Change* (ACE, 2014), *ACE Fitness Nutrition Manual* (ACE, 2013), *Family Fit Plan: A 30-Day Wellness Transformation* (American Academy of Pediatrics, 2019), *The Picky Eater Project: 6 Weeks to Healthier, Happier Family Mealtimes* (American Academy of Pediatrics, 2016), *"Eat Your Vegetables!" and Other Mistakes Parents Make: Redefining How to Raise Healthy Eaters* (Healthy Learning, 2012), the textbook *Sports Nutrition for Allied Health Professionals* (F.A. Davis, 2014), and several chapters in the *ACE Diabetes Prevention Lifestyle Coaching Handbook* (ACE, 2019). She holds a Bachelor of Science degree in psychology and physiological science from UCLA, and a Master of Public Health and Medical Doctor degree from the University of North Carolina-Chapel Hill.

JAN SCHROEDER, PHD, is a professor in the Department of Kinesiology at California State University, Long Beach. She is the coordinator of the Bachelor of Science degree in fitness as well as past department chair. Dr. Schroeder holds more than 20 licenses and certifications, from Certified Group Exercise Instructor to Certified Exercise Physiologist to X-Ray Technician – Bone Densitometry, and she has published more than 60 research and applied articles and prepared more than 40 presentations. She also owns Garage Girls Fitness, both an online and in-person training platform. Her degrees include a bachelor's degree in Movement and Exercise Science from Chapman University, a master's degree in Physical Education/Exercise Physiology, and a doctorate in Physical Education/Exercise Physiology with a specialization in Gerontology from the University of Kansas.

Foreword

The breadth and complexity of the senior population cannot be overstated. Just as with younger clients, these individuals present a spectrum of health status, fitness level, disease state, and experience with exercise and nutrition. *Coaching Senior Fitness* presents the content professionals need to work with senior clients and empower them to take charge of their long-term function, health, and fitness.

For those of us who make our living advocating for healthy and physically active lifestyles, it may come as a surprise to realize how little many older adults know about physical activity. However, most older adults were educated at a time and in a culture during which little was known about the health benefits of physical activity and both professionals and members of the public were skeptical about the need to remain physically active after retirement. In the pages of this book, you will find a succinct and easy-to-read summary of the current evidence base in the area of exercise and physical activity for older adults. As an exercise professional or health coach, one of the most important things you can do for your clients is to help them understand that there are many different ways to be active. By following some of the strategies and suggestions presented in this book, you can help your older clients realize the many benefits associated with a physically active lifestyle.

Many years ago, when I was a young assistant professor, my mother called me from her home in England and asked me to help her become more physically active. At that time, my mom was in her early 60s, a widow living alone, working full-time as a teacher. Mom told me that she knew that she was supposed to do 30 minutes of aerobic exercise on most days of the week, but by the time she got home from a long day at school she was much too tired to even imagine doing that much exercise. For her, the physical-activity guidelines seemed like an impossible mountain to climb. In my advice to Mom, I suggested that when she got home from work, before she took off her coat, she should ask herself a simple question: "Do I have the energy to walk to the shops at the end of the road?" The shops were about 100 yards from her home and she often walked there to buy milk and other groceries. If the answer to the question was "yes," she simply had to walk to the shops and come back. If the answer was "no," it was perfectly fine to take off her coat and relax. I asked her to mark her wall calendar each day that she decided to walk to the corner store. We agreed that I would call back in a couple of weeks (this was before the era of Skype, Facetime, and Zoom). When I called back two weeks later, the first words out of her mouth were, "I had three check marks on the calendar last week and four this week." She was ecstatic; she had broken through a barrier. A few weeks later, I suggested that when she got to the corner store, she should ask herself another question: "Am I ready to go back home, or do I want to walk around the block?" For the next 20 years my mom maintained an active daily routine that she credits for her independence and high quality of life. Today, she is 90 years old and continues to live independently in her own home. I am not suggesting that the strategy I used with my mom will work for all seniors. However, it is clear that if we are to be successful in supporting sedentary individuals to change their behavior, we will need to pay close attention to their goals and preferences as we work with them to develop a program that is meaningful and that helps them overcome their personal obstacles and barriers.

What sets this text apart is that in addition to the science-based content focusing on physical activity and nutrition that ACE is well known for, behavior-change strategies are woven throughout. The ACE Mover Method™ philosophy and ACE ABC Approach™ will enable the health coach or exercise professional to empower their clients to make behavioral changes to improve their health, fitness, and overall quality of life by recognizing that clients are the foremost experts on themselves and are resourceful and capable of change.

This combined approach to the art and science of behavior change, as well as nutrition and exercise, makes *Coaching Senior Fitness* an essential part of your library. Whether you are a relatively inexperienced exercise professional in a club setting who occasionally works with older adults or a manager of a hospital-based fitness facility, this textbook is an indispensable tool that you will return to throughout your career.

Wojtek J. Chodzko-Zajko, PhD
Dean, Graduate College
Shahid and Ann Carlson Khan Professor
University of Illinois at Urbana-Champaign

Introduction

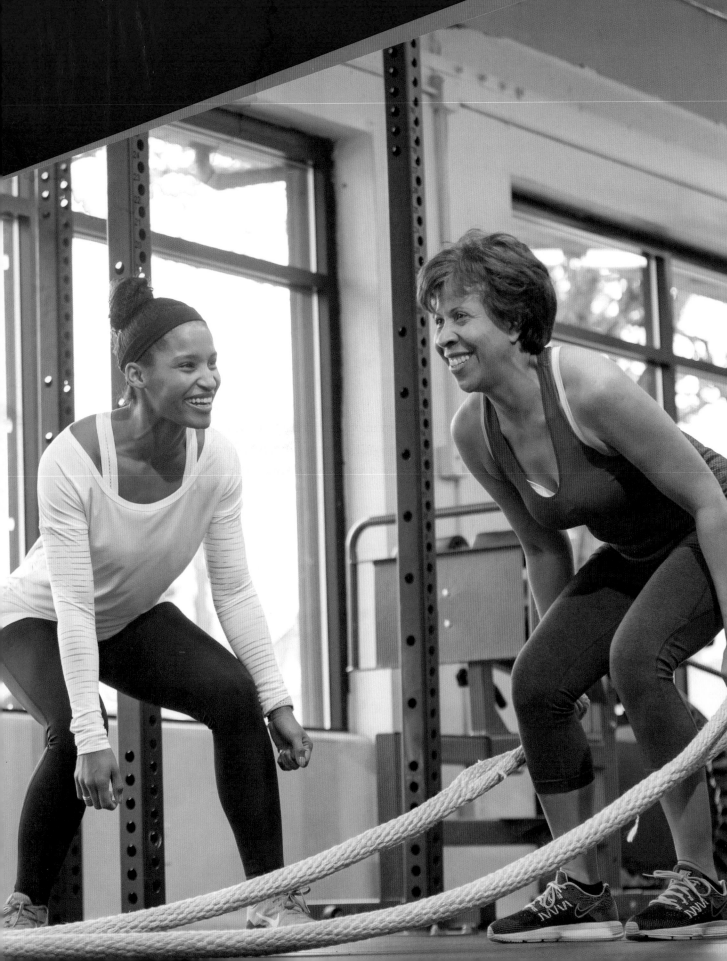

Coaching Senior Fitness is the most current, complete picture of the behavior-change and exercise-science knowledge and techniques that health coaches and exercise professionals can use to empower their older clients to reach their goals through safe, effective, and personalized exercise programming. This text takes an application-based approach that will enable professionals to offer client-centered coaching and training and to better understand and communicate with their senior clients.

Features are included throughout—including Apply What You Know, Think It Through, Expand Your Knowledge, and the ACE Mover Method™—that bring theoretical concepts to life and ask you to pause to gauge your understanding of the topic being discussed, as well as your comfort level with utilizing that knowledge in your everyday work with senior clients. We encourage you to take advantage of these application-based tools so that you will be better prepared to thrive in real-world situations.

Chapter 1: An Introduction to the Senior Population introduces one of the overarching themes of this text—the importance of treating every client, of every age, as an individual. This chapter covers the unique needs of the senior population as well as techniques for communicating to effectively learn about each client's individual needs and goals—including the ACE Mover Method and ACE ABC Approach™. Finally, this chapter closes with a discussion of how to create a safe physical and psychological environment for older clients.

Chapter 2: Motivation and Adherence introduces several theories of behavioral change and then offers practical tips for turning these theories into actionable steps for clients. It is essential that exercise professionals do not assume that all clients are at the same stage of readiness, and this chapter provides the tools that professionals need to identify where their clients stand and then set and pursue appropriate and meaningful goals.

Chapter 3: Physiology of Aging and Exercise explains the physiology of the aging process and covers the physiological and psychological benefits of participating in regular physical activity as one grows older, which range from reversing age-related changes in cardiovascular and musculoskeletal function to improving cognitive function and relieving depression and anxiety.

Chapter 4: Senior Nutrition begins by outlining the physiological changes associated with aging that affect nutrition choices, including sensory changes and structural changes in the various systems of the body. In addition, the relationship between nutrition and various chronic diseases of older adulthood, including osteoporosis and sarcopenic obesity, is discussed. This chapter also teaches the nutrition and hydration guidelines that all health coaches and exercise professionals who work with older adults should know.

Chapter 5: Preparticipation Health Screening and Interview is an extension of the theme of personalization that carries throughout this text. The process outlined in this chapter—which features several forms and questionnaires that health coaches and exercise professionals can use as models when developing their own paperwork—is the starting point from which all client–exercise professional relationships must develop. Finally, the chapter closes with a discussion of common medications and how they may impact the body's response to exercise.

Chapter 6: ACE Integrated Fitness Training Model introduces ACE's comprehensive training model, which covers both cardiorespiratory and muscular training. The ACE IFT Model allows for truly individualized fitness programming for older adults. This chapter also covers special considerations specific to working with older clientele on balance and flexibility, as well muscular and cardiorespiratory exercise.

Chapter 7: Conducting Assessments begins with several health-related resting measures, including anthropometric measurements, heart rate and blood pressure checks, and a static postural assessment. This is followed by fitness assessments, including the Senior Fitness Test as well as balance and gait assessments, cardiorespiratory assessments, core function assessments, and movement assessments. The techniques and protocols learned in this chapter will help you determine where on the broad spectrum of function, health, fitness, and performance each individual client falls.

Chapter 8: Exercise Programming goes into tremendous detail in outlining how to utilize the knowledge gained through screening and assessments when training clients of any level of ability. This chapter goes through the three phases of each component of the ACE IFT Model and presents exercises and techniques specific to each.

Chapter 9: Common Health Challenges Faced by Older Adults covers many of the health challenges that health coaches and exercise professionals are likely to encounter when working with senior clients. The chapter is organized into cardiovascular and cerebrovascular disorders, pulmonary disorders, musculoskeletal conditions, metabolic disorders, neurological disorders, and visual and auditory disorders.

It can be easy for many health coaches and exercise professionals to buy into misconceptions or make assumptions about older people without taking the time to get to know them, both in terms of their goals and personalities as well as in terms of their capabilities and exercise experiences. As is made clear throughout this book, there is no homogeneous "senior population," as this group includes everyone from a highly fit woman in her 50s seeking to improve her tennis game to a man in his 90s working to gain the leg strength to stand up from a chair on his own. This book is designed to help health coaches and exercise professionals effectively coach each client along that broad continuum and then develop safe and appropriate exercise programs that help clients reach their individual goals.

Sabrena Jo, MS
Director of Science and Research

Daniel J. Green
Senior Project Manager and Editor for
Publications and Content Development

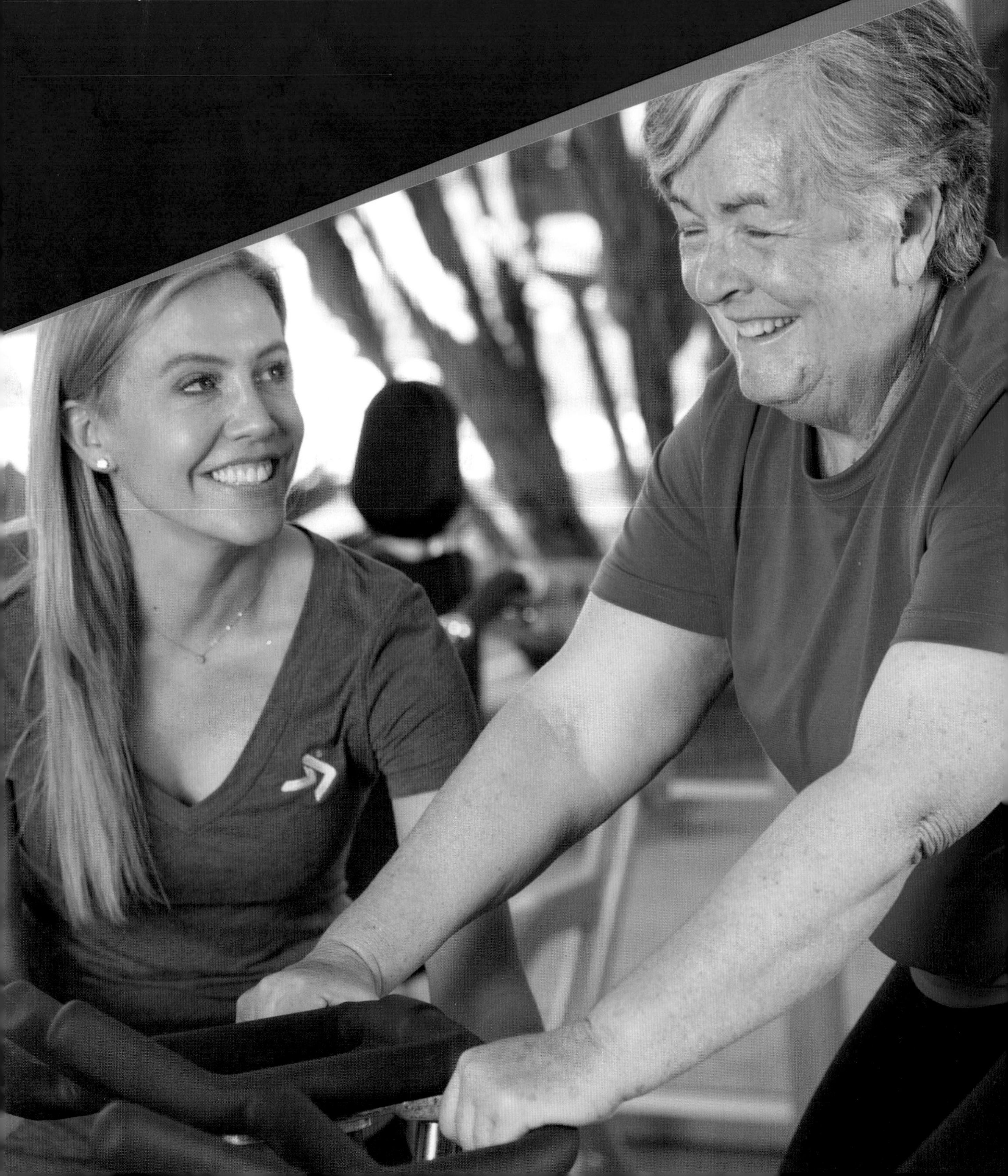

CHAPTER 1

An Introduction to the Senior Population

LEARNING OBJECTIVES

After reading this chapter, you will be able to:

▸ Dispel myths that are commonly ascribed to older adults regarding fitness, communication, attitudes, and learning ability

▸ Briefly describe unique characteristics of older clients regarding memory, fitness status, and self-efficacy

▸ Apply strategies to enhance communication with senior clients

▸ Create a fitness environment that is safe, both physically and psychologically, for older adults

While defining and making generalizations about a generation is always ill-advised, it is especially problematic in a textbook presenting training guidelines and recommendations, as there is clearly no "one size fits all" approach when it comes to designing a lifestyle-modification program for such a broad population. Considering that the senior population potentially includes everyone from 50 to 100+ years old, it becomes obvious that any statement about this population as a whole is a gross generalization. The terms "seniors" and "older adults" encompass multiple generations. The oldest members of Generation X, those born in 1965, now make up the youngest element of the senior population, while baby boomers (born 1946–1964) make up the largest segment of the older adult population. The oldest seniors are from the GI generation (born 1901–1924) and the silent generation (born 1925–1945). As time marches on, these generations will sadly die off as new generations begin to age and bring their own uniqueness to the marketplace.

Most health coaches and exercise professionals would never pretend to know everything about a 30-year-old client based simply on their age, yet many are prone to making assumptions about older adults without really getting to know them. As is discussed throughout this textbook, there is a broad spectrum of health status, fitness level, disease state, and experience with exercise and nutrition among the senior population. When utilizing the screening and assessments presented in Chapters 5 and 7, exercise professionals will observe the tremendous differences among the most fit and most frail members of this group of clients. As when working with clients of any age, exercise professionals must take a client-centered approach to understanding older adults' health history, program goals and preferences, past exercise experiences, preferred methods of tracking progress, and readiness to change to determine whether it may be helpful to administer certain assessments before designing a personalized exercise program. It is necessary for the exercise professional to assess each client's function to discover any movement compensations or dysfunctions, regardless of age.

EXPAND YOUR KNOWLEDGE

Myths about Senior Clients

The following myths should be dispelled when working with seniors:

▸ *Chronological age dictates how an older adult behaves:* The process of aging varies widely and is affected by many factors, including personality, belief system, experiences, habits, health, **social support,** the physiological and psychological responses to aging, and the loss of friends, loved ones, and meaningful relationships. Thus, exercise professionals should take this into account and treat their older clients as individuals with their own unique contexts, histories, and circumstances. It is important to remember that there are master athletes over 100 years of age and **sedentary** individuals in their 30s.

▸ *The older one is, the harder it is to learn new things:* Intelligence is both crystallized (from lived experiences that build wisdom) and fluid, which involves learning new skills on the spot. Research suggests that **neuroplasticity** has the potential to take place at any age and **cognitive** functions can improve with a combination of physical and cognitive activities (Bamidis et al., 2014).

▸ *As one ages, one naturally becomes older and wiser:* Stereotyping, both positive and negative, can be detrimental. Believing that most seniors are wiser is simply not accurate, just as it is not true that most older clients will experience **dementia.** There is overwhelming evidence that the way in which people think about aging can have a significant impact on a wide array of health and well-being outcomes (Robertson, 2016).

▸ *Older adults become more resistant to new ideas as they age:* Many older clients may be very receptive to new information, especially if it involves their health, fitness, and well-being—depending in large measure upon how the concepts are presented. Adults learn continuously from life experiences and therefore are often open to pursuing new interests and goals.

▸ *Older adults' work productivity declines:* Between 2016 and 2026, the number of Americans in the workplace over the age of 65 will increase from 35.7 to 42.1 million, representing nearly one-quarter of the labor force (U.S Senate: Special Committee on Aging, 2017). From 2000 to 2016, employment rates for older adults had outpaced the overall growth of the labor force and are projected to grow by 4.2% annually for individuals 65 to 74 and by 6.7% for workers 75 and older. Interestingly, one in three Americans over the age of 50 plans to work full-time past the age of 65 and many men and women will transition from full-time to part-time work before leaving the workforce altogether, whether from economic need or the satisfaction derived from the work (U.S. Senate: Special Committee on Aging, 2017). Unretirement, or a return to work after being retired for some time, is also an increasingly common phenomenon among older adults.

▶ *Older adults prefer quiet and tranquil daily lives:* It would be a mistake for exercise professionals to believe that older adults prefer a sedentary lifestyle. A hallmark of the baby boomer generation, which makes up the majority of older adults, is that they stay active as a key to health and well-being.

❋ EXPAND YOUR KNOWLEDGE

Bridging the Digital Divide

Ted Vickey, PhD, ACE Senior Advisor for Fitness Technology and member, ACE Scientific Advisory Panel

There is a misconception that older adults are averse to technology. However, a poll by the Pew Research Center found that there has been a dramatic shift in the adoption of technology in recent years. From smartphones to social media, tech use has become the norm across all generations. As of 2019, nine in 10 U.S. adults say they go online, 81% say they own a smartphone, and 72% say they use social media (Hitlin, 2018).

Once online, most seniors make the internet a normal part of their daily routines. Roughly 75% of older internet users go online at least daily, including 17% who say they go online about once a day, 51% who indicate they do so several times a day, and 8% who say they use the internet almost constantly—and these numbers are even higher among cell phone users (Pew Research Center, 2017).

Pew Research Center surveys have found that the oldest adults face some unique barriers to adopting new technologies—from a lack of confidence in using new technologies to physical challenges that make it difficult to manipulate devices (Anderson & Perrin, 2017). Despite these concerns and challenges, there are a number of areas in which seniors hold relatively positive views of technology and technology-related topics. For instance, at a broad level, 58% of seniors feel that technology has had a mostly positive effect on society, while just 4% feel the impact has been mostly negative (Anderson & Perrin, 2017).

All generations will interact with health, fitness, and wellness technology, but not all generations will interact with that technology in the same way. Younger generations may want to track outdoor activities using GPS or have a virtual visit with a physician, whereas the older population may use technologies to measure **blood pressure** or communicate with family and friends using video chats. In either case, technology, if used well, can contribute to an individual's overall health, fitness, and well-being.

Research suggests that the baby boomer generation is open to using wearables, apps, and other connected health technologies to manage their health, and are interested in sharing such collected data with their healthcare teams (Wang et al., 2019). Once seniors are online and using technology, they engage at high levels with digital devices and content (Pew Research Center, 2017).

One of the major benefits for the older population to adopt the use of health technology is to allow seniors to "age in place" in their homes and live as long as possible outside of an assisted-care facility. Technology can be used to monitor movement, alert for falls, and remind people to take medication, which can allow them to live in the comfort of their own homes without the expense and potential anxiety of moving into an assisted-care facility. This use of technology can allow seniors to live with a sense of independence and pride and delay the need to move into an adult care facility in the later years of their lives.

Exercise professionals should empower clients to decrease the digital divide and help people of all ages live healthier lives through the effective use of technology.

Unique Needs of the Senior Population

MEMORY

One of the most common problems among older adults is memory loss, ranging from minor lapses that a client may find annoying or frustrating to dementia that can be truly debilitating. It is important for exercise professionals to have advanced education and certifications in cognitive training if they are working with this population. Neurological disorders, including **Parkinson's disease** and **Alzheimer's disease,** are discussed in detail in Chapter 9. To help clients who are struggling with memory issues, exercise professionals can do the following:

> ▶ Learn the level of cognitive impairment of each client.

> ▶ Be sure to provide a review of information from one training session or class to the next.

> ▶ Provide a written summary of workout routines and information for the client and/or caretaker.

> ▶ Focus on short-term, brief, and frequent information sharing, observing levels of both frustration and mastery.

> ▶ Understand that older clients may need time or clues to retrieve previously learned information.

> ▶ Use multimedia content, various forms of delivering information (showing, telling, and doing, while layering to add new information slowly), and ways to associate new information for memory retention. Combine cognitive and physical activities for a synergistic approach to brain health.

HEALTH AND FITNESS STATUS

Older adults often cope with various health conditions (see Chapter 9). It is important that exercise professionals properly screen for these conditions (see Chapter 5) and work with physicians and other healthcare professionals as appropriate. In addition, the physical-fitness assessments presented in Chapter 7 will allow the exercise professional to determine where on the fitness spectrum each client resides. It is imperative when

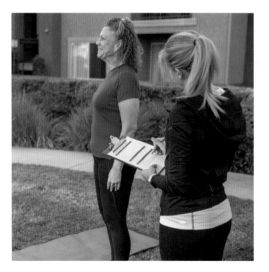

performing assessments that the safety of the client is considered and the proper assessment is chosen, even if it is subjective or through observation. Considering that the senior population includes everyone from Senior Olympians to frail older adults who may be restricted to chair-based exercise, it is clear that the use of assessments and screenings may be helpful in determining the best plan for each client. Keep in mind that the program is a collaborative plan that considers not only the physical aspects of the client, but also the mental and emotion aspects.

The health conditions covered in this textbook include:

▶ Cardiovascular and cerebrovascular disorders (**coronary artery disease, peripheral artery disease, hypertension,** and **stroke**)

▶ Respiratory problems [**Chronic obstructive pulmonary disease (COPD),** including **asthma, chronic bronchitis,** and **emphysema**]

▶ Musculoskeletal disorders (**arthritis** and low-back pain)

▶ Metabolic conditions (**diabetes, sarcopenic obesity, osteoporosis,** and **menopause**)

▶ Neurological disorders (dementia, Alzheimer's disease, and Parkinson's disease)

▶ Visual and auditory problems

In addition, **stability** and **mobility** issues (both how to assess them and how to address them via exercise program design) are discussed, as improving joint health and **balance** may improve the quality of life for many older adults.

SELF-EFFICACY

With older clients, **self-efficacy** (the degree to which an individual believes they can successfully perform a given behavior) often centers on reappraisals and misappraisals of their capabilities, given that the biological conceptions of aging typically focus on declining physical function (see Chapter 3). Tips for cultivating self-efficacy in older clients are presented later in this section. Exercise professionals should also be aware that beliefs about self-efficacy are a prime predictor of health-related behavior change and that targeted physical-activity interventions for older adults should focus on mastery experience, a decrease in negative mood states, and verbal persuasion in the form of self-persuasion (Warner et al., 2014). Strategies for helping older adults adopt healthy new behaviors and then maintaining these important lifestyle choices are covered in Chapter 2.

📖 APPLY WHAT YOU KNOW

Approaches for Working with Clients with Issues Related to Memory, Health and Fitness, and Self-efficacy

Memory:

▶ Learn and understand the level of cognitive impairment for each client.

▶ Discuss observations with the client and refer out when needed for further testing and diagnosis.

▶ Design exercise programs that are challenging, fun, purposeful, and appropriate without being frustrating.

▶ Gather further information and education on training clients with cognitive impairment and develop specific combined cognitive and physical activities for a synergistic approach to brain health.

Health and fitness:

▶ Screen and assess all clients using a thorough health-history and lifestyle questionnaire (see Figure 5-7, pages 145–148) and appropriate preparticipation assessments.

▶ Identify all risk factors and health conditions, including compensation patterns and other issues that negatively impact health and independence.

▶ Prioritize program design using the results of assessments to develop personalized programs designed to meet the physical and emotional needs of each client.

▶ Create additional programs (homework) for clients to accomplish on their own, thereby enabling enhanced progress and self-efficacy, which may lead to improved **adherence.**

Self-efficacy:

▶ Build a trusting, empathetic, and open communicative relationship with the client.

▶ Understand what stage of change clients are in and meet them at that level, using the ACE Mover Method™ to break down barriers and collaborate on goal setting.

▶ Collaborate on creating an appropriate program design to ensure a willingness and desire to participate.

▶ Continue collaboration and social support when progressing the program, while assuring that program enjoyment, positive experiences, and skill mastery are taking place.

Communication

Effective communication requires two willing parties, but the parties must do more than merely speak. They must be able and willing to listen carefully and respond in respectful, constructive ways. Exercise professionals need to be particularly responsive to the communication needs of their older adult clients. Because older adults often are stereotyped or patronized by others, they may be especially appreciative of attentive listening and understanding. The better the communication between an exercise professional and their clients, the more likely it is that the exercise professional will learn about potential barriers that could both physically and emotionally interfere with the program's success.

Unfortunately, younger people who have not spent much time around older adults may feel intimidated about communicating with them and rely upon familiar stereotypes to guide interactions. This type of **ageism,** when reflected in communication, can unfortunately have a negative impact on the quality of care received and ultimately impact the client's health and well-being (Burnes et al., 2019). These negative stereotypes and discrimination based on age can contribute to communication problems and misunderstandings between people and harm the client–professional relationship.

⚫️⚫️⚫️ **EXPAND YOUR KNOWLEDGE**

The Impact of Ageism on the Health of Older Adults

According to the World Health Organization (Officer & de la Fuente-Núñez, 2018), ageism is the stereotyping, prejudice, and discrimination against people based on their age and is believed to be the most socially normalized of any prejudice. But what influence do these attitudes and beliefs have on the health and well-being of older adults? A review of the literature evaluated the impact of age discrimination, negative age stereotypes, and negative self-perceptions on health (Chang et al., 2020). The results of this systematic review suggest that there is an association between ageism and poor quality of life and well-being, poor social relationships, mental and physical illness, cognitive impairment, reduced longevity, and risky health behaviors (e.g., unhealthy diet, smoking, excessive drinking, and medication noncompliance).

This review also showed a connection between ageism and exclusion from health research, lack of work opportunities, denied access to healthcare and treatments, and devalued lives of older persons. Interestingly, ageism was found to impact health across geography and time, as it was observed in 45 countries and across six continents and appeared in every year studied. Overall, ageism led to significantly worse health outcomes in 95.5% of the 422 studies reviewed (Chang et al., 2020). Therefore, it seems probable that ageism in the health and exercise setting could also contribute to a negative effect on the health and well-being of older adults. It is imperative to be understanding and build a positive **rapport** when working with older individuals who have experienced ageism. Once a mutually trusting relationship has been established, an optimistic and collaborative program can be created.

One especially common stereotype is that all older adults have problems communicating based on hearing loss, poor memory, or other factors. The reality, though, is that while some older clients may have hearing impairments, comprehension problems, or difficulties in finding the right words to express themselves, others may have excellent communication skills.

Younger adults and many caregivers of seniors with health problems often use what is known as "patronizing speech" or "elderspeak" when addressing older adults. This speech style is characterized by simplification strategies (e.g., speaking more slowly and using very simple grammar) and clarification strategies (e.g., speaking loudly and articulating very carefully) in addition to basing content on stereotypes of aging (Williams et al., 2018). While adjustments in speech patterns may be well-intentioned, older adults may feel they are being "talked down to." Exercise professionals must be aware of this type of speech pattern and avoid using it when working with older clientele.

On the other hand, people who use effective communication techniques with older adults can promote an environment that enhances their cognitive and functional abilities, as well as the client–professional relationship. Achieving optimal communication environments may contribute to higher levels of well-being for older adults and lead to increased quality of life. The major keys to effective communication are **attending, active listening, and empathetic responding.** In the fitness setting, attending refers to the exercise professional focusing their attention on the client rather than on internal thoughts or things going on in the external environment. Active listening requires focusing on both the spoken content and feelings or other messages to which the client is only alluding. Active listening can be difficult because it necessitates that professionals stay quiet and instead use body language to demonstrate that they are listening. In addition, the professional needs to become comfortable in the silence to allow the client to think and feel while communicating.

Empathetic responding can be more challenging. **Empathy** refers to understanding a person's experience from their perspective. Asking, "How would I feel in my client's situation?" is a good way to understand their point of view. Next, the exercise professional's response should accurately acknowledge the client's experience. Ideally, empathetic responses increase the client's awareness of their experiences.

Consider the case of Vivian, a 68-year-old client who said to her personal trainer, Joe, "These weight machines are so complicated. I still get confused about how to use them and have to ask for help, even after three weeks in the program!" Joe simply agreed that some of the machines are complicated and then immediately proceeded with reviewing their proper use. While his technical review may have been helpful to Vivian in some ways, Joe's response, which focused on only technical issues, could have left her feeling somewhat misunderstood and unsupported.

Now imagine that Vivian made the same statements to a different personal trainer, Tim. Before responding, Tim asked himself how he would feel in her situation and decided that he would probably feel embarrassed and/or discouraged. Tim then acknowledged these feelings in the empathetic response, "The weight machines can take quite a while to get used to, especially if you haven't used them before. It sounds like you feel badly about having to ask for help after three weeks, but it's great that you ask questions. You are doing a good job of learning the machines—you'll probably find that it will get easier with practice. If you ever have any questions, we are here for you and want you to feel comfortable with the exercises and set-ups. Remember, the more confident you are with your program, the more likely it is that you will do it."

Tim's understanding of Vivian's feelings, his reassurance that she was not a failure, and praise for asking questions increased her confidence in being able to master the machines, as well as her comfort with asking questions. Once Vivian indicated that she was ready, Tim reviewed the use of the problematic machines. This technical review was important to Vivian's safety and success, and it was of even greater value because it followed an empathetic response, which relieved some of her anxiety and allowed her to continue her efforts with greater ease and success.

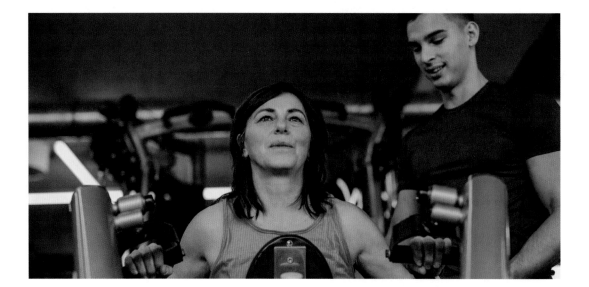

📖 APPLY WHAT YOU KNOW

Communication Considerations for Working with Older Adults

▸ *Listen without interruption to your clients' questions and statements before responding:* Exercise professionals often think they must have all of the answers to appear competent but may miss part of what a client is saying because they are busy thinking about how they will answer. To avoid this problem, hear all of what your client has to say before commenting. If needed, remind yourself to take your time and think about what is being said. If you are at a loss for a response, tell your client that you need to think about the question for a moment, then formulate your answer. If you are "stumped," assure the client that you will consider the question and get back to them. If you do this, be sure to follow up with an answer as soon as you have researched one.

▸ *Tune out distractions:* Distractions can occur in the environment (things we see or hear around us), within ourselves (our state of mind or physical condition), or from the speaker (mannerisms or a communication style that make it difficult to pay attention). Because your clients should be the focus of your attention, eliminate or minimize distractions that make it hard for you to listen. Move to a quiet location if surrounding noise or activity is disruptive. If your mind keeps wandering to a personal issue, silently repeat to yourself everything the speaker says. If the speaker's style makes it hard to listen, respectfully work with the speaker to solve the problem (e.g., ask a soft speaker to speak more loudly). It is appropriate to take notes when needed. Whether you circle back to the notes to reveal habits and trends you see in behavior or choose to study the notes for the following session, note-taking can be very helpful.

▸ *Avoid overusing filler words:* Sometimes, exercise professionals feel uncomfortable with brief silences and attempt to fill pauses with words. While it often is helpful to acknowledge that you are listening with an occasional "uh-huh," overuse of filler words can become distracting and should be avoided. If you find yourself using too many filler words, take a deep breath and remind yourself that some pauses and brief silences are natural and productive. Smiling and nodding in a supportive manner can show your interest without being disruptive (effective active listening).

▸ *Avoid patronizing language:* Too often, older adults are spoken to as if they are children, with little regard for their dignity. For example, if a small-framed elderly female fits the "little old lady" stereotype, some adults may unthinkingly address this woman as "dear" or "honey." While the speaker may consider these terms of affection, others may find this approach condescending and offensive. Address older adults as you would anyone—with respect—in the manner they request. It is not uncommon for older persons to prefer being addressed in a more formal manner (e.g., Mr. Smith, rather than Bill.) If in doubt about addressing an older client by first or last name, ask for their preference.

▸ *Avoid using slang:* Slang often is age-, gender-, and/or culturally specific. It is best to use mainstream language. If you are working with an individual or with group members who are from a similar age group and background as yourself, the use of some slang may be acceptable. Be careful, however, not to patronize clients by attempting to use slang terms you would not otherwise use.

▸ *Make eye contact:* This demonstrates your interest in each client. Frequently making brief eye contact with clients shows concern and interest. If you are leading a group, be sure to make eye contact with each participant.

▸ *Speak at an appropriate volume and pace:* Nervous and/or enthusiastic leaders tend to speak rapidly, often not allowing time for listeners to ask about what was said. If you are a rapid speaker, be conscious of slowing your pace. Additionally, the volume of speech must be loud enough for clients to hear, especially if there is background noise. Note that hearing aids amplify all noise—not just your voice—so the volume of any background music must be low when working with clients who use these devices. Ask your clients about volume and pace until you become familiar with their needs and adjust accordingly. For hearing-impaired clients, it often is beneficial to slow down the rate of your speech, use some gestures or demonstrations to emphasize points, and look at clients so they can pick up visual cues about what you are saying.

▸ *Teach new material at an appropriate pace:* It has been noted that although the ability to learn new information remains relatively stable over time, the speed of learning may slow with aging, especially when older adults are learning new physical tasks by imitating their sequence (e.g., hitting a golf ball or square dancing). There may be large variation from one client to another, but a good rule is to allow clients to learn at their own pace and to tell you when they are comfortable with what you have taught them and when they are ready to move on. Periodically ask individuals to demonstrate new moves or explain what you have just said. Inquire whether additional practice is desired or if they would like homework. If the majority of a class is ready to move on, reassure those who want more practice that you will review the information again, making sure to let them know when. In groups, give clients the option of using a familiar move until they become comfortable with the new one. Provide opportunities for older clients to meet with you or peers to work on new steps or exercises.

▸ *Visual communication should be easy to read:* Older adults' visual health may vary widely. To meet the needs of those with vision difficulties, it is best to make lettering on boards, signs, flyers, and instruction sheets easy to read. Keep visual material uncluttered and brief. Color combinations that give maximal contrast should be used, while varying shades of the same colors (like grays) should be avoided. Pictures or diagrams can enhance some messages, but they should be simple and clear.

▸ *The best way to determine if you are meeting clients' needs is simply to ask:* Most clients will appreciate your concern and will tell you how to help them. It is less important to know all the answers than to ask the right questions. Remember, this is a collaborative experience and the client needs to be an integral part of the program design.

THE ACE MOVER METHOD

The greatest impact that health coaches and exercise professionals can regularly have on the lives of their clients is to help them to positively change health-related behaviors and establish positive relationships with exercise. For this reason, the client–exercise professional relationship is the foundation of the ACE Integrated Fitness Training® (ACE IFT®) Model. This relationship is built upon rapport, trust, and empathy, with the professional serving as a "coach" to the client throughout their physical-activity and health behavior-change journey. This approach starts with realizing that the client is the central person in the client–exercise professional relationship.

The ACE IFT Model is designed to help exercise professionals competently navigate the process of working with clients, beginning with the initial meeting and continuing throughout the client–exercise professional relationship (Chapter 2).

ACE→ MΩVER™ METHΩD

Introducing the ACE Mover Method Philosophy and ACE ABC Approach™

A key element of using the ACE IFT Model to empower clients to make behavioral changes to improve their health, fitness, and overall quality of life is the adoption of the ACE Mover Method, which is founded on the following tenets:

▸ Each professional interaction is client-centered, with a recognition that clients are the foremost experts on themselves.

▸ Powerful **open-ended questions** and active listening are utilized in every session with clients.

▸ Clients are genuinely viewed as resourceful and capable of change.

ACE→ ABC APPROACH™

Exercise professionals can easily apply the ACE Mover Method through the ACE ABC Approach:

▸ Ask open-ended questions

▸ Break down barriers

▸ Collaborate

Every client–exercise professional interaction offers an opportunity to utilize coaching skills to help build rapport while positioning the client as an active partner in the behavior-change journey. Asking questions leads to the identification of goals and options for breaking down barriers, which in turn leads to collaborating on next steps. The ACE Mover Method provides the foundational skills for communicating effectively with clients, but it is not the equivalent of a health coaching certification. Exercise professionals should work in concert with other professionals, such as health coaches, **registered dietitians,** and other allied health professionals whenever appropriate, to take a team approach to improving their clients' health and wellness.

Step 1 involves asking powerful questions to identify what the client hopes to accomplish by working with an exercise professional and what, if any, physical activities the client enjoys. Open-ended questions are the key to sparking this discussion.

Step 2 involves asking more questions to discover what potential barriers may get in the way of the client reaching their specific goals. Questions like "What do you need to *start* doing now to move closer to your goals?" and "What do you need to *stop* doing that will enable you to reach your goals?" can be very revealing.

Step 3 involves collaboration as the client and exercise professional work together to set **SMART goals** and establish specific steps to take action toward those goals. Allowing the client to lead the discussion of how to monitor and measure progress empowers them to take ownership of their personal behavior-change journey.

Throughout this textbook, look for ACE Mover Method features to learn more about effective strategies for employing a client-centered approach to working with older adults.

Creating a Safe Environment

To facilitate the success of older clients in meeting exercise goals, exercise professionals must create an environment that is safe, both physically and psychologically. In a review of the barriers to physical activity for older adults, researchers reported many factors that may influence an individual's decision to initiate or maintain a physical-activity program. These barriers included pain, risk of injury, lack of professional guidance, and being unsure of appropriate guidelines (Bethancourt et al., 2014). Research has suggested, however, that while fear of injury may increase with age, older adults generally are not more injury-prone than younger adults (Stathokostas, 2013). However, good judgement and sound practices are imperative for the safety of all clients.

Increased psychological comfort with exercise programs can dramatically improve program adherence. Help older adults safely exercise at or near their physical abilities by accurately identifying and minimizing both physical and psychological risks of exercise. Making sure

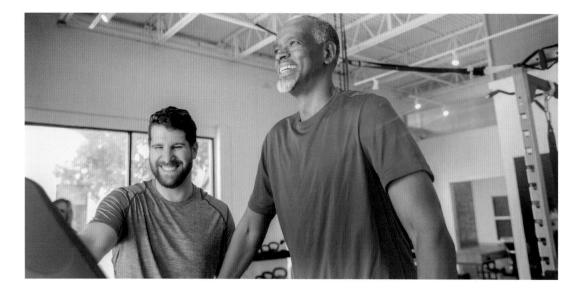

that the client has mastery of the exercises and is self-sufficient over time ensures proper progressions and self-efficacy, which will improve adherence. Chapters 6 through 8 suggest specific components of program design intended to minimize the risk of physical injury to older clients. The following list presents a few common psychological risks of exercise for older adults, as well as suggested strategies for helping older clients overcome each of the risks (Bethancourt et al., 2014):

▸ *Risk of embarrassment or ridicule:* This risk may be especially relevant for older adults who have never been **physically active,** have had a negative exercise experience, or who are attempting to engage in exercise after an extended break. All clients may be susceptible to embarrassment, but older adults may be attempting to engage in an exercise plan despite societal messages that exercise is most appropriate for younger adults, and that older adults may be too frail for exercise or too old to develop new skills. It is no wonder that some older adults fear criticism.

- **To help older clients:** Acknowledge clients' wisdom and courage in committing to improving their health or physical fitness by exercising. Reassure them that most people in exercise programs are preoccupied with their own performance, leaving little time to worry about what others are doing. Establishing rapport to ensure the acceptance of a new program design and progressions will lead to improvement, action, and confidence.

▸ *Risk of facing diminished endurance and balance:* This problem can be especially difficult for former athletes or former regular exercisers who have not remained physically active. Some older adults may compare their current performance to what they could do when they were younger or prior to a medical problem. Discovering that they can no longer do what they once did can be demotivating. Older clients who note declines in their abilities may be reluctant to continue exercise activities that remind them of these changes.

- **To help older clients:** Encourage them to measure progress from their present starting point. Additionally, remind clients that individuals of any age have plenty of room for substantial gains in physical abilities. With time and consistent participation in their exercise routine, they may be pleasantly surprised at how much they can improve.

▸ *Risk of intimidation:* Given society's obsession with youth, older people may feel acutely self-conscious while exercising. Some clients may not like to exercise in settings or participate in group activities that make them feel embarrassed about their appearance. Additionally, a competitive atmosphere in group settings may lead to apprehensions about not being able to keep up or even slowing down the group.

- **To help older clients:** Encourage them to concentrate on the benefits of participating in an exercise program. Point out, too, that by actively taking steps to improve their health, they are improving their own physical fitness and abilities.

These are just a few of a wide variety of psychological risks that clients may associate with physical-activity programs. By supportively encouraging them to come to terms with these and other risks, exercise professionals can free their clients of restrictive barriers to exercise and fears that may impact many aspects of their lives.

📖 APPLY WHAT YOU KNOW

Is Your Facility Senior Friendly?

Facility type, size, and location, as well as accessibility for anyone with functional impairments, are significant factors in establishing inclusive participation in your exercise programming. The type of equipment available for exercise sessions and the existing atmosphere of a facility also are important considerations.

Type

Exercise programming for skilled nursing and assisted-living facilities consists of routines primarily for older adults with lower functional capacities. Senior centers and residence facilities catering to independent older adults may require exercise programming that meets the needs of frail to physically fit seniors. Fitness facilities catering to the general public would most likely provide programming for seniors from the independent to the more physically fit and elite categories of function (see Chapter 3).

Size

Facility size largely determines programming options. Sizes range from very large facilities with access to extensive equipment, to small fitness centers with very little equipment. In senior housing complexes, an exercise facility can range from one small room to a large wellness center complete with a swimming pool, weight room, and group exercise room. Community-dwelling seniors have more options, including home exercise plans or programs held at local fitness facilities or studios. Regardless of the size of the facility, the exercise professional should use what is available to create safe and effective exercise programming.

Location and Accessibility

The facility's location is also important. Facilities in a central area that can easily be reached on foot or by public transportation have the advantage of attracting older adults who no longer drive. In contrast, hard-to-reach facilities, regardless of the amenities offered, will be underutilized.

Equally as important as location is the accessibility of the facility itself to those with mobility impairments. Parking areas that are far from the building or facilities with excessive stairs make it difficult for many lower-functioning older adults to participate in exercise programs. Poorly maintained parking lots and sidewalks, and areas where snow and ice are a problem, also serve as barriers to participation. If the client has a difficult time coming to the facility, the exercise professional should consider whether it is appropriate to go to the client's home for sessions.

Another aspect of accessibility concerns the times the facility is available for programming. Some seniors are early risers and prefer to get up and complete their exercise routines before proceeding with the rest of the day. Others enjoy exercise later in the day. To reach the largest percentage of seniors, consistently offer sessions throughout the day, if possible.

Equipment and Facility Systems

Equipment options within the facility are a consideration when programming for seniors. Resistance-training machines should be fully adjustable to body size and allow for increasing resistance by small increments [2.5 pounds (1.1 kg) or less]. Take time to learn which activities the client is having concerns with, such as **activities of daily living** (both inside and outside the house) or specific movement patterns. Exercise sessions may include machines, body weight, and tubing as resistance, along with various movement patterns.

Exercise facilities lacking appropriate heating or cooling systems can pose a risk to seniors whose bodies often do not regulate heat as efficiently as those of younger adults. Evaluating these aspects of the facility in advance allows the exercise professional to make the necessary adjustments for safe programming.

Evaluating the advantages and limitations of a facility helps the exercise professional identify what types of programs are appropriate within that environment, if in-home training would be more appropriate, and for which segments of the senior population safe and effective programming can be provided.

◀ **SUMMARY** ▶

The senior population covers a broad range of individuals included beneath that umbrella term, from competitive athletes to the mobility impaired. It is essential that exercise professionals, whether they specialize in working with members of this population or simply have a handful of older clients or class participants, respect all individuals and take the time to learn about them without making assumptions. Exercise professionals must stay within their **scope of practice** and refer clients out if necessary, or if there are questions or concerns. As with all clients, the goal when working with older adults is to perform a proper screening and assessment of their health and fitness levels and then create personalized programs that meet their needs and help them reach their goals.

REFERENCES

Anderson, M. & Perrin, A. (2017). *Barriers to Adoption and Attitudes towards Technology.* https://www.pewresearch.org/internet/2017/05/17/barriers-to-adoption-and-attitudes-towards-technology/

Bamidis, P.D. et al. (2014). Gains in cognition through combined cognitive and physical training: The role of training dosage and severity of neurocognitive disorder. *Frontiers in Aging Neuroscience,* 7, 152.

Bethancourt, H.J. et al. (2014). Barriers to and facilitators of physical activity program use among older adults. *Clinical Medicine & Research,* 12, 1–2, 10–20.

Burnes, D. et al. (2019). Interventions to reduce ageism against older adults: A systematic review and meta-analysis. *AJPH Open-Themed Research,* 109, 8, e1–e9.

Chang, E-S. et al. (2020). Global reach of ageism on older persons' health: A systematic review. *Plos One,* 15, 1, e0220857.

Hitlin, P. (2018). *Internet, Social Media Use and Device Ownership in U.S. Have Plateaued after Years of Growth.* https://www.pewresearch.org/fact-tank/2018/09/28/internet-social-media-use-and-device-ownership-in-u-s-have-plateaued-after-years-of-growth/

Officer, A. & de la Fuente-Núñez, V. (2018). A global campaign to combat ageism. *Bulletin of the World Health Organization,* 96, 4, 295–296.

Pew Research Center (2017). *Roughly Three-quarters of Internet Users Ages 60 and Up Say They Go Online Daily.* https://www.pewresearch.org/internet/2017/05/17/tech-adoption-climbs-among-older-adults/pi_2017-05-17_older-americans-tech_2-04/

Robertson, G. (2016). Attitudes towards ageing and their impact on health and wellbeing in later life: An agenda for further analysis. *Working with Older People,* 20, 4.

Stathokostas, L. et al. (2013). Physical activity-related injuries in older adults: A scoping review. *Sports Medicine,* 43, 955–963.

U.S. Senate: Special Committee on Aging (2017). *America's Aging Workforce: Opportunities and Challenges.* https://www.aging.senate.gov/imo/media/doc/Aging%20Workforce%20Report%20FINAL.pdf

Wang, J. et al. (2019). Mobile and connected health technology needs for older adults aging in place: Cross-sectional survey study. *JMIR Aging,* 2, 1, e13864.

Warner, L.M. et al. (2014). Sources of self-efficacy for physical activity. *Health Psychology,* 33, 11. DOI: 10.1037/hea0000085.

Williams, K.N. et al. (2018). Person-centered communication for nursing home residents with dementia: Four communication analysis methods. *Western Journal of Nursing Research,* 40, 7, 1012–1031.

SUGGESTED READINGS

American Council on Exercise (2019). *The Professional's Guide to Health and Wellness Coaching.* San Diego: American Council on Exercise.

National Institute on Aging (2017). *Tips for Improving Communication with Older Adults.* https://www.nia.nih.gov/health/tips-improving-communication-older-patients

Rivera-Torres, S., Fahey, T.D., & Rivera, M.A. (2019). Adherence to exercise programs in older adults: Informative report. *Gerontology and Geriatric Medicine,* 5, 1–10.

CHAPTER 2

Motivation and Adherence

LEARNING OBJECTIVES

After reading this chapter, you will be able to:

▸ Explain important theories of behavior change and how they relate to helping older adults begin a new behavior, such as starting an exercise program, and then maintaining that newly adopted behavior

▸ Discuss the different stages of change as described in the transtheoretical model of behavior change and provide practical strategies for how to work with older clients in each of those stages

▸ Effectively interview senior clients to obtain pertinent information about their desires, needs, and lifestyles in order to promote motivation and adherence to a program of regular physical activity

▸ Build rapport with senior clients that ultimately affects desired actions and outcomes

▸ Work with senior clients to help them establish and achieve SMART goals that build self-efficacy

▸ Develop relapse-prevention strategies with senior clients to facilitate long-term maintenance of a physical-activity program

Most people understand that physical activity and exercise, when performed regularly, are highly beneficial for both physical and psychological health. Yet, only a minority of adults report engaging in physical activity at a level compatible with public health guidelines. For example, in the United States, nearly 80% of all adults do not achieve recommended levels of both cardiorespiratory and muscle-strengthening exercise and only about 50% of adults reach key guidelines for cardiorespiratory exercise (U.S. Department of Health & Human Services, 2018). While many people may lack sufficient **motivation** to be active, personalizing the benefits of regular physical activity based on values, setting personal goals that allow for the attainment of valued benefits, and developing the skills and knowledge to achieve goals may increase a person's motivation to participate in the recommended 150 minutes of moderate-intensity exercise or physical activity per week (U.S. Department of Health & Human Services, 2018).

Lack of motivation is a complex concept caused by a variety of factors specific to each individual. People may not be sufficiently interested in exercise or value the benefits enough to make it a priority in their lives. For many, competing demands from career and family obligations use up time and resources that could be invested in exercising regularly. Some people may not feel competent at physical activities, perceiving themselves as either not physically fit enough or skilled enough to exercise, or they may have health limitations that present a physical or emotional barrier to activity. Simply increasing clients' knowledge of health benefits from physical activity provides insufficient motivation to bring about behavior change. It may be more beneficial to emphasize the positive relationship between regular physical activity and a fulfilling and purposeful life. For older adults specifically, feeling connected to others and finding a sense of purpose may provide greater motivation to change (Morgan et al., 2019). Physical activity can be meaningful to older adults due to a variety of important factors, including the following (Morgan et al., 2019):

- The need to feel needed (responsibility and duty)
- Building self-esteem and self-belief
- Companionship, intimacy, and support
- Feelings of rejuvenation, vitality, energy, and youthfulness
- Pleasure, fun, laughter, and enjoyment
- Belonging to a group and having a shared identity
- Creating and strengthening feelings of togetherness, community, and belonging
- Change and disruption during the transition to older age
- Challenging established attitudes about aging

It is important to note, however, that factors that may motivate individuals to start exercising are not the same factors that will keep them participating in an exercise program over the long haul. While getting people to start a new program can be challenging, it is only part of a larger battle that health coaches and exercise professionals will face. The true challenge involves creating programming and exercise environments that maximize the likelihood that a person will stick with the program, avoid the potential for **relapse,** and adopt an active lifestyle as they age. It is important to remember that senior clients are the most diverse clients in multiple domains. **Specificity** in programming is imperative, both physically and emotionally, to build client commitment.

Theories of Health Behavior Change

Beginning or modifying an exercise program requires making lifestyle changes and replacing old habits with new ones, which is often difficult. A regular exerciser may have to increase the intensity, duration, or frequency of exercise, add another type of exercise to address a new component of fitness, or modify, remove, or add new exercises to address injuries, degeneration, or other health issues. Non-physically active individuals may have to incorporate a new set of activities into their routines, which may require decreasing sedentary pursuits like watching television or reading and/or setting aside time for exercise despite an already busy schedule.

To help others make desired behavioral changes, exercise professionals must first understand those factors that encourage or hinder those behaviors. Various health, exercise, and psychology researchers have developed useful theories about how and why people engage in physical activity.

HEALTH BELIEF MODEL

The **health belief model** suggests that the major factors influencing behavioral change include perceptions of susceptibility to a health threat, combined with the perceived seriousness of the threat (Figure 2-1). A client with a family history of heart disease who feels personally vulnerable and recognizes the seriousness of the disease, for example, might be highly motivated to improve their **cardiorespiratory fitness** as a means of decreasing their chance of having a heart attack. The individual must also believe that the proposed action (such as regularly walking) will help prevent the health threat. Additionally, the perceived benefits of a health behavior must outweigh the perceived barriers to changing (e.g., time spent away from family or the cost of new walking shoes). This model also suggests the use of cues as reminders to be active, such as placing walking shoes by the front door. Furthermore, this theory posits that clients must have a minimum degree of confidence in their ability to start and maintain the healthy behavior. For example, a review of the literature showed that people with low-back pain presenting with positive recovery expectations were more likely to recover from pain, return to work, and demonstrate an increase in the number of activities they are able to perform (Hayden et al., 2019). Therefore, it seems important for exercise professionals who work with

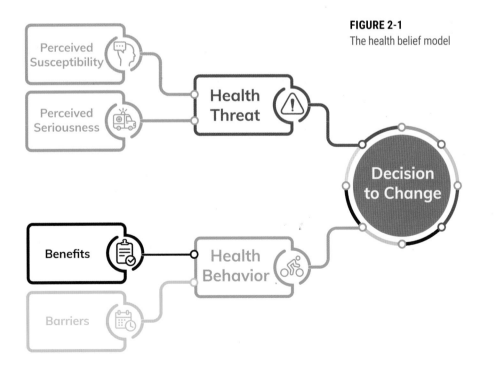

FIGURE 2-1
The health belief model

clients who have **chronic** ailments—which are common among the senior population—to bolster their clients' positive beliefs about their present or future health conditions and their functional ability.

SELF-EFFICACY

Self-efficacy refers to a person's belief that they can perform a given task or change a behavior. While self-efficacy is similar to self-confidence, it is always situation- or behavior-specific. For example, a client may be very confident in their ability to reduce caloric intake but have low self-efficacy in terms of sticking to an exercise program. Self-efficacy predicts how much effort clients will exert in sticking to their exercise programs, as well as how hard clients will persist in their behavior-change efforts when facing difficulties.

Much of an exercise professional's work with senior clients in the beginning stages of behavioral change will be focused on helping them believe that they can modify their lifestyles and change problematic behaviors. One way in which exercise professionals can help promote self-efficacy is to provide opportunities for clients to achieve early success in their exercise programs through appropriate goal setting and personalized program design. Empowering clients to set realistic goals that they can reasonably accomplish, while also providing continued positive reinforcement, will help clients feel like they are being successful. Introducing exercise programming that is commensurate with the fitness level and abilities of an older adult will help to ensure successful completion of individual workouts, as well as the mastery of new exercise skills that are required to progress to the next phase of the program.

The key to continued self-efficacy is to assist clients so they can do the exercises on their own, which will help encourage them to take responsibility for their own actions and health. This can be accomplished through activities that are performed on days when clients are not with the exercise professional and then following up to ensure competence and follow-through.

Another method for increasing self-efficacy in clients is to expose them to a variety of role models. Observing people of a similar size, age, gender, and ethnic background who exercise regularly and have adopted a physically active lifestyle encourages the belief that, "If they can do it, so can I." If an older client feels "different" from everyone else in the group or at the

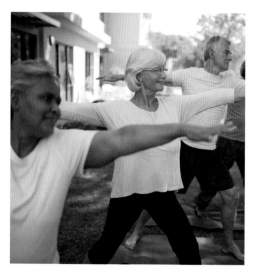

fitness center, self-efficacy may decline. The key to enhancing self-efficacy is to uncover the defining variables that make the client feel "different." For example, if a client is older than most other gym members, they may lack self-efficacy because they think they are too old. Observing people at the gym who are about the same age as the client could be a way for them to see potential role models. To expose new clients to inspiring role models, exercise professionals could introduce former clients, friends, or acquaintances who could serve as appropriate role models to talk to the client. Role models might be willing to exercise with the client or perform their own workouts at the same time as the client. This will give the client the opportunity to observe the desired behavior first-hand and may ultimately lead to performance of the new behavior. Recommending an exercise class or group that includes people with whom the client identifies, or starting a group for older clientele, is an effective option for introducing role models to clients. If role models are difficult to find, exercise professionals can direct clients to videos, articles, books, and websites featuring people similar to the client.

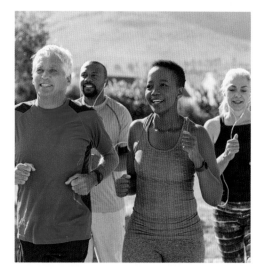

Exercise professionals can use the following six sources of self-efficacy to help influence client self-efficacy levels and promote exercise adoption and continued adherence.

▸ **Past performance experience** is an influential source of self-efficacy information. Exercise professionals may ask clients about their previous experiences with exercise, fitness facilities, and personal trainers or other exercise professionals. Both positive and negative past performance experiences will strongly influence current self-efficacy levels. It is imperative for exercise professionals to learn from these experiences to collaboratively create positive and meaningful programs that lead to enjoyment, generate feelings of accomplishment, and build self-efficacy.

▸ **Vicarious experience** is important for clients who are new to exercise and who have little previous personal experience with a supervised program. The observation or knowledge of someone else who is successfully participating in a similar program—or has done so in the past—can increase self-efficacy. This is particularly true if the person being observed is perceived by clients to be similar to themselves (e.g., in terms of age, chronic illness status, sex, and/or fitness level).

▸ **Verbal persuasion** typically occurs in the form of positive and constructive feedback and encouragement from important individuals, such as exercise professionals. Affirmative statements from others are most likely to influence self-efficacy if they come from a credible, respected, and knowledgeable source. Different clients will require different amounts and various styles of verbal encouragement.

▸ **Physiological state appraisals** related to exercise participation are important because a client may experience **emotional arousal,** pain, or fatigue. The types of appraisals clients make about their physiological states may lead to judgments about their ability to participate successfully. It is essential to educate clients about appropriate sensations during an exercise. Many clients do not know the difference between muscle pain and joint pain, nor do they know the intensity at which to work. With proper training, clients will have a better understanding of what is happening physiologically, which will help them create realistic and positive interpretations. By teaching clients to appropriately identify muscle or joint fatigue, soreness, and tiredness, as well as the implications of these states, exercise professionals can help clients perceive and control the sensations experienced while exercising, which leads to improved self-efficacy.

▶ **Emotional state and mood appraisals** of program participation can also influence self-efficacy. Negative mood states and emotional beliefs associated with exercise, such as fear, anxiety, anger, and frustration, are related to reduced levels of self-efficacy and lower levels of participation. On the other hand, positive mood states and emotional beliefs, including mastery, are related to higher levels of self-efficacy. Hence, giving encouraging coaching cues and tailoring client programs that are sufficiently challenging, yet simply achieved, contribute to elevated moods and positive emotional states.

▶ **Imaginal experiences** refer to the imagined experiences (positive or negative) of exercise participation. It is important to understand a client's preconceived notion of what exercise will be like, as this information will influence their self-efficacy levels. The exercise professional may encourage positive imagined experiences by asking open-ended questions such as, "How do you imagine you'll feel when you reach your goal of being able to walk on the treadmill for 20 minutes without stopping?"

With this information, the exercise professional will be better able to design and deliver a program that sets up the client for success. In an exercise program, self-efficacy levels will influence the types of tasks individuals want to engage in, how hard they will try, and if they will persist. Specifically, people with high self-efficacy will choose challenging tasks, set goals, and display a commitment to master those tasks. They will display maximal effort to reach their goals and will even increase their effort when challenges arise. Highly self-efficacious clients tend to work hard to overcome obstacles and recover from setbacks, and ultimately, are much more likely to adhere to a program (Bauman et al., 2012).

On the other hand, people with low self-efficacy will be more likely to choose nonchallenging tasks that are nonthreatening and easy to accomplish. They will display minimal effort to protect themselves in the face of a challenge—since failing when not working hard will be a lesser blow to their self-efficacy than failing when doing their best—and, if faced with too many setbacks, are more likely to give up and drop out of the program. There is a significant relationship between self-efficacy and physical activity, which indicates a need to focus on psychological factors such as self-efficacy to improve health and self-care (Daniali et al., 2017).

RELAPSE-PREVENTION MODEL

As mentioned in the chapter introduction, factors that motivate a person to start a new behavior such as exercise are different from those that spur continued adherence to the behavior. This section introduces concepts surrounding the maintenance of behavioral change versus the initiation of a new behavior.

The **relapse-prevention model** was derived from research on how individual and environmental factors can influence relapse risk and why people stop abstaining from undesirable behaviors such as substance misuse (Bowen et al., 2014). The concept of relapse prevention also has been applied to understanding why individuals stop healthy habits. Some clients who are struggling with behavioral change may find that making the initial change is not as difficult as maintaining behavioral changes over time. Factors such as negative emotional states, limited coping skills, social pressure to cease desired behaviors, interpersonal conflicts, limited social support, stress, and encountering "high-risk" situations can contribute to the cessation of desired behaviors. The broad aim of the relapse-prevention model is to minimize the impact of high-risk situations by increasing awareness and building coping skills, and to limit how prone a client is to relapse by promoting a healthy and balanced lifestyle (Hendershot et al., 2011).

When individuals do experience a setback (a temporary **lapse** in activity), they often believe it will lead to complete failure. Belief in their ability to succeed may be lost after only one slip-up, leaving them feeling out of control, guilty, discouraged, and ashamed. This negative thinking can interfere with resuming the desired behaviors. Preparing clients to cope with high-risk situations can prevent relapses. Helping clients understand that relapses are normal, and even likely, can help them to better cope with setbacks when they do occur, and to resume physical activity as soon as possible. Research suggests that relapse-prevention strategies (such as the ones presented later in this chapter) may increase long-term adherence to physical-activity and weight-management programs (Middleton, Anton, & Perri, 2013).

TRANSTHEORETICAL MODEL OF BEHAVIOR CHANGE

The **transtheoretical model of behavior change (TTM)** is different from previous models discussed in that it suggests an individual's readiness to engage in behaviors can be described on a continuum known as the stages of change (Figure 2-2). Although this theory was originally developed to refer to psychotherapy processes and later, to smoking

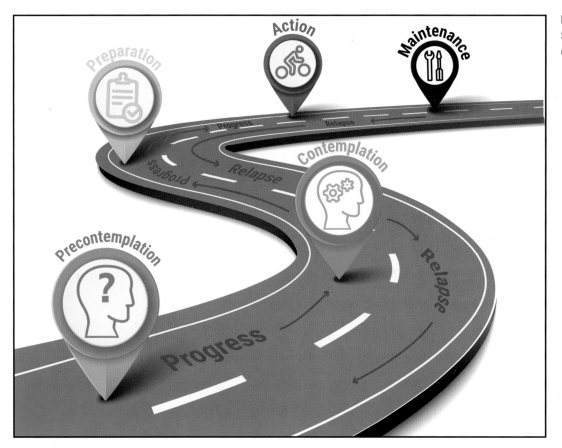

FIGURE 2-2

Stages of behavior change

cessation, others have adapted the model specifically to physical activity. A review of the literature suggests that as long as exercise interventions are matched to an individual's stage of change, there is support for using the TTM in promoting adoption of, and adherence to, physical-activity programs.

A number of processes of change are important in moving people from one stage to the next (Table 2-1). These processes were incorporated into the TTM by looking at important mechanisms from other theoretical models. Therefore, the TTM can be thought of as an integration of a number of different motivational theories, and it incorporates many of the theorized determinants described in the prior models. As mentioned earlier, self-efficacy and outcome expectancies are also thought to be important determinants of physical activity in the TTM.

TABLE 2-1
Processes of Change

Processes of Change	Description
Consciousness raising	Finding and learning new facts, ideas, and tips that support healthy behavior change
Dramatic relief	Experiencing negative emotions because the negative behavior (e.g., being physically inactive or eating fast food) is perceived to be problematic, then feeling relief from deciding to change
Self-reevaluation	Realizing behavior change is an important part of one's identity as a person
Environmental reevaluation	Realizing how the behavior influences the environment, especially the person's social environment
Self-liberation	Deciding to change and experiencing a new belief in the ability to change
Helping relationships	Seeking and using social support for behavior change
Counter-conditioning	Substituting healthier behaviors and cognitions for the unhealthy behavior
Reinforcement management	Increasing rewards for healthy behavior change and decreasing rewards for unhealthy behavior
Stimulus control	Removing reminders and cues to engage in unhealthy behaviors and replacing them with reminders/cues for healthy behavior
Social liberation	Taking advantage of opportunities to be with people who model the new behavior, noticing the social norms that reinforce the new behavior

The TTM is especially helpful to exercise professionals because it acknowledges individual differences in readiness to exercise at any particular point in time. Goals and program strategies must be tailored to the readiness of each individual. It is imperative that the exercise professional appropriately address clients at each stage. This means that the client's goals must match the type of information given to the client, as will be discussed later in this chapter for each stage of change (Prochaska, Norcross, & DiClemente, 2013). It would be inappropriate, for example, to expect a person in the **precontemplation** stage to commit to an exercise program. Instead, interventions with individuals in this stage would ideally validate their lack of **readiness to change,** clarifying that the decision is theirs, encouraging self-exploration and reevaluation of current behaviors, exploring personal values, and sharing information to increase awareness.

In contrast, a person who has been in the **maintenance** stage of engaging in physical activity for three years has already discovered the benefits of exercise. This exercise "maintainer" might be interested in discussing ways to add excitement to their well-established routine, a topic that clearly would not be appropriate for a person just beginning a physical-activity program. Because people can move back and forth between stages due to either progression or relapse, exercise professionals should remain alert for potential changes in clients' stages and adjust interventions accordingly (Table 2-2).

TABLE 2-2
The Stages of Behavior Change

Stage	Traits	Goals	Strategies
Precontemplation	▸ Unaware or under-aware of the problem, or believe that it cannot be solved	▸ Increase awareness of the risks of maintaining the status quo and of the benefits of making a change ▸ Focus on addressing something relevant to them ▸ Have them start thinking about change	▸ Validate lack of readiness to change and clarify that this decision is theirs ▸ Encourage reevaluation of current behavior and self-exploration, while not taking action ▸ Explain and personalize the inherent risks ▸ Utilize general sources, including media, Internet, and brochures, to increase awareness ▸ Explore the client's personal values
Contemplation	▸ Aware of the problem and weighing the benefits versus risks of change ▸ Have little understanding of how to go about changing	▸ Collaboratively explore available options ▸ Support cues to action and provide basic structured guidance upon request from the client and with permission	▸ Validate lack of readiness to change and clarify that this decision is theirs ▸ Encourage evaluation of the pros and cons of making a change ▸ Identify and promote new, positive outcome expectations and boost self-confidence

Continued on the next page

TABLE 2-2 *(continued)*

Stage	Traits	Goals	Strategies
Preparation	▸ Seeking opportunities to engage in the target behavior	▸ Co-create an action plan with frequent positive feedback and reinforcements on their progress	▸ Verify that the individual has the underlying skills for behavior change and encourage small steps toward building self-efficacy ▸ Identify and assist with problem-solving obstacles ▸ Assist the client in identifying social support and establishing goals
Action	▸ Desire for opportunities to maintain activities ▸ Changing beliefs and attitudes ▸ High risk for lapses or returns to undesirable behavior	▸ Establish the new behavior as a habit through motivation and adherence to the desired behavior	▸ Use behavior-modification strategies ▸ Empower clients to restructure cues and social support toward building long-term change ▸ Increase awareness of inevitable lapses and bolster self-efficacy in coping with lapses ▸ Support clients in establishing systems of accountability and self-monitoring
Maintenance	▸ Empowered, but desire a means to maintain adherence ▸ Good capability to deal with lapses	▸ Maintain support systems ▸ Maintain interest and avoid boredom or burnout	▸ Reevaluate strategies currently in effect ▸ Plan for contingencies with support systems, although this may no longer be needed ▸ Reinforce the need for a transition from external to internal rewards ▸ Plan for potential lapses ▸ Encourage reevaluation of goals and action plans as needed

The models previewed in this section help explain the motivation for, and continued adherence to, physical activity. Generally, models of physical-activity behavioral change take into account some combination of expected outcomes (including benefits and costs), perceived ability to engage in the physical activity, and positive and negative social influences. The TTM can be especially useful because it incorporates ideas from a number of other models and considers when and for whom each of these potential determinants is important, based on the individual's readiness to change.

From Theory to Practice

Motivation refers to the internal processes that energize, direct, and sustain a given behavior. More simply, it can be thought of as wanting change. Often, people talk about motivation as if it were a completely stable, enduring characteristic. Some people just seem motivated to accomplish great things and appear to stay motivated against all odds. In reality, motivation varies over time and according to the task.

Motivation impacts decisions to exercise as well as the likelihood of stopping or maintaining exercise over the long run. A review of the literature reveals that common barriers to participation in physical activity among older adults include chronic health ailments, lack of knowledge, fear of falling or injury, time constraints, and lack of transportation (Table 2-3) (Bethancourt et al., 2014).

TABLE 2-3

List of Barriers to, and Facilitators of, Physical Activity and Program Participation Based on a Social-ecological Framework

BARRIERS	FACILITATORS
Intrapersonal Level Factors	
Physical or Mental Health	
▸ Pain ▸ Decreased endurance and balance ▸ Increased recovery time ▸ Risk of injury ▸ Risk of failing	▸ Potential prevention of health problems ▸ Management of existing conditions ▸ Maintenance of balance, strength, and mental acuity ▸ Potential weight loss ▸ Mood boost
Individual Preferences	
▸ Dislike of physical activity, gyms/indoor physical activity ▸ Dislike of organized/group physical activity ▸ Lack of motivation ▸ Intimidation/embarrassment ▸ Unsure of appropriate physical activity ▸ Preference for sedentary activities ▸ Boredom with physical activity ▸ Not accustomed to doing physical activity	▸ Enjoyment of physical activity ▸ Belief that physical activity is important ▸ Feeling guilty when not active ▸ Awareness of benefits ▸ Physical activity as part of a routine ▸ Sense of self-efficacy ▸ Proactive pursuit of programs ▸ Daily activities provide physical activity ▸ Physical activity combined with enjoyable/useful activities
Interpersonal Level Factors	
▸ Lack of guidance from a professional ▸ Not motivated by instructors ▸ Not receiving or able to access information on physical-activity programs ▸ Being pushed too hard ▸ Presence of others perceived as intimidating	▸ Encouragement from others ▸ Companionship of others ▸ Camaraderie in classes ▸ Guidance from a professional ▸ Social contact ▸ Others as role models or incentives ▸ Support from dog companions

Continued on the next page

TABLE 2-3 *(continued)*

BARRIERS	FACILITATORS
Physical Environment Factors	
▸ Hills and stairs ▸ Uneven sidewalks ▸ Bad weather ▸ Unsafe neighborhood ▸ Physical-activity location not aesthetically pleasing ▸ Inconvenient physical-activity locations ▸ Difficult parking	▸ Living in a walkable area ▸ Proximity of stores ▸ Places to rest ▸ Even walking surfaces ▸ Alternatives in bad weather ▸ Physical-activity options at home ▸ Convenient/nearby physical-activity locations ▸ Pleasurable weather
Structural and Organizational Factors	
▸ Expense to drive to or use facilities ▸ Limited SS and EF facilities ▸ Being ineligible for SS and EF ▸ Inadequate information ▸ Lack of quality instructors ▸ Programs that are not engaging or too challenging ▸ Providers who are not knowledgeable about programs	▸ Free, low-cost programs ▸ High-quality instructors ▸ Flexible program schedule ▸ Engaging classes ▸ Programs appropriate for different fitness levels and physical limitations ▸ Distribution of information

Note: SS = Silver Sneakers; EF = EnhanceFitness

Reprinted with permission from "Barriers to and Facilitators of Physical Activity Program Use Among Older Adults," *Clinical Medicine & Research*, vol. 12, no. 1–2, pages 10–20. ©2014 Marshfield Clinic. Full article available at: http://www.clinmedres.org/content/12/1-2/10.full.pdf+html

---

◈ EXPAND YOUR KNOWLEDGE

Motivational Interviewing

Motivational interviewing (MI) focuses on the client's own ability to overcome **ambivalence** to behavioral change. Miller and Rollnick (2013) define MI as a client-centered, directive method for enhancing **intrinsic motivation** for change by exploring and resolving ambivalence. As the client and exercise professional collaboratively move toward a particular goal, the professional will sometimes observe ambivalence in the client about behavioral change. The task of the exercise professional is to help clients resolve their ambivalence in the direction of positive change, meaning that the professional prompts them to come up with solutions to their own barriers to change. In fact, if the conversation is not specifically about change in a collaborative manner that respects the **autonomy** of the client, it is not motivational. Engaging, guiding, and evoking are the key elements of MI.

The MI approach readily works with the TTM, which is reflected in the sample interviews between clients and exercise professionals presented throughout this chapter. A more detailed approach to using MI strategies with clients can be found in *The Professional's Guide to Health and Wellness Coaching* (ACE, 2019).

Physical-activity research involving older adults suggests that there are behavior-change strategies that can help people initiate exercise and stay motivated to continue. Physical-activity programs may increase long-term behavior change by increasing client self-efficacy and motivation, and by giving clients a sense of control over the program by working together to set meaningful goals, enhancing social support, using a personalized approach, and implementing self-regulatory strategies (Lachman et al., 2018; McAuley et al., 2011).

Consistent with the TTM, some strategies are more effective at different stages of motivational readiness. Each strategy presented here is followed by an example of how it might be implemented with an older adult.

STRATEGIES FOR OLDER ADULTS IN THE PRECONTEMPLATION STAGE

Clients in the precontemplation stage do not intend to begin a program of physical activity within the next six months and they may discount the importance of becoming physically active. Therefore, teaching them ways to set goals or strategies for reminding them to exercise is not appropriate. Instead, these clients can benefit from reevaluation of current behaviors, discussions about inherent risks of being **physically inactive,** and the exploration of personal values. Once they are motivated, more specific strategies about how to increase physical-activity levels are relevant. Individuals in the precontemplation stage may encounter exercise professionals during a routine physical or exercise stress test or while accompanying or transporting friends or family to exercise programs. However, encounters with these potential clients can be rare; therefore, it is important to make the most of these opportunities. This is a fragile stage in which rapport and education are essential. It is important that the client feels supported, guided, and encouraged. In addition, the strategies discussed in this section may be used in advertising campaigns to encourage potential clients to set up an initial appointment.

Potential Costs and Benefits of Beginning an Exercise Program

It is basic human nature to want to engage in activities that produce more benefits than costs. Who wants to toil away at a job that offers no pay and no other rewards? The perceived "costs" of physical activity vary from person to person, but could include the time it takes to exercise; the hassle of getting to the exercise location; muscle soreness; feeling tired after exercise; feeling self-conscious about exercising in front of other people; the expense of a fitness facility membership, special equipment, or clothing; and having to miss out on preferred activities.

The perceived benefits of physical activity also vary with the individual. Although certain physiological benefits might be expected for most or all people, only the benefits that are personally valued will serve as motivators. For example, if a client does not care about their improved ability to climb stairs without losing their breath, reminding them of this benefit will not be helpful. On the other hand, if they value being able to sleep better and having to take less medication to control their high blood pressure, these are more potent motivators worth discussing. Values are principles that motivate people and indicate

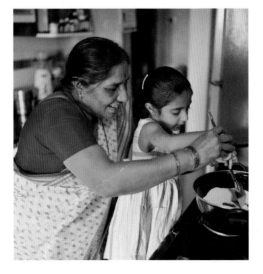

their preferences and choices. Values influence attitudes and behaviors, which dictate actions and outcomes. Finding out what people value and deem as important through the initial interview process helps exercise professionals guide clients with programs that are relevant and meaningful.

Why discuss anything negative such as the costs of exercise with clients? To help clients maintain a physically active lifestyle over the long run, it is necessary to be realistic about their negative expectations about physical activity. Ignoring the drawbacks of engaging in an exercise program will not make these costs disappear. In fact, negative expectations that are never addressed may eventually lead clients to drop out of their programs. Through effective communication, the clarification of long-held myths and beliefs and the building of a trusting relationship, exercise professionals can help relieve much unneeded stress and anxiety during this early stage of change. By discussing clients' objections to their exercise routine up front, it is possible to work with them to decrease or eliminate the costs before they give up on exercise. Although people in the precontemplation stage are not currently engaging in any exercise, it is likely that they have done so before, or at least exerted themselves physically at some time in the past. If a client hates working out alone, for example, perhaps they can find an exercise partner or try some group activities. If feeling tired after exercise is a complaint, perhaps they could schedule gentle exercise, such as restorative yoga, in the evening, when feeling relaxed would encourage better sleep. Barriers and obstacles need to be addressed, as they may lead to relapse at any stage, especially the earlier ones.

Many people do not like to have to expend physical effort when it is not necessary. Discussing this drawback of exercise lets clients know that their perception of exercise as requiring excessive effort is not abnormal, but a natural step in developing new, healthy exercise habits. This is important, as people who spend a majority of their time in sedentary behaviors may mistakenly assume that people who exercise regularly are fundamentally different from themselves—that regular exercisers stick with it because they love every minute of working out. The realization that even physically active people encounter difficulties—but have learned ways to overcome them—will help clients see that they too can overcome barriers and learn new skills that will help them stay active.

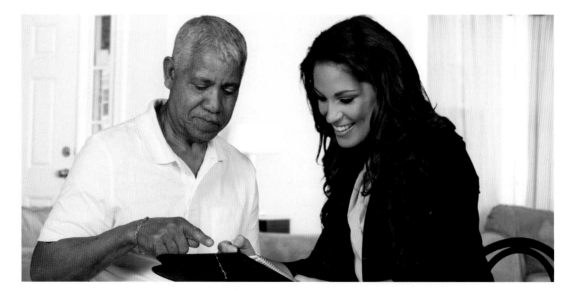

While addressing client concerns over the costs of exercise, it is also necessary to discuss the benefits they may reap from being active. Some of these may be immediate, such as feeling more alert or experiencing a boost in self-esteem after an exercise session. Others may be long-term, such as living longer or decreasing the loss of **bone mineral density** associated with **osteoporosis.** Helping clients maximize their expected benefits improves the ratio of expected benefits to costs, which will make them more likely to initiate physical activity. If a client identifies increased energy and weight management as the greatest benefits of exercise, they could consider scheduling their workout in the morning on their busiest days to help them to tackle those days with more energy. Once again, the specificity of the program is essential to meet the goals, preferences, and needs of the new exerciser.

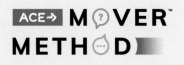

The Benefits-to-Costs Ratio of Exercise

Loretta is a 67-year-old client with whom you have been working for the past four months. She has been regularly attending private personal-training sessions and has just shared with you that she has not followed through with her goal of exercising at the gym two times per week on the days that she is not scheduled for personal training. Loretta lets you know that she enjoys exercising and has been feeling like her daily activities are less fatiguing since becoming more physically active but is not sure she wants to spend more time at the gym.

ACE→ ABC APPROACH

The following is an example of how the ACE Mover Method™ and the ACE ABC Approach™ can be used to address the benefits-to-costs ratio of exercise.

Ask: Asking powerful open-ended questions during this conversation will allow the exercise professional to find out more about why the client does not want to spend more time at the gym even though she has more energy and it makes daily activities feel easier. In addition, powerful questioning will allow the client to be more insightful and have more clarity about her thoughts and actions.

Exercise Professional: On the days you exercise you have more energy, and daily activities feel easier since becoming more physically active. In a perfect world, how many days per week would you exercise?

Client: That's right. My energy levels have been noticeably higher and I don't feel as tired after doing work around the house or even after a whole day of running errands. Beginning and sticking with an exercise program is really making a difference in my life. In a perfect world, I could see myself exercising five to six days per week, including my scheduled sessions with you.

Break down barriers: Ask more open-ended questions to find out what barriers are getting in the way of the client making it to the gym on the days she is not scheduled for personal-training sessions.

Exercise Professional: Exercise has become important for you and ideally you could envision yourself exercising five to six days per week. What is preventing you from adding more exercise to your week?

Client: Yes. Exercise has become important to me. To be honest, I don't come to the gym on my own because I feel like the more athletic and fit gym members are always watching me while I am doing my exercises. I am very self-conscious and the thought of being watched has been enough of a barrier that it has prevented me from reaching my weekly goal of coming to the gym twice per week on my own. Even though I want to exercise, the thought of the more fit people watching me makes me embarrassed and so I choose not to exercise at all.

Collaborate: Working together with the client to come up with solutions is the next step now that the client has expressed her perceived benefits (e.g., increased energy and ease of doing daily activities) and costs (e.g., embarrassment) and the desire to exercise five or six days per week.

Exercise Professional: Exercise feels good and you would like to do more of it, but the thought of being watched at the gym is embarrassing to you. What other options are there?

Client: I have been thinking about this question lately and have come up with some alternatives. The two options that seem the most realistic to me are to either exercise at an alternate location outside of the gym or to find a time to come to the gym when it is not as crowded. Both options seem like good ideas to me.

Exercise Professional: I can see you have put some thought into coming up with these solutions. What do you think you will do?

Client: To start, I want to come to the gym during off-peak hours. I found out that the gym is not that crowded during the middle of the day Monday through Friday. I want to stick with my original goal of going to the gym twice per week on my own but now I will go midday.

In this scenario, the client worked through her perceived costs and benefits to exercising regularly. The ACE ABC Approach can be used to explore the perceived costs and benefits of exercise and other health-related behaviors in a nonjudgmental and collaborative way while guiding clients toward their future vision. There are multiple long-lasting benefits to using the ACE ABC Approach, some of which include: identifying obstacles and barriers, discovering options and choices, collaborating with others, being proactive, and taking action, all of which build self-esteem and self-efficacy.

📖 APPLY WHAT YOU KNOW

Decisional Balance Worksheet

Another helpful tool for exercise professionals to use with clients who are weighing the pros and cons of beginning an exercise program is a **decisional balance** worksheet (Figure 2-3). The balance sheet recognizes that both gains and losses can be consequences of a single decision. The balance sheet is a place to record the advantages and disadvantages of different options facing an individual. Clients can use this tool to detail everything that could affect their decision to make changes. The client writes down all of their positive and negative perceptions about exercise (or any other health-related behavioral change), which helps them connect with the benefits of change and become more aware of barriers to change and then remove them.

FIGURE 2-3
Decisional balance worksheet

Instructions:

▸ Work with the client to document the gains and potential losses that they might experience when making a lifestyle change.

▸ Identify and list the recommended implementation strategies needed to achieve the gains and list coping strategies that can be used to deal with the potential losses or obstacles associated with the change.

DECISIONAL BALANCE WORKSHEET

Perceived gains associated with adopting desired behaviors

1. _____
2. _____
3. _____
4. _____

Perceived losses associated with adopting desired behaviors

1. _____
2. _____
3. _____
4. _____

Strategies to maximize potential for achieving gains

1. _____
2. _____
3. _____
4. _____

Strategies to minimize potential of perceived losses

1. _____
2. _____
3. _____
4. _____

STRATEGIES FOR OLDER ADULTS IN THE CONTEMPLATION STAGE

Clients in the **contemplation** stage are still not physically active but have begun thinking about participating in physical activity and intend to begin a physical-activity program in the near future (within the next six months). These clients may understand some of the benefits of physical activity but may need further encouragement with respect to how physical activity might be beneficial for them in the short-term. Evaluating the pros and cons of becoming more physically active is important in this stage, as ambivalence about change is explored to make the implications of being inactive more apparent. In addition, validating the client's lack of readiness to change and making it clear that the decision to change rests with them while exploring new positive outcome expectations and boosting self-confidence will foster progress toward the next stage of change. Again, do not discuss specific goal-setting strategies at this point, as too much specific planning may overwhelm clients, sending them back to the precontemplation stage.

The Social Connection: Using Social Support to Assist with Motivation for Exercise

Support from other people is an important resource that may help clients of all ages maintain physical activity. Many older adults are faced with the challenge of coping with multiple losses that often restrict the amount and nature of social contact. Spouses, siblings, or treasured friends now may be deceased, while others may have moved away to retirement or assisted-living communities. Physical disabilities or illnesses may prevent friends or other family members from being able to engage in previously enjoyed activities, such as long walks or shopping excursions. Retired individuals who relied upon the work setting as a primary source of social contact may now experience distress over the loss of that environment. Children and other relatives may live in distant cities and be unable to visit regularly.

However, rather than disengaging from society, many older adults desire to rebuild and keep nurturing social connections. If older clients want to maintain social connections with others and do not already have sufficient opportunities to do so, their physical-activity programs can serve a dual function by meeting both exercise and social needs. Exercise programs that take into account the value of social interaction, in addition to the physical benefits of exercise, can be especially valuable to older adults.

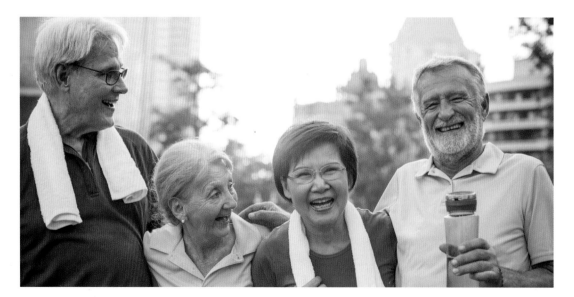

APPLY WHAT YOU KNOW

Social-support Strategies

How can social support be employed to help clients? One way is to suggest that they seek support from others on an ongoing basis. The following are some social-support strategies to suggest to clients:

▶ Find an enjoyable and reliable exercise partner. If partners are not readily available in the exercise setting, look to community agencies or programs offered by organizations such as churches, social groups, or university-based senior programs.

▶ Ask friends and family members to be encouraging and positive about the exercise program. Find out if they have a similar interest in becoming more physically active and invite them to join in the program.

▶ Ask for reminders from friends and family members about physical-activity goals or appointments.

▶ Set up fun "contests" with a friend as well as rewards based upon meeting a **process goal,** such as attending a water aerobics class 10 times without an absence. (The friend's goal does not have to be exercise-related, although mutual support for exercise is beneficial for everyone. The main objective is to use accountability to someone else as a source of motivation for meeting exercise goals.)

▶ Add a social element to the exercise program. For example, arrive at class a little early if it affords the opportunity to chat with other class members.

▶ Find an enjoyable activity that is based on being physically active with a group or club, such as dancing, bowling, or hiking.

Exercise professionals can facilitate social support for exercise by fostering interaction in their programs. Speak with as many clients as possible, even in a large class or group. Introduce clients to one another. Incorporate brief exercise activities that require a partner or small groups. Allow clients the space to meet before or after classes to socialize and encourage participants to plan social events if desired. Over time, clients may develop rewarding friendships with other exercise participants, thereby enhancing their sense of belonging and improving their commitment to the program.

It also should be noted that social influences can sometimes make exercise more difficult. Common examples include a spouse who makes negative comments about an exercise program or friends who try to persuade a client to go to lunch rather than exercise. A client's participation in an exercise program may require adaptation on the part of others, which may or may not be forthcoming.

📖 APPLY WHAT YOU KNOW

Helping Clients Deal with Negative Social Influences

Although friends and family ultimately may only want the best for the client, they may be experiencing some feelings of neglect or jealousy, or other interpersonal issues that need to be resolved. If you hear clients discussing negative influences, work with them to evaluate the impact of such instances on their exercise motivation level. Help clients take greater control over the situation by suggesting that they:

▸ Schedule their contact with unsupportive people after they exercise for the day.

▸ Try to balance out time with unsupportive people by increasing time with supporters.

▸ Set clear limits for how much time they will spend with unsupportive people, or avoid such contact altogether.

▸ Mentally prepare to respond to negative comments so they do not provoke negative behaviors and lack of adherence.

▸ Mentally review why their exercise program is important prior to spending time with unsupportive peers as well as understand the reasons behind negative responses from peer pressure.

▸ Explain to an unsupportive person why exercise is important and ask for the person's encouragement. If the person is willing to try to be more supportive, the client should say specifically what the client would and would not like the person to do. (For example, "It would help me a lot if you wouldn't say, 'Are you off to the gym *again*?' each time I leave the apartment for a while. But asking how I am progressing in my program every now and then would be nice.") It is important to have an honest discussion with the saboteur to discover the deeper underlying motives and emotions behind the negative actions. This can make both parties feel more comfortable and lead to better communication.

Helping clients recognize the impact that others' responses may have on their motivation can prepare them to use positive social support to their advantage, and to decrease the impact of discouraging influences. Recruiting social support is almost always an effective strategy for physical-activity promotion; however, it can be most effective during the contemplation and **preparation** stages when clients are attempting to establish regular patterns of physical activity.

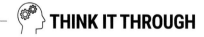 **THINK IT THROUGH**

Social Support

What strategies will you use in your practice to help older adults connect with others and fulfill their social outcome expectations?

STRATEGIES FOR OLDER ADULTS IN THE PREPARATION STAGE

Clients in the preparation stage have decided that they want to begin a physical-activity program and have begun to engage in some activity while mentally and physically preparing to be physically active on a regular basis. Activity in this stage may be described as inconsistent and sporadic, as clients are not yet regularly active. This is a good time to reinforce the benefits of engaging in regular physical activity, ensure the client has the skills needed for behavior change, encourage small steps to build self-efficacy, determine and plan for potential obstacles, identify sources for and establish social support, and collaborate on setting specific physical-activity goals.

Using Reminders to Exercise

"Cues" are simply influencers—either planned or coincidental—that remind people to engage in certain kinds of behaviors. Seeing walking shoes by the front door can remind a client of plans to walk that day, while keeping a fitness facility ID card on one's key ring can provide an ongoing reminder about an exercise commitment. Setting a calendar notification or cell phone alarm as a reminder to leave for an exercise class can be quite helpful.

Unfortunately, some influences also make it harder to exercise. Starting an engaging new book can make it difficult to start watching a live-stream exercise class. Having friends drop by unexpectedly can make it hard to go outside for a walk. Teach your clients to intentionally use cues to remind themselves to exercise. Whenever possible, also encourage them to avoid cues that make it difficult to exercise until after they have met their physical-activity goal for the day.

Using Rewards as Motivators

Eventually, clients may find exercise rewarding in and of itself and move from being physically active to gain a reward or avoid a consequence (**external regulation**) to being physically active because the behavior is consistent with their goals (**integrated regulation**). Over time, new behaviors may become internalized as they become more autonomous and self-regulated in nature. Focusing on intrinsic aspirations such as health, personal growth, and meaningful relationships compared to extrinsic aspirations (e.g., wealth and image) may lead to greater autonomy, relatedness, and physical and mental well-being and vitality. Note that **autonomous regulation** predicts exercise participation across all settings, with personally valuing the outcomes of exercise leading to initial program adoption, while intrinsic motivation (i.e., valuing the experience itself) is more important for long-term exercise adherence (Teixeira et al., 2012).

Intrinsic motivation is derived from a sense of autonomy, wherein people act as a result of their own free will and because they want to. Long-term exercisers typically find that many inherent aspects of physical activity give them pleasure and motivate future exercise behaviors (e.g., a sense of accomplishment as they are exercising or post-workout relaxation). Exercise professionals sometimes expect clients to enjoy the intrinsic rewards of exercise, just as they do. The reality, however, is that it often takes time to begin enjoying exercise for its inherent benefits. Until clients sufficiently develop their physical abilities to focus on pleasurable aspects of their workouts rather than how difficult their exertion feels, they cannot be expected to necessarily enjoy working out. Motivational, desirable outcomes such as improved muscle strength or weight loss may not occur for several months. For some clients, a genuine, internally generated love of exercise may never develop.

Externally motivated people perform a behavior because they feel pushed by an external force to do so. For example, when a person engages in exercise to gain a tangible or social reward (e.g., a discounted health insurance premium or the approval of friends who belong to a gym) or to avoid disapproval (e.g., from a spouse or loved one), they are extrinsically motivated. Externally regulated behaviors can also be controlled and driven by self-approval (e.g., exercising regularly because a person knows it will help them reach a weight-loss or fitness-related goal). Controlled forms of **extrinsic motivation** are expected to sometimes regulate (or motivate) short-term behavior, but not to sustain maintenance over time (Teixeira et al., 2012). Clients who do not find exercise internally rewarding still can develop and maintain regular exercise routines, but they will need to continue using external rewards. Until clients begin to report internal rewards, it is worthwhile to employ external rewards to keep motivation levels high. Such rewards can be planned in conjunction with setting physical-activity goals.

External rewards for exercise can take many forms. Clients can establish their own reward systems, such as allowing themselves to enjoy a relaxing soak in the spa immediately after they exercise or treating themselves to a movie each week they meet their exercise goals. Exercise professionals can provide external rewards in the form of praise for achievements (see Chapter 1) or tangible rewards such as prizes for meeting short-term goals. Rewards also can be linked to program monitoring, as in the case of a prominently posted attendance chart documenting each client's attendance, with a gift certificate given for every 10 classes attended. Rewards should be designed to coincide with the accomplishment of goals. Rewards can also vary in size based on the duration and perceived difficulty of the goal.

One word of caution: Too much focus on external rewards can foster a reliance upon such rewards, which could be problematic if the rewards are not always available. To minimize this risk, provide more external rewards when clients are new to exercise and gradually decrease them when clients begin to express internal motivation to exercise.

STRATEGIES FOR OLDER ADULTS IN THE ACTION STAGE

Clients in the **action** stage have been engaging in regular physical activity, but for less than six months. At this stage, it is helpful to review the initial goals and adjust them as necessary, empower clients to restructure cues and social support, increase awareness of inevitable lapses, bolster self-efficacy, and support clients in establishing systems of self-monitoring and accountability. In addition, clients may be looking for additional ways to motivate themselves, especially on days when social support is unavailable. Now that the client has some experience with exercise, introducing the use of environmental cues and self-talk strategies can be helpful and is appropriate at this stage.

Revising Short-term Goals as Needed

Patterns of exercise successes and difficulties contain a wealth of information that can be used to help clients. Try to review goals with clients on a weekly or biweekly basis. Congratulate them on all successes, including partially met goals. Clients may feel like failures when they do not meet 100% of their goals and they may not give themselves credit for what was accomplished. Clients should understand that all effort put toward meeting their long-term objectives and improving their health or fitness is valuable.

Ask successful clients what helped them to succeed. Did they discover especially helpful strategies such as exercising with a friend or attending fitness classes at a certain time of day? Congratulate them on their ingenuity and note the strategies that were helpful for them. If a client begins to have difficulties with exercise, encourage them to employ these strategies again.

Clients who are unsuccessful at meeting their goals can share valuable personal experiences that will facilitate problem solving. In an understanding manner, ask what factors made it difficult for them to meet their goals. Listen for possible patterns. Once major problems have been identified, work with them to generate solutions or modify goals. Exercise professionals can help increase clients' ownership of overcoming future obstacles by allowing clients to come up with realistic solutions for tackling potential program barriers. Praise clients for talking about their obstacles—even if they do not meet their goals—and remind them that this is a critical step toward eventual success with behavioral change.

The first concern should be helping clients feel good about what they have accomplished. This will give them the confidence to meet future goals. Explain that it is only through trying to meet exercise goals that they can discover which strategies do or do not help them succeed. Explain that instances they perceive as failures can be helpful if they learn from the experience.

After evaluating successes and challenges, clients should commit to a new set of short-term goals. They may opt to keep the same exercise goals, decrease goals that were overly ambitious, or challenge themselves with new or intensified goals. In any case, all the previous goal-setting steps still apply. The exercise professional may make recommendations for revision, but the final selection of the next short-term goals should ultimately rest with the client. As clients become regular exercisers, a formal review of goals may occur less often (perhaps monthly or every two to three months, depending on the client). Ideally, clients will become quite good at tracking their own progress and revising their own goals.

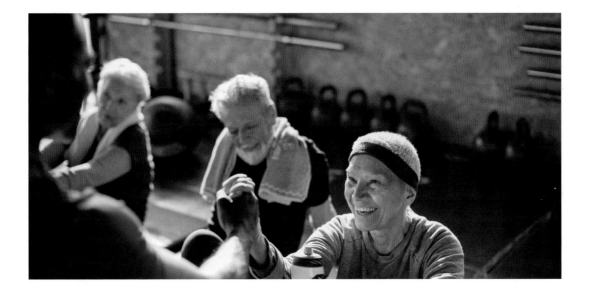

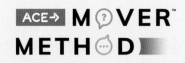

Evaluating Original Goals and Setting New Ones

Anna, a client with whom you have been working once every other week for the past six months, has arrived at the fitness facility for her session with you. During the warm-up portion of the exercise session, she lets you know how things have been going regarding her goals.

ACE→ ABC APPROACH

The ACE Mover Method and ACE ABC Approach can be used to revisit the client's current goals and work together to identify any successes or challenges to determine how the client would like to proceed. This will be accomplished by using active listening and asking open-ended questions that draw upon the client's own expertise.

Exercise Professional: Great job with performing your warm-up exercises today! You asked some good questions and I can tell you really want to understand why these exercises are important.

Anna: Thank you. I have been looking forward to our session all week! Asking questions to understand the purpose of each exercise seems to motivate me.

Ask: Taking the time to ask powerful open-ended questions during an exercise session will not only continue the rapport-building process, but also create an environment where the client has a safe space for sharing information and potentially build more self-efficacy.

Exercise Professional: We have a few more minutes left before moving on to the conditioning segment of today's workout. Before we do that, tell me what your experience has been related to your health goals over the past two weeks.

Client: Thank you for always following up with me on the goals that we set at the end of each session. I feel like you are genuinely interested in how I am doing. Knowing that we will be discussing my goals makes me want to have something good to tell you. As you may recall, I had set a goal of working out one additional time per week on the weeks we have meetings and working out twice per week on the weeks when we do not meet. In total, my goal has been to exercise twice each week. I am happy to tell you that I am still achieving this goal. After consistently exercising twice per week for the past five months, I feel like I have this routine under control, and it feels good!

Exercise Professional: Your hard work is really paying off. You intend to work out two times per week and you consistently reach your goals and that feels good.

Client: Yes. It feels good in two ways. It feels good to know that I can set goals around exercise and achieve them, and it physically feels good to exercise. I am on a roll! In fact, I have been thinking about expanding my current exercise routine.

Exercise Professional: Feeling good physically and achieving your goals is important to you and you feel ready to set a new goal. What would you like to do?

Client: Exercise has become important to me and something I look forward to. For the past two months, I have been considering adding a third day of exercise to my routine. I have made a few friends at the gym and they have been encouraging me to join them for a weekly circuit training class. I have observed the class before from afar and it looks fun. The class time and day work with my schedule. My only hesitation is that the class may not be right for me.

Break down barriers: It is time to ask more questions to find out what perceived or actual barriers the client has regarding the new short-term goal.

Exercise Professional: Adding a third day of exercise to your routine has been on your mind for a few months and you found a group class you want to try. What are your hesitations about taking the class?

Client: Well, I am not sure I am physically ready for the demands of the class. Even though I recognized some of the movements being performed when I observed the class, it just seems different. I am so glad to have made friends at the gym and am thankful that they invited me to join them, but they are younger than me and probably in better shape.

Exercise Professional: How have you handled situations like this in the past?

Client: I have never been in a situation like this before when it comes to exercise but I have experienced insecurity like this during my career and with family and friends when they have invited me to try new things. Previously, in situations like this I would research the new thing I would be doing and I would practice it to build up my comfort and confidence.

Collaborate: The next step involves working together with the client on solutions for overcoming barriers and reaching a new goal. It is important that the client remains in control of the goals she wants to set.

Exercise Professional: Feeling comfortable and confident with circuit training before attending the class is important to you. What will you do to build confidence in this type of exercise?

Client: Good question. Is it possible for us to do a circuit training workout together? I trust your expertise and would appreciate it if we could do this type of workout together so I can feel what it will be like when I take the class. Also, my goal of exercising three days per week is independent of this class, so I would like to start implementing that right away. Is circuit training something I can do on my own?

Exercise Professional: Yes. Circuit training is something you can do on your own. Tell me more about what you would like to do and how you would like to go about implementing that plan.

Client: Starting next week, I would like to begin exercising three days per week and I would like for one of the three days to be circuit training either in the class or on my own until I feel comfortable joining the class. Can you teach me how to turn my existing routine into a circuit or work with me to create a circuit?

Exercise Professional: Yes. I would be happy to do this. In fact, if you would like we can do today's workout in circuit format and you can use this same workout next week for your third day of exercise if you like.

Client: That sounds great!

This scenario explored the importance of evaluating original goals and setting new ones. During this process, clients may decide they would like to stick with their existing goals, decrease the intensity of their goals, or expand on their goals. In any case, it is important to use active listening skills and open-ended questioning to understand what your clients want to accomplish and what they need in order to increase their chances of success.

Using Self-talk as an Exercise Motivator

Self-talk can help clients meet exercise goals if it is positive or otherwise motivating. Statements such as "I can do it" or "I'll feel much less stiff once I've done my exercises" can help clients begin or continue exercising. Self-talk also can be discouraging, as in the case of people who say to themselves, "I don't know why I should bother with all of this effort; it's never going to pay off" or "I'll never be able to keep up with the rest of this class." Promote motivation by teaching clients how to identify and take control of self-talk related to their exercise goals.

To identify self-talk, encourage clients to ask themselves what is "going through their minds" when they are feeling discouraged about exercise or having difficulty meeting physical-activity goals. This should help them pinpoint the negative thinking that is interfering with their success. They also can learn from positive experiences. Thoughts that help them feel good about exercising can be recalled when they feel discouraged.

Next, negative self-talk should be corrected. This does not require becoming oblivious to reality or trying to think only "happy thoughts." Instead, encourage clients to try to make their self-talk realistic, rather than unduly harsh, by assessing the accuracy of self-talk. Acknowledging that such statements as "I always mess up" or "I'll never be able to succeed" are exaggerations and should be changed to more accurate statements will help clients regain a more realistic perspective.

Sometimes, negative statements will be accurate (e.g., perhaps the client is not in the mood to exercise or finds a particular exercise difficult). In these cases, suggest that they work to find solutions, such as determining a way to make the program more appealing or substituting other exercises for ones that are currently frustrating. When negative thoughts arise, ask clients to try shifting their attention to understanding what is feeling negative and why. Once this is understood, negative thoughts can be changed to positive and motivating thoughts and self-talk that emphasize the positive effects of exercise: "This will help me improve my balance" or "I will be so proud of myself when I finish my workout today." Using affirmative self-talk to their advantage is a way for clients to motivate themselves to adhere to their exercise routines. As with goal setting, positive self-talk can be an effective strategy during any stage of change. It is imperative that exercise professionals encourage clients to become aware of their inner thoughts and to reflect on how this inner commentary may influence behavior. Be aware of any negative self-talk at any stage of change and bring it to the client's attention.

📖 APPLY WHAT YOU KNOW

Cognitive Restructuring

Cognitive restructuring refers to the process by which people attempt to replace habitual unproductive thinking with more helpful thoughts. Cognitive restructuring means learning to perceive and think about a situation in a new way. Exercise professionals can help clients notice and challenge unhelpful thought patterns in several ways. Professionals might try these approaches with clients who bring up their tendencies to experience negative self-talk that interferes with their behavior-change plans. The following suggestions focus on food choices, but the same ideas can be used with exercise, smoking cigarettes, and other health behaviors.

- ▸ Encourage clients who are interested to keep a record of negative thoughts and self-talk that "cause" them to eat fast food. Give clients one to two weeks to observe and record these thoughts. If clients have trouble becoming aware of their thoughts, instruct them to pay special attention to what is going through their minds when they are feeling stressed or conflicted about their food choices or what thoughts prompt them to eat fast food.

- ▸ Spend part of a session looking at these thoughts together. Which statements reflect real problems that clients might wish to discuss? Let the clients suggest ways that they could deal with these problems. Which statements tend to be "excuses"?

- ▸ Suspend judgment and allow clients to evaluate their self-talk. If clients feel that their problems are valid and not excuses, the exercise professional should express empathy. If clients feel the professional is belittling their problems, they may become defensive and no longer be open to guidance and cognitive-restructuring efforts.

- ▸ Examine misconceptions that may underlie negative thoughts. Clients may express some common irrational beliefs, such as, "It is selfish to take time to go to the grocery store and prepare healthy meals when my family would be happier going out for fast food." In this example, the exercise professional might ask an open-ended question, such as, "What does having healthy meals instead of fast food mean to you?" This may reveal the client's values, such as the importance they place on the health and well-being of their family. The professional can then utilize a double-sided reflection to capture what the client has shared, such as, "It feels selfish to take time to go to the grocery store and it's important to you to provide meals that support the health and well-being of you and your family." This can help to elicit **change talk** and support the client in reframing their perspective.

- ▸ Empower clients to rephrase negative self-talk. The new self-talk should be less negative, but also realistic. Consider one of the most common thoughts: "I'm too tired to make dinner tonight." One could say instead, "I am going to prepare a simple meal this evening, even though I feel tired. I know I'll feel better and have more energy if I eat well." Another example of unhelpful thinking is, "This approach to eating is a waste of time. I've got more important things to do." Clients may challenge this thinking and reframe their perspective by saying, "I need to eat well to stay healthy. Staying healthy is just as important as my work, and by making time each day to eat well, I can stay healthy and work as effectively as possible."

▸ Help clients anticipate and cope with common unhelpful thoughts. Once clients have uncovered and rephrased unhelpful thoughts, the exercise professional can ask them to imagine feeling tired at the end of the day, with the negative thoughts springing up in their minds. Clients can imagine themselves restructuring the negative thoughts and then eating as planned. Clients might finish this visualization by imagining how good they feel because they are eating well.

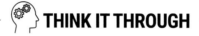 **THINK IT THROUGH**

Self-talk

For 24 hours, practice listening to your own self-talk. Pay attention to your thoughts as they relate to you performing your daily tasks. Is your self-talk mostly negative? Were there positive examples of self-talk that occurred? Practice replacing any of your own negative self-talk with positive statements. Think about how you can use this experience to help your clients become more effective at changing their unproductive self-talk. It is important for the client to remember that thoughts create emotions, emotions drive actions, and actions lead to outcomes. This is another reminder of why individuals who desire positive outcomes should have positive self-talk and thoughts.

STRATEGIES FOR OLDER ADULTS IN THE MAINTENANCE STAGE

Clients in the maintenance stage have been participating in regular physical activity for at least six months. Reevaluating current strategies and goals while planning for contingencies with social-support systems and potential lapses can help prevent these lapses (brief periods of inactivity) from turning into relapses (extended periods of inactivity). Clients in the maintenance stage should find ways to transition from external to internal rewards for continuing to exercise even when not intrinsically motivated. Clients at this stage can also benefit from strategies that keep physical activity interesting to avoid boredom and burnout.

Planning for the Future: Relapse-prevention Skills

Knowing the factors that contribute to a relapse can help individuals predict and plan for future high-risk situations. Factors such as illness or injury, social pressure not to engage in activity, a lack of support from friends or family, highly stressful or busy times, and an inability to cope with high-risk situations are just a few of the problems that may hinder progress toward activity goals. Such factors can be difficult for exercisers of all ages.

Exercise professionals should prepare clients to cope with tough situations that are likely to interfere with their exercise programs. Clients must first learn to identify their own high-risk situations. Then they can develop the crucial skills of predicting potential problems and proactively develop plans to deal with them. For example, Mike has difficulty swimming regularly and knows that this will become even harder for him when his family arrives for a three-week visit. He realizes there will be plenty of distractions. Nevertheless, he wants to try to stick to his swimming routine.

Mike could work together with an exercise professional to turn this challenge into a victory by collaborating on, and implementing, an action plan. Perhaps Mike can reschedule his swim sessions at the time of day when his grandchildren typically nap, so he will not miss out on time with them. Maybe he could arrange to meet a friend at the pool at predetermined times for added accountability, so he will feel compelled to go. Mike is likely to have some good ideas about what will help him keep swimming. Encourage him to generate his own ideas and respect his autonomy by recognizing that he is the foremost expert in himself.

Teaching clients to distinguish between a lapse and a relapse can also be helpful. After missing one or more planned activity sessions, it is common for people to start feeling guilty and ashamed, and to experience decreased self-confidence in their ability to exercise regularly. Additionally, some people will engage in all-or-none thinking, labeling themselves as "quitters" or failures. However, if clients have acknowledged in advance that lapses are common and temporary setbacks rather than catastrophic failures, they can more easily forgive themselves and get back on track with their activity plans. Encourage clients to start anew as soon as possible after a lapse, even if they must again start slowly. The sooner they resume some sort of physical activity, the better they will feel about themselves, and the easier it will be to get back into their desired exercise routine.

Balancing Convenience and Enjoyment

As mentioned earlier, it is easier to quit an activity that carries more costs than benefits. If an activity is too inconvenient, it will be stopped as soon as the effort outweighs the rewards. Many people do engage in highly inconvenient activities with some regularity. There are snow skiers, for example, who buy expensive and specialized equipment, drive for hours to reach a ski area, wait in line for lift tickets, brave even the harshest of weather conditions on the slopes, ski to the point of exhaustion, and willingly opt to do it all again as soon as they have another chance. This inconvenient exercise occurs because the people who engage in it are having fun. But if every trip to the fitness facility or every daily walk were as inconvenient as a ski trip, most people simply would not bother. The difference is that people are willing to deal with hassle if an activity is extremely enjoyable or rewarding in other ways.

Therefore, there are two very important lessons to teach clients:

▸ **Engage in exercise plans that are convenient.** This applies to a regular exercise routine that can be done even on days when clients have little time or energy for elaborate plans. Going to a nearby fitness facility for a regular class held at a convenient time or streaming an exercise video at home are good examples of such activities. Hopefully, these will be somewhat enjoyable, but they do not have to be blissfully fun if they are relatively easy to do.

▸ **Engage in inconvenient but fun exercise activities but be realistic about how often they can be done.** For example, one client may love to dress in formal attire and go ballroom dancing, while another is willing to drive for an hour to a favorite hiking spot.

Clients should be taught to engage in inconvenient but treasured activities when it is realistic to do so, but also to have a set of very convenient exercise options to employ on a daily basis.

Consider enjoyment and convenience when reviewing client progress. Clients who are having trouble meeting exercise goals may need help to increase convenience. If they hate traffic and driving to the fitness center, perhaps they can carpool with someone or participate in a home exercise program. If they dislike early-morning obligations, they should attempt to take fitness classes in the afternoon or evening or find a time that they can build into their daily schedule that is more suitable, such as a lunchtime walk with a friend.

THINK IT THROUGH

Behavior-change Strategies

The behavior-change strategies described in this chapter are useful in promoting exercise adherence among all clients. Some, however, may be particularly helpful when working with older adults. Think about your own experiences as an exercise professional, and about times that you used—or could have used—these strategies with your clients. How would you introduce these behavior-change topics to your clients? What recommendations would you make to those clients based upon these behavior-change principles? Visualizing yourself using these techniques will help you become comfortable enough with them to incorporate them into your work.

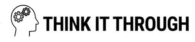

Exercise Convenience

Bill is meeting with you after following his initial exercise program for four weeks. Bill's initial program goals were to meet with you three days per week, on Tuesday, Thursday, and Saturday, and to play nine holes of golf on Wednesday and Friday each week.

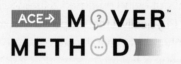

The ACE Mover Method philosophy can be used with clients in all stages of the behavior-change process. In this instance, the ACE ABC Approach is used to discuss the status of a current exercise program to understand the client's definition of success and to identify what changes the client may like to make.

Ask: Asking powerful open-ended questions allows the client to express what is going well with his current plan and what areas exist for improvement. This step will open the door for a productive conversation.

Exercise Professional: Hello, Bill. It's good to see you. It has been four weeks since we started working together and I am curious to hear an update on progress toward your goals.

Client: It's good to see you, too. I did pretty well the first week. I came to the gym for our scheduled sessions each day and completed the routine three times, just like we planned. But the second, third, and fourth week, I got to the gym only twice. I was also able to play golf twice the first week on my planned days and only once per week on weeks two through four. Overall, it does not feel like I accomplished much over the first month of this program.

Exercise Professional: It was not that long ago when you were not going to the gym at all. You tried really hard this month!

Client: That's true. Prior to us working together, I was not going to the gym or exercising at all, aside from playing golf. I guess working out even twice per week is a big step from where I was four weeks ago. I do feel like I have been giving my health-related goals my best effort, but I did not hit the intended target. It seems like things continued to get in the way as the week went on and by the time Saturday rolled around I was not prepared to show up for our session and it was too much of a hassle to make it to the gym and golf course.

Break down barriers: Asking more open-ended questions at this time will help the client be more specific with identifying the obstacles that got in the way.

Exercise Professional: What does being prepared to show up for a workout look like to you?

Client: I guess what I mean about being prepared is feeling like I am mentally and physically ready for exercise. Physically, I feel prepared, but mentally I am thinking about how Saturday is my only day to sleep in, go to the grocery store, and actually have some fun. When I think about the time commitment to drive to and from the gym, plus the actual workout time and showering, it seems like half the day is gone. This is what has been going through my mind when I make the decision not to show up for our Saturday sessions.

Exercise Professional: You are prepared both mentally and physically for exercise on Tuesday and Thursday and even make it to sessions early and sometimes stay in the gym afterward, socializing with new friends. How have you been successful with being prepared on Tuesdays and Thursdays?

Client: Monday through Friday I have a very set routine and have been able to incorporate our exercise sessions into that routine because there are no other commitments pulling me in other directions. In fact, after 1:00 pm on Tuesdays and Thursdays I have nothing planned except our appointments. I plan ahead regarding meals, clothes, and daily activities to make sure I am all set for the gym.

Collaborate: Now that the barrier of conflicting priorities and convenience has been identified, the client and exercise professional can work together on goals and solutions for moving forward.

Exercise Professional: Prioritizing your commitments Monday through Friday allows you to stay on track with your weekly goals, while on Saturdays your exercise goals seem inconvenient

Client: That's it. It's not that exercise is not important to me. It's just the way I like to spend my time on Saturdays and the things I need to get done seem incompatible with getting my workout done. I still want to find a way to exercise three days per week, but it has to be convenient.

Exercise Professional: What options can you think of?

Client: I have been thinking about checking with you to see if you are available to meet with me on another day during the week or to see if we can cut the workout time in half on Saturdays. That said, other than Tuesday, Thursday, and Saturday I am not sure what other days will work with my golf schedule. I also am not that excited about cutting the workout time down, as my goal is to achieve more exercise in my life.

Exercise Professional: Are there any other options?

Client: One theme that keeps coming up for me is what if I did not have to travel to the gym. That would save me quite a bit of time. I actually like this idea the best but am not sure where to begin.

Exercise Professional: Having a plan for a home workout to complete on Saturdays would be a good option to try.

Client: Yes. If I had a specific plan to follow, I think shortening the time commitment by removing the travel and not reducing the exercise time is something I would like to try. If you can help me create a home exercise plan for one day per week, I think I would like to adjust my goal to making it to the gym twice per week and exercising at home once per week.

In this scenario, the exercise professional used the ACE ABC Approach to check in on program goals and make adjustments based on the client's perception of convenience as an obstacle. Ultimately, following this approach led to a client-centered, nonjudgmental conversation that left the client in control of his goals and exercise program.

Setting Exercise Goals with Older Adults

Goal setting is important for anyone attempting to change a behavior. Exercise professionals can play a pivotal role in teaching clients how to set and evaluate their physical-activity goals.

Setting goals is an important process for initial and continued behavioral change. It is an integral part of all exercise programs. The best thing about goal setting is that it is relatively simple to employ and extremely effective when done properly. Goal setting must be used systematically and should be an active part of the program to maximize adherence. The following are a few key considerations to keep in mind during the goal-setting process:

▸ *Avoid setting too many goals:* Keep the number of goals manageable and attainable so that the client is not overwhelmed with all that they need to accomplish.

▶ *Avoid setting negative goals:* If the client wants to set a goal of not missing any workouts, the exercise professional should help the client reframe this goal in a positive way: "I will attend every scheduled workout session." Setting negative goals puts the focus on the behavior that should be avoided, not the behavior to be achieved. It is important that the client is thinking about achievement, not avoidance.

▶ *Set short- and long-term goals, as well as process and product goals (also called performance goals):* Long-term goals can be thought of as the client's "North Star" or the guiding light that ensures the program is moving in the right direction, while short-terms goals are the incremental milestones to be reached while moving closer to the North Star. Process goals are the actionable steps taken to reach short-term goals (e.g., walk for 50-minutes on Monday, Wednesday, and Friday to meet physical-activity guidelines) and **product goals** include things such as reaching a desired body weight. Long-term and product goals are important to maintaining program direction and focus, while short-term and process goals are particularly helpful when progress toward achieving the long-term goal is slow. Clients should be achieving successes in each workout because the workout itself is the "process" that will lead to **performance goal** achievement.

▶ *Include the client in the process:* For a client to optimize success in attaining a desired outcome—to achieve one's vision of what life will be like after a behavior change has been made—it is important that the client's values inform the development of their goals. Thus, collaboration between the client and the exercise professional during the goal-setting process will strongly influence the potential success of client achievement.

▶ *Revisit the goals on a regular basis:* This is the most important thing that an exercise professional can do to maximize the effectiveness of the goal-setting process. Goals need regular adjusting and should be consistently reviewed to help direct attention and effort, and to promote persistence.

An important note about health, fitness, and exercise goals: Goal-setting with clients should be contingent upon whether they are seeking health or fitness benefits, or both (see Chapter 6 for information on the ACE Integrated Fitness Training® Model and how it can be applied to older adults). Although vigorous activity may be desirable for certain fitness gains, moderate-intensity physical activity is quite sufficient for attaining health benefits. Most older adults (and most clients in general) will need to be informed that the "no pain, no gain" mantra is not accurate, and that moderate-intensity activity provides substantial health benefits. Similarly, unrealistic weight-loss goals should be addressed early on so that clients are less likely to quit exercising if they do not experience significant weight loss. While exercise is certainly a key to long-term weight loss, it is necessary to decrease caloric intake below caloric expenditure to lose weight. Therefore, for most people, an adjustment in dietary intake also is necessary to achieve weight-loss goals. Clients may need some information about guidelines to assist them with goal setting. The *Physical Activity Guidelines for Americans* acknowledge that regular physical activity is crucial for people of all ages to improve health and that individuals can reduce their risk of developing chronic disease by participating in regular physical activity (U.S. Department of Health & Human Services, 2018). The *Guidelines* suggest that adults (including older adults) should move more and sit less, as performing any amount of physical activity may lead to some health benefits. For substantial health benefits, key guidelines for adults include participating in cardiorespiratory physical activity at a moderate intensity (such as brisk walking) for at least 150 minutes per week, a vigorous intensity (such as running) for at least 75 minutes per week, or some combination of the two. In addition, it is recommended that adults incorporate muscle-strengthening activities of a moderate intensity or higher for all major muscle groups on at least two days a week.

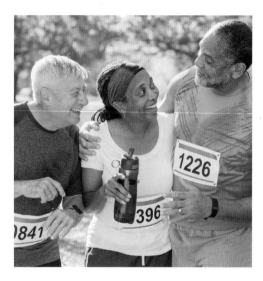

While the physical-activity guidelines for older adults mirror those of younger adults, it is important to note a few key guidelines specific to older adults. It is recommended that older adults participate in multicomponent physical activity that includes balance training. Further, there should be an understanding of how chronic conditions may influence their ability to safely perform regular physical activity. If the presence of chronic conditions limits the ability to achieve recommended levels of physical activity, older adults should be as physically active as possible. There are several options for attaining the recommended amount of moderate-intensity physical activity, including performing 30-minute sessions or breaking up activity into multiple short bouts on at least five days per week. Program recommendations should be personalized to the type of benefits sought or needed, as well as client interests and lifestyle. Be sensitive to the fact that for some older adults, goal setting may need to revolve exclusively around increasing lifestyle activity—a very worthy goal in its own right.

Effective goals can be collaborated upon and developed using the concept of SMART goal setting. SMART goals are:

- *Specific:* Goals must be clear and unambiguous, stating precisely what should be accomplished.

- *Measurable:* Goals must be trackable so that clients can see whether they are making progress. Examples of measurable goals include performing a given workout two times a week or losing 5 pounds (2.3 kg).

- *Attainable:* Goals should be realistically achievable by the client. The tasks related to the achievement of goals reinforce commitment to the program and encourages the client to continue exercising.

- *Relevant:* Goals must be pertinent to the particular interests, needs, and abilities of the client.

- *Time-bound:* Goals must contain estimated timelines for completion. Clients should regularly monitor progress toward goals.

Goals must be specific so that plans for meeting them are not left to chance. Vaguely stated intentions such as "mall walking three times this week" are easy to forget or put off (indefinitely). In contrast, people often feel much more committed to meeting specifically defined goals such as "mall walking at XYZ Mall at 8:30 a.m., Monday, Wednesday, and Friday, for at least 30 minutes each day." To encourage clients to think through their plans and increase their commitment, supportively ask them to explain the "what, when, where, and how" of meeting their exercise goals.

Goals must be measurable so that there is a clear and objective way to determine whether they have been met. Take vague goals and find one or two quantifiable ways to track progress. For example, a goal of "working out" is hard to measure, but a goal of completing a preplanned workout routine in the gym six times over the next two weeks is measurable. It is crucial to have clients track their exercise behaviors. This can be accomplished in various ways, including writing in a personal notebook or on structured forms, or electronically, using exercise-tracking software or an app.

Collect high-quality screening and assessment data from clients, which may be used to determine whether their goals are attainable. Goals also must be appropriate for the client's current fitness level, stage of readiness, and lifestyle. Chapters 5 and 7 detail the specifics of preparticipation health screening and fitness assessment. It is helpful to develop short-term goals that are slightly challenging, so the person feels a genuine sense of accomplishment when they are met. At the same time, these goals should be designed to produce success and, as such, be within the client's ability. Early successes help to increase a client's confidence (both in the ability to perform physical activity and to incorporate the exercise routine into their life), thereby encouraging adherence to exercise programs.

Even though the client may want to set multiple goals right away, it is advisable to initially focus on only one or two short-term goals. If necessary, explain to the client that new habits—even healthy ones like exercise—take time to develop. Encourage clients to focus their energy on one or two main goals and allow clients to succeed in meeting those goals for a period of time before adding new goals. This is far more productive than having an overly ambitious client try to do too much too soon and then experience the frustration and disappointment of failing.

An important note about selecting short-term goals: It can be very motivating to track and record physical outcomes, or performance goals, such as changes in body measurements. However, try to ensure that a client's short-term goals focus on the actual behaviors they are doing, rather than solely on outcomes. This is especially important for older adults who may no longer experience rapid physiological or performance improvements. If the primary focus is on the process of completing their exercise routine properly and regularly, clients can feel good about these very important accomplishments, even if they do not see rapid gains in stamina or strength. Of course, tangible physical or physiological measurements are valuable for tracking a client's response to the program and for helping improve health and fitness. To facilitate motivation, have clients set some small, short-term goals focused on personal behaviors under their control (e.g., participating in a walking program or completing their **flexibility** exercises), rather than performance outcomes, which can vary widely from one person to the next.

THINK IT THROUGH

Goal-setting Strategies

Your new client, Grace, comes to you with a goal of "losing a few pounds and having more energy to play with the grandkids throughout the day." How might you help Grace rewrite her goal in a way that best facilitates long-term success?

It also is important that clients explicitly agree to meet their exercise goals within a given timeframe (e.g., two weeks, four weeks, or three months) so that it is clear when they will be evaluated to check on progress. This may take the form of a verbal commitment. Some exercise professionals prefer to put such commitments into writing with a "behavioral contract" that defines physical-activity goals and states that the client agrees to make every effort to meet the goals (Figure 2-4). Written contracts should be signed by both the exercise professional and the client, and each should keep a copy for subsequent reference. Such contracts assist in keeping track of client goals and underscore the importance of their exercise plans.

Behavioral contracting is an effective behavior-modification strategy. In behavioral contracting for lifestyle change, the client and the exercise professional set up a system of rewards for adopting a new behavior. Rewards are most effective when they are outlined by, and meaningful to, the client. If the rewards are not meaningful, the client may not find them to be worth pursuing. Behavioral contracting works differently for each individual and exercise professionals have to be careful not to push certain rewards on clients. Behavioral contracts may not be motivating for all clients and should not be used unless the client is in full agreement and feels that it would be an appropriate tool for motivation and adherence. Additionally, behavioral contracting is most effective when it is used consistently. Once certain goals are met, contracts can be revisited and modified throughout the duration of program participation.

Goal setting is a vitally important strategy for clients in the preparation, action, and maintenance stages. However, as clients move into the action and maintenance stages and learn how to set and readjust goals on their own, the exercise professional may end up spending less in-session time with them on goal setting.

FIGURE 2-4

Sample behavioral contract

I Will: (Do what) _____

(When) _____

(How often)_____

(How much)_____

How confident am I that I will do this? _____ (on a scale of 1 to 10, with 1 being not at all confident and 10 being completely confident)

If I successfully make this positive lifestyle change by _____, I will reward myself with _____

_____

_____.

If I fail to successfully make this positive lifestyle change, I will forfeit this reward.

I, _____, have reviewed this contract and I agree to discuss the experience involved in accomplishing or not accomplishing this health-behavior improvement with _____ on _____.

Signed (Client): _____

Signed (Exercise professional):_____

APPLY WHAT YOU KNOW

Effective Goal Setting

Strategies for setting effective health and fitness goals are described below (Brehm, 2004). An example of the implementation of each strategy with Bill (the client from the ACE Mover Method feature on pages 48–50) accompanies each description.

Strategy 1: Listen carefully to understand what clients hope to accomplish with an exercise program.

Ask the client what he wants to accomplish over the long run (months or years) by engaging in an exercise program. He may want to decrease blood pressure, lose weight, improve appearance, perform daily tasks such as carrying groceries or climbing stairs with more ease, decrease stress, meet new people, relieve boredom, improve balance, prevent or manage certain medical conditions, improve mood, or obtain other positive outcomes. Often, a person's reasons for developing an exercise plan will be discussed during the first meeting. In this case, it is appropriate to review Bill's general long-term objectives when developing specific goals.

Exercise Professional: How will your life be different when you reach your physical-activity goals?

Bill: When I start exercising regularly, I will be in better shape and will not be so tired after working on home repair projects.

Strategy 2: Help define specific, measurable goals.

Although conceptually it is fine to have general, long-term goals (such as improving golf performance, losing 100 pounds, or transforming from a sedentary person to a marathon runner), it is difficult to stay motivated with only general long-term goals in mind. Work with clients to set specific and measurable daily or weekly goals so they can experience smaller, motivating successes on the way to meeting their long-term objective.

Exercise Professional: Exercising regularly will help you get in shape and have more energy. What does exercising regularly mean to you and how will you know when it is happening?

Bill: For me, exercising regularly means making it to the gym three times per week for 45 minutes. In fact, I know right now I would like to work out on Tuesdays, Thursdays, and Saturdays. I have attempted exercising regularly before and this time a success will mean going for three months and making it to the gym three times per week.

Strategy 3: Suggest additional goals that clients may not have thought of, such as feeling more energetic and less stressed.

Exercise Professional: You also mentioned getting in shape. What does this mean to you?

Bill: Well, I like to play golf and I feel tired after playing nine holes. I often leave without finishing the entire course even though I want to keep playing. I guess getting in shape means I can play a full 18 holes of golf and have energy left afterward.

Exercise Professional: Having more energy and playing more golf are important to you. What goals might you set around these things?

Bill: Now that we are talking about it, these things are important to me. It would mean a lot to me if I had enough energy to golf for longer. This is the main activity I do with my youngest daughter and would love to spend more time with her.

Strategy 4: Break large goals (reachable in more than six months) into small goals (reachable in three to six months) and even weekly goals (such as completing a certain number of exercise sessions).

Bill: In one year, I would like to be able to play a complete 18 holes of golf without using a cart and while carrying my own bag to spend more time with my daughter.

Exercise Professional: What steps will you take over the next three months to work toward this long-term goal?

Bill: Over the next three months, I will stick with my exercise program and continue to play golf each week.

Strategy 5: Include many process goals, such as the completion of exercise sessions. In other words, simply completing workouts accomplishes a goal.

Exercise Professional: Being as specific as possible, what will the process be for sticking with your plan?

Bill: I will meet with you two days per week on Tuesday and Thursday, and will work out at home on Saturday. I will also play nine holes of golf on Wednesday and Friday each week.

Strategy 6: Record goals and set up a record-keeping system to record workouts and track progress toward goals.

Exercise Professional: How will you know if you are on track with reaching your long-term goals and achieving your short-term goals?

Bill: I plan to use an app I added to my phone to track my progress. Initially, I want to ensure that I can actually be physically active five days per week. This will be a really big victory for me if I can actually just show up for these sessions and make it to golf each week.

Strategy 7: Be sure clients understand what types of exercise will help them reach their health and fitness goals.

Exercise Professional: Now that we have decided what days will work best for us to work together, tell me what you already know about the types of exercise that will help you reach your goals.

Bill: I don't know much about the science of exercise, but if I had to guess I would say that I need to do some combination of lifting weights and aerobics. Am I missing anything?

Exercise Professional: We will work together to determine a baseline for your current fitness levels and collaborate on a varied approach that includes cardiorespiratory exercise, muscular training, flexibility exercise, and balance work to implement a well-rounded program that prepares your body for the demands of becoming more physically active. Does that make sense to you?

Strategy 8: Reevaluate and revise goals and exercise recommendations periodically to prevent discouragement if large goals are not being met.

Bill: It has been five months since we first started working together and I am not sure if I am on track or have moved any closer to reaching my goals.

Exercise Professional: What changes have you noticed over the past five months?

Bill: Well, the most important observation I have made is that I have been consistently showing up for my exercise sessions and I have not missed a day of golf in more than three months. I feel like I have more energy and feel stronger when I am getting in and out of the car.

Exercise Professional: What else?

Bill: My golf game has improved a bit and my body seems to handle the demands of hitting the ball better.

Exercise Professional: Your consistency has led to more energy, feeling stronger, and improved golf performance. Since it has been five months since we first did our baseline assessments, would you like to revisit those same assessments and see what other observations we can make?

SUMMARY

An older client's exercise-program satisfaction and participation are often directly related to their relationship with the exercise professional. Applying behavior-change principles can help clients develop and sustain new exercise habits. This includes various methods described in this chapter, including meeting the client at their stage of change, building rapport, promoting collaboration, developing self-esteem, fostering social support, and creating an awareness of, and an ability to cope with, negative self-talk. Showing interest and frequently giving sincere affirmations are especially motivating to older adults. Be sure to incorporate the ACE Mover Method and the ACE ABC Approach. Because older clients may not have recent exercise experiences or physically active peers to help them understand what to expect, support from an exercise professional may be even more important when older adults are just beginning to exercise.

REFERENCES

American Council on Exercise (2019). *The Professional's Guide to Health and Wellness Coaching.* San Diego: American Council on Exercise.

Bauman, A.E. et al. (2012). Correlates of physical activity: Why are some people physically and others are not? *The Lancet,* 380, 9838, 258–271.

Bethancourt, H.J. et al. (2014). Barriers to and facilitators of physical activity program use among older adults. *Clinical Medicine & Research,* 12, 1–2, 10–20.

Bowen, S. et al. (2014). Relative efficacy of mindfulness-based relapse prevention, standard relapse prevention, and treatment as usual for substance use disorders: A randomized clinical trial. *JAMA Psychiatry,* 71, 5, 547–556.

Brehm, B.A. (2004). *Successful Fitness Motivation Strategies.* Champaign, Ill.: Human Kinetics.

Daniali, S.S. et al. (2017). Relationship between self-efficacy and physical activity, medication adherence in chronic disease patients. *Advanced Biomedical Research,* 6, 63.

Hayden, J.A. et al. (2019). Individual recovery expectations and prognosis of outcomes in non-specific low back pain: Prognostic factor review. *Cochrane Database of Systematic Reviews,* 11, Art. No.: CD011284.

Hendershot, C.S. et al. (2011). Relapse prevention for addictive behaviors. *Substance Abuse Treatment, Prevention, & Policy,* 6, 17. DOI: 10.1186/1747-597X-6-17.

Lachman, M.E. et al. (2018). When adults don't exercise: Behavioral strategies to increase physical activity in sedentary middle-aged and older adults. *Innovation in Aging,* 2, 1, 1–12.

McAuley, E. et al. (2011). Self-regulatory processes and exercise adherence in older adults: Executive function and self-efficacy effects. *American Journal of Preventive Medicine,* 41, 3, 284–290.

Middleton, K.R., Anton, S.D., & Perri, M.G. (2013). Long-term adherence to health behavior change. *American Journal of Lifestyle Medicine,* 7, 6, 395–404.

Miller, W. & Rollnick, S. (2013). *Motivational Interviewing: Helping People Change* (3rd ed.). New York: Guilford Press.

Morgan, G.S. et al. (2019). A life fulfilled: Positively influencing physical activity in older adults – A systemic review and meta-ethnography. *BMC Public Health,* 19, Art. No. 362.

Prochaska, J.O., Norcross, J.C., & DiClemente, C.C. (2013). Applying the stages of change. *Psychology in Australia,* 19, 2, 10–15.

Teixeira, P.J. et al. (2012). Exercise, physical activity, and self-determination theory: A systematic review. *International Journal of Behavioral Nutrition & Physical Activity,* 9, 78. DOI: 10.1186/1479-5868-9-78.

U.S. Department of Health & Human Services (2018). *Physical Activity Guidelines for Americans* (2nd ed.). www.health.gov/paguidelines

SUGGESTED READING

American Council on Exercise (2019). *The Professional's Guide to Health and Wellness Coaching.* San Diego: American Council on Exercise.

Marlatt, G.A. & Donovan, D.M. (2008). *Relapse Prevention: Maintenance Strategies in the Treatment of Addictive Behaviors* (2nd ed.). New York: Guilford Press.

Miller, W. & Rollnick, S. (2013). *Motivational Interviewing: Helping People Change* (3rd ed.). New York: Guilford Press.

CHAPTER 3

Physiology of Aging and Exercise

LEARNING OBJECTIVES

After reading this chapter, you will be able to:

▸ Explain three different biological theories of aging

▸ Define aging and explain what it means to age successfully

▸ Understand the diversity in aging and how chronological age does not necessarily determine functional age or the ability to remain independent

▸ Briefly explain the effects of aging on cardiovascular and pulmonary function, blood pressure, muscular strength and endurance, and flexibility

▸ Describe the physiological, psychological, and sociological benefits of physical activity as they apply to older adults

Aging is a universal phenomenon that affects everyone. Provided someone lives long enough, they will eventually experience significant sensory, motor, and cognitive changes in response to advancing age. However, although everyone is aging, people do not age at the same rate. While some people experience relatively rapid declines in physiological and cognitive functioning as they grow older, others undergo significantly less pronounced changes over time.

A major focus of **gerontologists** continues to be understanding the factors responsible for individual differences in the rate and extent at which people age. Clearly, hereditary factors play a role in determining the pattern of changes observed in **senescence** (the process of deterioration with age). However, family studies demonstrate that about 25% of the variation in human longevity is due to genetic factors (Passarino, De Rango, & Montesanto, 2016). Healthy aging and longevity in humans are modulated by a combination of genetic and non-genetic factors.

This genetic component of human aging is largely beyond anyone's control and gerontologists often joke that the single best way to ensure longevity and healthful old age is to choose one's parents wisely. However, in addition to the genetic factors influencing human aging, there is strong evidence that many aspects of the aging process are related to environmental factors, such as nutrition, stress, smoking, and physical activity (Sgarbieri & Pacheco, 2017).

The need to develop effective lifestyle interventions that have the potential to improve the quality of life for older persons is especially apparent when one considers the growing proportion of older adults in today's society. The following statistics illustrate some aspects of the enormous demographic shift observed worldwide (United Nations, 2019; United Nations, 2017):

▸ In the year 2017, an estimated 962 million people were age 60 and older. This number is twice as much as in 1980 and is expected to double again by the year 2050.

▸ By 2030, it is projected that there will be more older persons (≥60 years old) than children under 10 years old.

▸ By 2050, there will be more older persons than adolescents and youth 10 to 24 years old.

▸ The number of persons aged 80 years and older is projected to increase from 137 to 425 million between 2017 and 2050.

▸ From 2015 to 2020, an individual aged 65 and older could expect to live an additional 17 years on average. By 2045 to 2050, this number will increase to 19 years.

There is little doubt that such a dramatic increase in the number of older adults will have far-reaching consequences for society. The past two decades have witnessed a remarkable expansion of interest in the physical-activity needs of older persons. Major medical and scientific organizations endorse the importance of physically active lifestyles for older adults [American College of Sports Medicine (ACSM), 2018; U.S. Department of Health & Human Services, 2018; Academy of Nutrition and Dietetics (AND), 2012]. It is now possible for students to specialize in the study of physical activity and aging, both through traditional academic programs offered at universities and specialized educational programs such as those offered by the American Council on Exercise.

This chapter examines some of the key issues influencing the relationship between physical activity and the aging process, beginning with a discussion of underlying biological mechanisms responsible for aging, including:

▸ What is aging?

▸ What causes people to age?

▸ What are the consequences of aging?

▸ Why do some people appear to age faster than others?

This chapter also examines the role that regular physical activity plays in physiological, psychological, and social functioning, and the extent to which lifestyle change promotes healthy aging. Throughout the chapter, a broad definition of physical activity is adopted, and the **acute,** or short-term, effects of a single bout of activity and the chronic, or long-term, benefits of extended participation are considered.

The Physiology of the Aging Process

AGING DEFINED

It may seem unnecessary to define aging, as age is typically defined as the number of years, months, or days that have elapsed since a person's birth. Similarly, the aging process is almost always defined by the passage of calendar time. However, many gerontologists believe that definitions of aging that focus exclusively on calendar time are incomplete, and that more complex definitions of both "age" and "aging" are needed to understand the intricacies associated with human aging.

Chronological age is the length of time—expressed by the number of years or months since birth—a person has lived. Its measurement is independent of physiological, psychological, and sociocultural factors. The presence of large differences in functional performance between individuals of the same chronological age, however, suggests that chronological age alone is an insufficient measure of senescence. Many experts believe that to increase the understanding of senescence, chronological age must be supplemented by other measures of aging designed to differentiate between individuals of the same chronological age. These measures are often described as indices of **functional age.** The most common measure of functional age is **biological age** or **physiological age,** although other functional ages, including **psychological age** and **social age,** have been identified.

Biological or physiological age characterizes senescence in terms of discrete biological or physiological, rather than chronological, processes. Research designs that emphasize chronological age typically focus on elements of calendar time (e.g., years and decades) as the principal units of analysis, whereas biological-age research focuses on senescent changes in biological or physiological processes and their subsequent effects on behavior. A common goal of all biological-age inventories is to determine **relative age,** or the extent to which an individual is aging faster or slower than an average person of the same chronological age. For example, an individual who is aging successfully may have a biological age 10 years younger than their chronological age. Conversely, a person experiencing multiple medical problems in old age may be older biologically than chronologically.

Because there is little consensus as to how biological age should be measured, it is difficult to summarize the research on the effects of physical activity on biological age. However, most studies suggest that, on average, people who exercise regularly have lower biological ages than people of the same chronological age who do not exercise (Duggal et al., 2018; Harridge & Lazarus, 2017; Tucker, 2017; Garatachea et al., 2015).

THINK IT THROUGH

Treating Senior Clients as Individuals

People have different patterns of aging and different life experiences, which contribute to the aging process. What will you do in your training or coaching practice to ensure that each of your senior clients is treated as an individual with unique needs and interests? That is, how will you avoid the "one-size-fits-all approach" to exercise programming for older adults?

In much the same way that people of the same chronological age can differ biologically, it also is possible for people to have different psychological ages. Psychological age refers to an individual's capabilities along a number of dimensions of mental or cognitive functioning, including self-esteem and self-efficacy, as well as learning, memory, and perception. The concept of psychological age is an important area of research because one element of **successful aging,** high cognitive functioning in midlife, is a future predictor of aging successfully (Bosnes et al., 2019).

Social age refers to the notion that society often has fairly rigid expectations of what is and is not appropriate behavior for a person of a particular age. Socialization is a tremendously complex process, and it is difficult to make broad generalizations about the acquisition of social roles in later life. However, the impact that social roles and expectations have on the lifestyle choices of older persons is of considerable interest in experimental **gerontology.** A number of studies have examined the extent to which later-life physical-activity choices are dependent on an individual's expectations regarding age (Andrews et al., 2017; Breda & Watts, 2017). For example, many older persons do not expect to age successfully, and these negative expectations may lead to an underestimation of physical capabilities (Breda & Watts, 2017). Additionally, age stereotypes around performance and the aging body that center on decreased physical health with age also contribute to decreased physical activity (Andrews et al., 2017). Nonetheless, older people should be encouraged to break away from such stereotypical perspectives about aging. Instead of "taking it easy" later in life, seniors should maintain social connections, as social engagement is an important correlate of health and well-being in older adults (Luo et al., 2020). When social participation is combined with physical activity, the physiological and psychological benefits can be even more pronounced.

⚛ EXPAND YOUR KNOWLEDGE

The Rate of Aging

The rate of aging is the change in function of organs and systems per unit of time. As an individual ages, the organ systems age at different rates within the body. For example, the cardiovascular system appears to age more rapidly than the gastrointestinal system (Khan, Singer, & Vaughan, 2017). People also age differently from one another due to factors such as genetics, environmental conditions, and developmental programming that occurs during pregnancy or the neonatal period (Lange et al., 2015).

There is convincing evidence that physiologic aging advances more rapidly with an accumulation of years of inactivity:

▸ Physical activity is strongly related to successful aging, a term used to represent the physical, psychological, and social success with which adults age. Dogra and Stathokostas (2012) found that those who spend less time in sedentary activities (<2 hours/day) are more likely to age successfully, regardless of their physical-activity levels, compared to those who engage in more sedentary time (>4 hours/day). For this study, sedentary behavior was defined as any waking behavior characterized by an energy expenditure ≤1.5 **metabolic equivalents (METs)** or by a sitting or reclining **posture.** For the psychological and sociological components of successful aging, the authors found that sedentary behavior lasting fewer than 2 hours/day is required for the highest levels of successful aging. These findings are in line with evidence that suggests that sedentary living may result in **functional capacity** losses that are as great as the effects of aging itself (Fielding et al., 2017).

▸ Exercise programming has been shown to have a positive effect on the functional performance of older adults through improved cardiorespiratory fitness, strength, mobility, balance, and the performance of activities of daily living (ADL) (Levy et al., 2020).

▸ **Sarcopenia** (age-associated loss of skeletal muscle mass and function) is associated with decreased physical activity and a selective decrease in **type II muscle fiber** size and amount. Evidence suggests that these changes are due to a reduction in high-intensity activities that recruit type II fibers, while **type I muscle fibers** are used for most ADL and during submaximal exercise (e.g., walking) (Cruz-Jentoft et al., 2019). In individuals over age 60, the effects of sarcopenia can show up as decreased strength and functional capacity, systemic inflammation and increased muscle protein breakdown, **insulin resistance** and **type 2 diabetes,** a fear of falling, and mild cognitive impairment, all of which can lead to further reductions in physical activity (Cruz-Jentoft et al., 2019). These findings highlight the need for older adults to regularly participate in some form of high-intensity exercise training. Chen et al. (2017) demonstrated that following a 12-week muscular-training program, older adults showed significant improvements in strength as well as **body-fat percentage.** Although sarcopenic effects cannot be fully reversed through physical activity, they can certainly be reduced through a program of appropriate, progressive exercise.

▸ Progressive declines in cardiorespiratory fitness and functional capacity as people age are associated with increased risk of frailty, dependency, loss of autonomy, and **mortality** from all causes (Paterson & Warburton, 2010). A meta-analysis of 10 research studies concluded that following cardiorespiratory training, older adults can improve their cardiorespiratory fitness levels, independent of health status (Bouaziz et al., 2018). This is further supported by Morente-Oria et al. (2020), who showed that cardiorespiratory fitness, as well as strength and **body composition,** can be improved following an eight-week cardiorespiratory-training program.

▸ Older adults experience declines in static and dynamic postural control of balance due to deteriorations in the sensorimotor and neuromuscular systems (Cruz-Jimenez, 2017). This loss of postural control can lead to changes in **gait** patterns and increased risk of falls. However, research consistently shows that performing activities such as interactive cognitive motor training can significantly improve overall gait performance and balance control (Kao et al., 2018).

▸ Furthermore, with aging comes a loss of flexibility, which has implications for muscle disuse, declines in functional abilities, and overall health status. However, older adults do maintain the ability to improve flexibility through stretching exercises (Inami & Shimizu, 2014). Thus, physical-activity interventions represent at least one strategy for possibly attenuating the effects of the aging process on functional limitations and disability and declines in quality of life.

Unfortunately, despite many years of research, there is no consensus on how best to quantify any of these alternative measures of aging. Thus, although it is apparent that chronological age is an inadequate measure of senescence and that alternative definitions of aging are necessary, no single unified definition of biological, psychological, or social aging exists. Nonetheless, an appreciation of chronological, biological, psychological, and psychosocial perspectives on aging is essential to grasp the true essence of aging.

A central tenet underlying physical fitness and aging research is that physically fit individuals may be functionally younger than less-fit individuals of the same chronological age. From this point of view, research studies examining the relationship between age, physical fitness, and behavior focus on both chronological and functional perspectives on aging are needed.

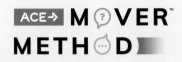

The Older Client Who Is Convinced Age Stereotypes Are True

You have been working with a 68-year-old client for three months. During a recent session, he mentions that he is enjoying meeting with you once per week but, according to his doctor and his family members, he should be doing more. He tells you that he is not against doing more exercise but does not think his body can handle a frequency of more than once per week because he is just too old. After he completes a set of step-ups, you decide to address his concerns about being too old for more exercise.

ACE→ /ABC APPROACH

Clients who express a desire to change but who are not doing so because of a perceived barrier present a unique opportunity for a client-centered interaction using the ACE Mover Method™ to address those concerns.

Exercise Professional: Great job with your last set of step-ups! You maintained good posture without bending forward for each repetition. Before that last set, you mentioned being encouraged to exercise more and that you are open to the idea.

Client: That's right. My doctor and my daughter have been encouraging me to exercise more often. They are both glad that I have started working with you, and they say doing more might help me maintain my current quality of life for longer. As you know, I don't currently have any major health issues and we all agree that the longer I can maintain my current health the better. I am having fun exercising and am enjoying coming to the gym. It gives me something to do and to look forward to. It really is too bad that I am 68 and too old to do more physical activity.

Ask: The use of powerful open-ended questions at appropriate times during an exercise session can be a great way to continue to build rapport and to explore more deeply a belief system (being too old to do more exercise) that is interfering with what the client wants and needs to do for his health.

Exercise Professional: I enjoy working with you also! Right now, you are enjoying your exercise program and would like to do more, but you believe you are too old to do more exercise. What is it about being 68 that makes you too old for more exercise?

Client: You know how it is. As you get older, you can't do as much, you're not as strong, and you can't keep up with what you used to be able to do. I feel like I can still do some of the things I did when I was younger, like going for a walk just for fun, hiking, or even shooting some baskets, but that's just not realistic for me and my older body. It sure does feel good when I do exercise, though. Over the past three months, I have been feeling stronger and more confident. It's a shame I did not start exercising 15 years ago when I had more energy.

Break down barriers: In this scenario, the client has clearly expressed the perceived barrier of "age" as a reason for not being able to be more active. Asking more open-ended questions at this point in the conversation will allow the client to more fully express what is holding him back.

Exercise Professional: You would like to exercise more because you enjoy it and if you were 15 years younger you would start doing more today. Being 68 feels too old but being 53 does not. What age is too old for more exercise?

Clients: Hmm. That's a good question. I am not sure what age is too old for exercise. For some reason, 68 feels too old but being in my 50s does not. I guess if my doctor is encouraging me to exercise, I must not be too old, but it just seems like I should be slowing down and not working too hard.

Exercise Professional: How would you know if you were working too hard for your age?

Client: I guess if I were doing things that hurt or did not feel safe, that might be a clue that it is not age appropriate. When we first started working together, I had these same concerns, but they dissipated as we continued with our program. In fact, it took me a while to work my way up to coming to the gym. It seemed like a place for young people. I had no idea how much it would benefit me and how much I would enjoy it. Maybe I could do some more exercise and see how I feel.

Collaborate: At this point, the client has worked his way through his own feeling of being old, determined that he is not sure why he thinks he is too old for more exercise, and knows that if an exercise hurts or does not feel safe, it may be inappropriate. Working together with the client to use his own expertise on how hard he feels he should be working can lead to next steps.

Exercise Professional: Doing more exercise because you enjoy it and like the results you are getting, plus the support from your doctor, makes you think it might be okay to do more. What do you think is an appropriate next step as it pertains to doing more exercise?

Client: After talking through this with you, I think I might like to increase the amount of physical activity I am doing. I think if I am not in any pain and I feel safe, I would really like exercising more.

Exercise Professional: Being as specific as possible, what does exercising more mean to you?

Client: Well, right now we are meeting once per week for about one hour and that feels good. I think exercising twice per week for a total of two hours each week for the rest of this month would be a realistic first step. I don't want to change things up too much at this point, but I would really enjoy working together twice per week instead of once if my body can keep up. What is your availability like for adding another session?

In this scenario, the exercise professional used the ACE Mover Method and the ACE ABC Approach™ during the exercise session to further explore a client's internal stereotypes about being too old to do more exercise. Through the use of active listening, **reflecting,** and open-ended questioning, the exercise professional effectively worked together with the client to explore barriers to change and collaborate on next steps.

✦ EXPAND YOUR KNOWLEDGE

Successful Aging

As longevity increases and more people are reaching their 90s, a discussion about successful aging is becoming more commonplace. Although there is no universally accepted definition for successful aging, four main areas are typically assessed: absence of disease or well-managed disease, minimal to no depressive symptoms, good physical and cognitive function, and active life engagement (being independent and socially engaged). Bosnes et al. (2019) have suggested that lifestyle factors are related to each component of successful aging, with not smoking and having social support being the most related to absence of disease. Good social support is a predictor for high physical and cognitive function, and not smoking is a predictor of active engagement with life. Interestingly, not smoking and performing moderate to high levels of physical activity are the only two lifestyle factors related to all criteria for successful aging.

BIOLOGICAL THEORIES OF AGING

Biological theories of aging examine the underlying mechanisms responsible for the structural and functional changes that characterize advancing age. Our understanding of the highly complex aging process has advanced over the past decades and, while there is not a single accepted theory that can stand alone, several contribute to our current understating of biological aging (Bwiza, Son, & Lee, 2020). As such, aging is probably not a single biological process, but rather a wide variety of age-related changes that occur simultaneously in many different systems throughout the body. Together, these changes decrease the body's ability to respond appropriately to the stresses of everyday life.

The complex nature of aging is reflected by the wide variety of theories proposed to account for the underlying mechanisms of aging. While many different classification schemes exist, the model proposed by the renowned biologist Leonard Hayflick is among the most straightforward (Hayflick, 1985). Hayflick was one of the first to demonstrate conclusively that cellular aging is influenced by both genetic and environmental factors. In his model of biological aging, Hayflick proposes that aging theories can be subdivided into three major classes: cellular theories, genetic theories, and control theories.

Cellular Theories of Aging

Cellular theories of aging focus on the degenerative changes that occur at the level of the individual cell. The most commonly proposed mechanism of cellular aging is **free-radical oxidation.** A free radical is a highly unstable molecule of oxygen with an uneven number of electrons in its outer shell. The presence of an unpaired electron causes the free radical to be both unstable and highly chemically reactive. To obtain the electron it needs to achieve stability, the free radical attempts to link up with other molecules. This process initiates a cascade of destructive chain reactions that may number in the thousands.

In healthy individuals, free radicals coexist in a state of equilibrium with a series of mixed-function oxidases that neutralize the destructive effects. The disruption of this equilibrium may be caused by a wide variety of intrinsic biological processes, as well as in response to environmental factors, such as exposure to radiation and chemical carcinogens. Damage to essential molecules, increased **deoxyribonucleic acid (DNA)** mutations, and reduced **mitochondria** or cell death are among the damages attributed to an excess of free radicals.

Although widely accepted, the free-radical theory of cellular aging remains mostly unproven because the evidence supporting it is largely correlative. That is, long-lived animals produce fewer free radicals and have lower oxidative damage levels in their tissues. However, this does not prove that free-radical generation determines lifespan, as the longest-living species of rodents produces high levels of free radicals within specific organs and has significant oxidative damage levels in **proteins, lipids,** and DNA (Saldmann et al., 2019).

Genetic Theories of Aging

Genetic theories of aging focus on the role of heredity in the regulation of senescence. The **Hayflick limit** has been replicated in numerous tissues from a wide variety of species (Hayflick, 1985), and suggests that cellular aging is, at least to some extent, preprogrammed. Hayflick's finding indicates that, although important, lifestyle changes alone will not allow us to overcome the genetically programmed factors responsible for human aging. Humans simply cannot escape the aging process indefinitely.

More recent research into the genetic components of aging has focused on structures called **telomeres,** which are the protective protein structures that cap the ends of **chromosomes.** When cells divide (**mitosis**), the end of the telomere cap may not be replicated properly. Therefore, telomeres tend to shorten with mitosis so that cells in older organisms have on average shorter telomeres than cells in younger organisms. Telomere shortening is associated with senescence and bodily aging, as well as age-related metabolic, inflammatory, cardiovascular, and neurological diseases and various cancers (Bernadotte, Mikhelson, & Spivak, 2016). Thus, a burgeoning trend in aging-related health research involves studying measures to slow the rate of telomere shortening through activities such as stress-reduction techniques and exercise (Nomikos et al., 2018; Arsenis et al., 2017; Law et al., 2016).

Control Theories of Aging

A third class of theories explains aging in terms of the function of specific systems known to be vital for the control of physiological functioning. For example, it is now accepted that advancing age often compromises immune system functioning. Older persons not only exhibit a significant decline in **T-cell** activity, but they also are more susceptible to **autoimmune disease.** This process is known as immunosenescence (Crooke et al., 2019; Pae, Meydani, & Wu, 2012).

In addition to the immune system, the **neuroendocrine system** and **central nervous system (CNS)** have been implicated in the regulation of degenerative changes in aging. Future research will likely confirm the importance of several different control systems in the regulation of aging at the molecular, cellular, and intact-organ levels.

Biological aging is a complex process regulated by numerous redundant mechanisms. It is unlikely that a single biological mechanism can be identified as the principal factor responsible for senescence. Rather, it is more probable that a complex combination of mechanisms, acting at several different levels throughout the body, brings about the structural and functional changes that characterize old age. Since biological aging does not appear to be caused by a single mechanism, it is extremely unlikely that experts will develop a "cure" for the aging process in the foreseeable future.

THE STRUCTURAL AND FUNCTIONAL CONSEQUENCES OF AGING

The structural and functional consequences of aging are surprisingly consistent across a broad range of physiological systems.

With advancing age, most physiological systems eventually exhibit **atrophy, dystrophy,** and **edema** at the cellular level. These disruptions in the integrity of the cell are, in turn, precursors of more gross morphological changes, such as decreased **elasticity** and **compliance, demyelinization,** and **neoplastic** growth. As expected, these structural changes are almost always associated with profound behavioral consequences (e.g., pain, inactivity, and a change in biomechanics).

In much the same way that structural changes exhibit similarities across physiological systems, the functional consequences are fairly consistent across different systems of the body. Aging organ systems, which are usually slower and less accurate, exhibit not only reduced strength and stability, but also decreased **coordination** and endurance. Although structural decay and functional decline are inescapable consequences of aging, both the rate and extent vary widely among individuals. Individuals may deviate from expected patterns of aging and, at least for some period of time, postpone the consequences of aging. For example, while measures of cardiovascular functioning usually decline with age, physically active individuals sometimes exhibit slower declines in age-related arterial and cardiac stiffening, along with decreased cardiovascular **morbidity** and mortality (Jakovljevic, 2018). Furthermore, epidemiological studies suggest that not meeting physical-activity recommendations is associated with an increased risk for ADL and **instrumental activities of daily living (IADL)** deficits in older adults (Crevenna & Dorner, 2019).

Studies suggest that even those older adults who have chronic health conditions can help improve their physical function by remaining active and physically fit (U.S. Department of Health and Human Services, 2018; ACSM, 2009). Figure 3-1 presents a physical-function continuum. The largest percentage (65%) of older adults 65 years of age and older are independent, but generally have a low fitness level. Those older adults in the dependent/frail category who have become more dependent on others for their care represent approximately

FIGURE 3-1
Physical-function continuum

Adapted with permission from Rikli, R.E. & Jones, J.C. (2013). *Senior Fitness Test Manual* (2nd ed.). Champaign, Ill.: Human Kinetics (p. 4).

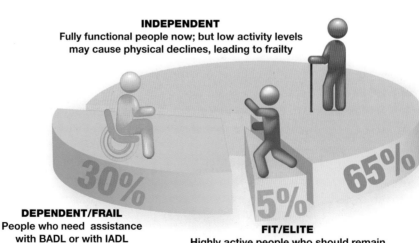

Note: BADL = Basic activities of daily living; IADL = Instrumental activities of daily living

30% of the older adult population. Moving older adults from the dependent/frail category to the independent category by increasing physical-activity levels and improving balance and mobility would improve their quality of life.

The physiological consequences of aging cannot be offset indefinitely. Nonetheless, there is increasingly strong evidence to suggest that aging need not occur at a uniform rate. Indeed, many age-related changes may be modified by specific lifestyle interventions, including regular physical activity.

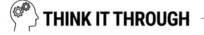 **THINK IT THROUGH**

Helping Frail Seniors

It is evident that many factors contribute to the aging process. Dependent, frail elderly are often cared for in long-term care facilities. How can you help senior clients move from the dependent/frail end of the physical-function spectrum to a more independent category and perhaps a higher level of fitness where quality of life can improve? What impact do you think this will have on rising healthcare costs related to the independence of the older adult?

Regular Physical Activity as a Lifestyle Intervention

Two often-cited reports strongly endorse participation in physical activity for individuals of all ages. In 2018, the U.S. Department of Health & Human Services released its second edition of the *Physical Activity Guidelines for Americans*. This report acknowledges that participation in regular physical activity is one of the most valuable actions people can take to improve their health by supporting normal growth and development, helping people to feel, function, and sleep better, and reduce the risk of chronic diseases (Table 3-1). Furthermore, the effect of exercise on adults and older adults is associated with a number of health benefits, including a decreased risk of all-cause and **cardiovascular disease (CVD)** mortality and reduced risks of CVD; **hypertension**; cancers of the bladder, breast, colon, endometrium, esophagus, kidney, lung, and stomach; and type 2 diabetes. In addition, regular participation in physical activity appears to reduce **depression** and **anxiety**; improve mood, cognition, bone health, and physical function; support healthy weight loss or slow, reduce, or prevent weight regain; and improve quality of life (U.S. Department of Health & Human Services, 2018).

The WHO's *Global Recommendations on Physical Activity for Health* (2011) offer a similarly strong endorsement for those aged 65 and older. The recommendations conclude that there is compelling evidence that regular physical activity can assist in avoiding, minimizing, and/or reversing many of the physical, psychological, and social hazards that often accompany advancing age.

In 2018, the WHO released a global action plan designed to ensure that people have diverse opportunities to be physically active in safe and enabling environments throughout their daily lives to improve both community and individual health and support the social, cultural, and economic development of all nations. *The Global Action Plan on Physical Activity 2018-2030: More Active People for a Healthier World* targets a 15% relative reduction to the global prevalence of physical inactivity in adults and adolescents by the year 2030. This document focuses on four key objectives considered essential to the achievement of this long-term

TABLE 3-1
Health Benefits Associated with Regular Physical Activity

Children and Adolescents

▸ Improved bone health (ages 3 through 17 years)
▸ Improved weight status (ages 3 through 17 years)
▸ Improved cardiorespiratory and muscular fitness (ages 6 through 17 years)
▸ Improved cardiometabolic health (ages 6 through 17 years)
▸ Improved cognition (ages 6 to 13 years)*
▸ Reduced risk of depression (ages 6 to 13 years)

Adults and Older Adults

▸ Lower risk of all-cause mortality
▸ Lower risk of cardiovascular disease mortality
▸ Lower risk of cardiovascular disease (including heart disease and stroke)
▸ Lower risk of hypertension
▸ Lower risk of type 2 diabetes
▸ Lower risk of adverse blood lipid profile
▸ Lower risk of cancers of the bladder, breast, colon, endometrium, esophagus, kidney, lung, and stomach
▸ Improved cognition*
▸ Reduced risk of dementia (including Alzheimer's disease)
▸ Improved quality of life
▸ Reduced anxiety
▸ Reduced risk of depression
▸ Improved sleep
▸ Slowed or reduced weight gain
▸ Weight loss, particularly when combined with reduced calorie intake
▸ Prevention of weight regain following initial weight loss
▸ Improved bone health
▸ Improved physical function
▸ Lower risk of falls (older adults)
▸ Lower risk of fall-related injuries (older adults)

Note: The Advisory Committee rated the evidence of health benefits of physical activity as strong, moderate, limited, or grade not assignable. Only outcomes with strong or moderate evidence of effect are included in this table.

*See Table 2-3 of the *Physical Activity Guidelines for Americans* (2nd ed.) for additional components of cognition and brain health.

Reprinted from U.S. Department of Health & Human Services (2018). *Physical Activity Guidelines for Americans* (2nd ed.) https://health.gov/paguidelines/second-edition/pdf/Physical_Activity_Guidelines_2nd_edition.pdf

goal: (1) creating active societies, (2) creating active environments, (3) creating active people, and (4) creating active systems (WHO, 2018).

Specific to older adults, the *Global Action Plan* reinforces the importance of physical activity to maintain physical, social, and mental health, prevent falls, and realize healthy aging. The action steps associated with objective 3 (creating active people) include enhancing the provision of, and opportunities for, appropriately created and implemented programs designed to increase physical activity and reduce sedentary behavior in older adults across all environments based on their needs and preferences. Other calls to action within this report include strengthening the implementation of national standardized protocols to assess physical-activity capacity in older adults and to improve national policies to strengthen the provision of affordable, accessible, and appropriate programs aimed at maintaining balance, **muscular strength,** and independent living.

The following sections provide a brief overview of some of the physiological, psychological, and social benefits of regular exercise. Whenever possible, an attempt is made to address both the acute effects of a single bout of physical activity, as well as the more persistent and long-term effects of sustained participation in exercise and physical activity. Because physical activity has been defined in many different ways, the WHO's broad and inclusive definition of physical activity, which includes all bodily movements produced by skeletal muscles and requiring energy expenditure, is adopted (WHO, 2011).

PHYSIOLOGICAL BENEFITS OF PHYSICAL ACTIVITY

The physiological benefits of participation in regular physical activity are well established. Among the short-term benefits attributed to regular physical activity are improved sleep quality (Wang & Boros, 2019), improved **glucose** regulation (Colberg et al., 2016), and increases in **catecholamine** activity (Laughlin, Bowles, & Duncker, 2012). Long-term adaptation to physical-activity participation includes improved cardiorespiratory fitness, increased musculoskeletal fitness, enhanced flexibility and **range of motion (ROM),** decreased **adiposity,** and improved lipid status (U.S. Department of Health & Human Services, 2018).

Several of the more common physiological adaptations associated with regular physical activity are discussed in the following sections. The immediate and long-term physiological benefits of physical activity are as follows (U.S. Department of Health & Human Services, 2018):

- ▸ Immediate benefits
    - *Improved insulin sensitivity:* Physical activity impacts peripheral tissues like muscle cells so they become better able to use available **insulin** to take up glucose during and after activity.
    - *Reduced feelings of short-term anxiety:* Physical activity has been associated with relieving short-term anxiety by serving as a positive distraction and affecting the levels of several **neurotransmitters** (e.g., **serotonin, norepinephrine,** and **dopamine**).
    - *Improved sleep:* Physical activity has been shown to enhance sleep quality and quantity in individuals of all ages.
    - *Blood pressure:* Physical activity has both short and long-term effects on blood pressure. A reduction in blood pressure following a single bout of physical activity is known as **postexercise hypotension.**
    - *Cognitive function:* Physical activity improves cognitive functions such as memory, executive function, attention, and processing speed.
- ▸ Long-term effects
    - *Cardiorespiratory fitness:* Substantial improvements in almost all aspects of cardiovascular functioning have been observed following appropriate physical training.
    - *Musculoskeletal fitness:* Progressive muscular training can have a significant impact on preserving and increasing muscle mass, **power,** and strength.

- *Flexibility:* Exercise that stimulates movement throughout the full ROM assists in the preservation and restoration of flexibility and may allow people to do activities requiring more flexibility.

- *Balance and coordination:* Regular activity helps prevent and/or postpone the age-associated declines in balance and coordination that are a major risk factor for falls.

- *Speed:* Reduced movement speed is a characteristic of advancing age. Individuals who are regularly active can often postpone age-related declines.

- *Depressive symptoms:* Engaging in regular physical activity reduces the risk of developing depression and may improve symptoms in those with depression.

In addition, it is equally important to recognize the value of incorporating a multicomponent physical-activity routine that includes cardiorespiratory, muscular, mobility, balance, and cognitive exercises to contribute to a successful aging process. Balance often is impaired as people age and causes mobility limitations and declines in functional independence. **Static balance** and **dynamic balance** are maintained by using multiple systems within the body—the sensory, musculoskeletal, and cognitive systems. Gradually building a foundation of good balance and mobility through deliberately designed progressive exercise routines creates a safer platform from which to build static and dynamic stability and other factors associated with quality of life, including memory and spatial cognition (Dunsky, 2019).

Cardiovascular Function

Maximal oxygen uptake ($\dot{V}O_2$max) during exercise is an excellent measure of cardiovascular fitness. $\dot{V}O_2$max was previously thought to decline at a constant rate with advancing age (about 10% per decade). This decline was considered to be relatively stable across individuals and, to a large degree, independent of physical-activity status. However, a number of studies suggest that age-related changes in $\dot{V}O_2$max may be more variable (Pollock et al., 2015). For example, highly trained individuals who maintain high activity levels often experience little or no decline in $\dot{V}O_2$max over periods of a decade or more (Gent & Norton, 2013).

Although the mechanisms by which exercise influences cardiovascular performance in older adults are complex, both central factors (increased **cardiac output**) and peripheral factors (increased oxidative capacity of the skeletal muscle) are involved. It is not possible to

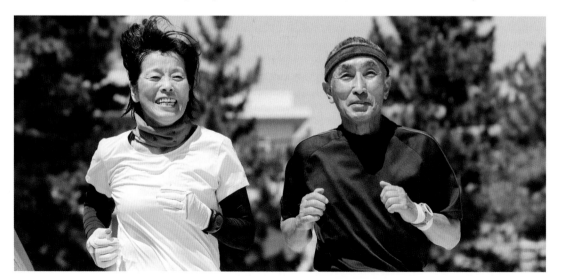

completely postpone age-related declines in aerobic power. Nonetheless, even modest levels of physical activity can result in significant increases in cardiovascular efficiency in old age.

Pulmonary Function

Pulmonary efficiency declines with age due to compromised lung elastic recoil and compliance (Roman, Rossiter, & Casaburi, 2016). Degenerative changes in the vertebral discs alter the shape of the thoracic cavity, with a resultant reduction in pulmonary volume. Decreased strength and mass of the respiratory muscles associated with changes in thoracolumbar curvature further compromise pulmonary efficiency, as do **calcification** and **ossification** of the **costovertebral** and **costochondral** joints (Rahman, Singh, & Lee, 2017).

In young and middle-aged individuals, cardiorespiratory exercise has minimal effects on vital capacity, expiratory volumes, and other measures of pulmonary performance. However, because regular exercise is associated with reduced vertebral degeneration rates and increased thoracic muscle strength, physical activity may help preserve adequate levels of pulmonary function in older adults (Sillanpää et al., 2014).

Blood Pressure

The incidence of hypertension increases with age, with approximately 70% of Americans over the age of 75 having hypertension (Mozaffarian et al., 2015). While both **systolic blood pressure (SBP)** and **diastolic blood pressure (DBP)** increase significantly with advancing age up to 60 to 70 years old, DBP may begin to decrease on its own with older age (Anker et al., 2018). Several exercise-training studies have shown that physical activity can reduce SBP and DBP in individuals of all ages with mild hypertension (Gambardella et al., 2020) and can reduce mortality in individuals with high blood pressure (Tun et al., 2017).

In middle-aged and older adult male subjects, Faselis and colleagues (2012) found that exercise capacity was a strong and independent predictor of the rate of progression from elevated blood pressure to hypertension (see Table 7-3, page 201). The adjusted risk for developing hypertension was observed to be 66% higher for the low-fit and 72% higher for the least-fit individuals (Faselis et al., 2012).

Blood Lipids

Aging is associated with increases in both total **cholesterol** and serum **triglycerides. Hypercholesterolemia** and **hyperlipidemia** are medical conditions that lead to the premature development of **coronary artery disease** and physical decline. Cardiorespiratory fitness is associated with a reduction of **coronary heart disease (CHD)** risk, and the American Heart Association (AHA) recognizes sedentary behavior as a modifiable risk factor for all-cause and CVD/CHD mortality (Lavie et al., 2019). A number of studies have shown that exercise promotes favorable biochemical profiles [increased **high-density lipoprotein (HDL)** cholesterol and reduced **non-high-density lipoprotein (non-HDL)** cholesterol] and may lead to reductions in **low-density lipoprotein (LDL)** cholesterol and total triglycerides, but HDL cholesterol is the most sensitive to exercise (Wang & Xu, 2017). Because almost all instances of favorable improvements in biochemical profiles are associated with coincident decreases in body weight, it is frequently difficult to dissociate the effects of exercise from the effects of weight loss. This problem notwithstanding, there is sufficient evidence to suggest that regular exercise is associated with a decrease in **body fat,** which, in turn, is associated with a decrease in circulating lipids. However, the effect of a single bout of exercise on blood lipids appears to be transient, and blood lipids return to pre-exercise values within a few days of cessation of physical activity. Compatible with recommendations from the *Physical Activity Guidelines for Americans* suggesting that health benefits are the result of an accumulated volume of physical activity (U.S. Department of Health & Human Services, 2018), a review of the literature showed no difference between continuous and accumulated patterns of exercise regarding cardiorespiratory fitness, blood pressure, lipids, insulin, and glucose metabolism (Murphy et al., 2019).

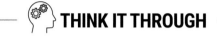 **THINK IT THROUGH**

Cardiorespiratory Training Strategies

How will you incorporate cardiorespiratory training into your senior clients' exercise programs? Think about a variety of options for older adults to complete their cardiorespiratory training, given that many may not be able to tolerate impact, long-duration, or high-intensity exercise due to functional decline or other health problems. Keep in mind that an accumulation of time throughout the week is important and even a short duration of exercise done more frequently can be beneficial to an individual's health. The progression must not only be tolerated physically, but emotionally and logistically as well.

Muscle Mass and Function

Muscle mass and function decline significantly with advancing age (Fragala et al., 2019; Wilkinson, Piasecki, & Atherton, 2018). Loss in muscle function is likely due to the muscle atrophy that accounts for a significant decrease in lean mass with aging. Muscle mass begins to decline at approximately age 30 and accelerates after age 60. Beginning around age 75, muscle mass is lost at a rate of 0.64 to 0.7% per year in women and 0.8 to 0.98% per year in men. Muscular strength, on the other hand, declines more rapidly, at a rate of 2.5 to 3% in women and 3 to 4% in men each year (Fragala et al., 2019; Wilkinson, Piasecki, & Atherton, 2018). Muscle atrophy that occurs as a natural part of the aging process is called sarcopenia and reflects both a decrease in the average fiber size and a decrease in the number of muscle fibers. Since the amount of force an individual can produce depends, in part, on the amount of working muscle mass, sarcopenia has a dramatic negative effect on strength, power, and function. Age-related decreases in muscular strength, particularly in the lower body, are associated with a decreased ability to maintain dynamic balance, walk, prevent falls, and move quickly (i.e., produce power). A client may also experience **dynapenia,** which is the loss of muscular strength not caused by neurological or muscular disease that typically is associated with older adults. Dynapenia is the loss of muscle strength, rather than muscle mass. In addition, age-related atrophy often coincides with increases in intermuscular **adipose** tissue infiltration and overall fat mass (i.e., **sarcopenic obesity**), systemic inflammation, **metabolic syndrome,** arterial stiffness, and glucose intolerance.

The causes of sarcopenia are multidimensional. In older adults, causative factors for skeletal-muscle atrophy include, but are not limited to, a loss of **fast-twitch muscle fibers** that exceeds the loss of **slow-twitch muscle fibers,** resulting in a loss of muscle power; a reduction of motor units, which hastens the loss of muscle strength; **hormone** imbalances, **anabolic** resistance, and an imbalance of pro- and anti-inflammatory **cytokines,** which lead to changes in body composition; and reduced levels of physical activity, vitamin D, and protein (Dhillon & Hasni, 2017; Wackerhage, 2017).

Researchers have reported that resistance exercise is an effective strategy to mitigate age-related declines in muscle mass and function. The results of a meta-analysis suggest that a strength-training program for an average duration of 20 weeks elicits an approximate 2.2-pound (1 kg) increase in lean body mass among older adults (Peterson, Sen, & Gordon, 2011). While this increase may appear modest, it is in contrast to the approximate 0.50-pound (0.18 kg) annual decline that may occur through sedentary lifestyles in those beyond 50 years of age (Melton et al., 2000). Moreover, volume of training and age of participation are important determinants of effectiveness, suggesting that higher dosages result in a greater adaptive response, and that aging individuals should consider starting a regimen of resistance exercise as early as possible, to optimize results.

Data from 16 studies establish both muscular strength and power as important predictors of physical function in older adults, and also provide evidence that muscular power is a marginally better predictor of function than strength. When viewed alongside evidence demonstrating the longitudinal decline in muscular power occurring at an earlier age and/or at a greater rate than muscular strength, it is reasonable to argue in favor of muscular power being the primary therapeutic target for resistance-training interventions aimed at enhancing physical function and preserving independence later in life (Byrne et al., 2016). Reid and Fielding (2012) concur that muscular power is a more discriminant indicator of functional performance in older adults than muscular strength and specify that power training has been found to be well-tolerated, safe, and effective, even among frail older adults. Therefore, choosing the appropriate exercise, speed, and load for each client to help develop power is imperative to ensure that the outcome is truly safe and effective.

THINK IT THROUGH

Muscular Strength and Power

The age-related combined loss of muscle size and fast-twitch muscle fibers results in weakness and reduced power in the elderly, which predisposes this population to traumatic falls. Loss of stamina and reduced physical activity further reduce muscle mass. As an exercise professional, how will you address these two issues (i.e., muscular strength and power) with exercise programming? Think about how training for strength, power, and even balance requires different approaches for each individual. How will you incorporate these various modalities into your sessions?

Flexibility

Aging is associated with changes in the elasticity and compliance of connective tissue, resulting in significant decreases in flexibility and ROM. These changes include **collagen** becoming more soluble and cross-linked; **cartilage, ligaments,** and **tendons** becoming stiffer and more rigid; connective-tissue cells becoming less able to repair their structure; and **synovial membranes** degrading and losing **viscosity** of the **synovial fluid.** On the other hand, regular physical activity (i.e., both stretching and muscular training) can improve flexibility by increasing collagen turnover in ligaments; lengthening skeletal muscle fibers; building up collagen fiber cross-linkage formation and synovial membrane structure; and increasing the viscosity of synovial fluid. Thus, muscular training may contribute to an increase in flexibility and can provide a stimulus for flexibility, as long as its action is through a full ROM that mimics the natural movement of a joint.

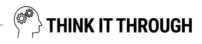 **THINK IT THROUGH**

Flexibility Training

Interventions to increase flexibility in older adults help them maintain their ability to perform various ADL and prevent falls. Think about how you will approach flexibility training in each of your sessions with older adults. Will you stretch with your clients? Will you do partner stretching with clients and, if so, what precautions will you take regarding intensity, communication, and compensation patterns that may develop due to overstretching? Will you provide them with a home stretching program so that they can get a daily dose of flexibility training? What precautions do you need to take to avoid contraindicated movements or specific limitations?

MENTAL HEALTH BENEFITS OF PHYSICAL ACTIVITY

In addition to its impact on physiological variables, physical activity also can have significant psychological effects, both positive and negative. Furthermore, neurodegenerative diseases become more prevalent as individuals age and, since inactivity is a prominent risk factor for many diseases, physical activity has become an emerging topic of interest for many investigators. Exercise might act as an efficient and low-cost adjunctive factor in the treatment and prevention of age-related neurodegenerative processes because of its positive relationship with the outcome of cognitive impairment, **dementia, Alzheimer's disease,** and depression, in that exercise improves not only patients' quality of life but the progression of the disease itself (Gallaway et al., 2017). Some of the more common psychological benefits associated with regular physical activity are discussed in the following sections. The following list is a summary of the long- and short-term benefits of physical activity for psychological functioning (U.S. Department of Health & Human Services, 2018):

- ▸ Immediate benefits
  - Reduced feelings of short-term anxiety
  - Improvements in sleep that increase with the duration of a single episode
  - Improved aspects of cognitive function
- ▸ Long-term effects
  - Decreased depressive symptoms
  - Improved quality of life
  - Reduced long-term anxiety for people with and without anxiety disorders
  - Improved aspects of sleep (e.g., sleep quality, efficiency, deep sleep, reduced daytime sleepiness, and reduced frequency of use of medication to aid sleep)
  - Improved cognition (e.g., memory, attention, executive function, processing speed, and the ability to retrieve and use information that has been acquired over time)

·:☀:· EXPAND YOUR KNOWLEDGE

Physical Activity and Cognitive Health in Older Adults

Improvements in physical fitness may facilitate brain plasticity (i.e., the ability of the brain to adapt as a result of experience), as well as improvements in cognitive function through increases in brain activation. Regular physical activity and management of cardiovascular risk factors (e.g., diabetes, obesity, smoking, and hypertension) have been noted to help reduce the risk of cognitive decline and may reduce the risk of dementia (Baumgart et al., 2015). Cardiorespiratory exercise was found to increase brain-derived neurotrophic factor (BDNF) in the hippocampus and improve memory and learning while lowering anxiety and depression. Cerebral blood flow is essential because the brain does not receive as much blood relative to the other organs in the body, and the blood it does receive is vital to bathe the tissues of the brain with oxygen, glucose, and other nutrients. Therefore, cardiorespiratory exercise becomes even more necessary as the body ages. Muscular training has been shown to help improve executive function and memory. Muscle mass stimulates immune-globulin factor 1 (IGF1), which is linked to immunity and health, including brain health. Resistance training is touted as a stand-alone cognitive exercise, as well (Tsai et al., 2015).

The question of how much exercise is needed to elicit adequate physical fitness to drive these improvements in cognitive health was explored by Sanders and colleagues (2019) in a review of dozens of studies on the dose-response relationship between exercise and cognitive function in older adults. What they found was that in healthy young and older adults, acute exercise was related to gains in executive functions such as processing speed and inhibitory control, and that these cognitive benefits may accumulate over time to yield greater and lasting cognitive improvements. Diamond and Ling (2016) established several basic guidelines to help with program design, which include the following:

▸ The exercises must be challenging, interesting, and effective without being too frustrating.

▸ The exercises must be specific and challenge the brain and body simultaneously.

▸ The exercises must be incorporated into daily life (homework).

▸ The more time spent on these exercises, the better the results (40 minutes vs. 20 minutes).

All older adults (i.e., those with and without cognitive impairments) should perform a combination of aerobic and anaerobic exercise on as many days of the week as is feasible, but at least three times per week, and they should integrate exercise into their daily lives as much as possible. For older adults with cognitive impairments, programs with shorter session durations and higher frequency may generate the best cognitive results. Finally, exercise professionals are advised to develop personalized exercise programs for their clients that maximize long-term adherence (Sanders et al., 2019). It has been proposed that doing physical and cognitive exercise simultaneously might induce larger functional benefits than performing the two types individually (Bamidis et al., 2014). Multicomponent exercise (i.e., performing multiple modes of training within a single session) was also shown to have a bigger (potentially synergistic) effect than doing the components independently (Suzuki et al., 2012).

In addition, it is imperative that exercise professionals continue to pursue advanced education and certification to obtain the knowledge and skills that enable them to create these specific cognitive programs.

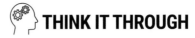

THINK IT THROUGH

Managing Cognitive Limitations

Careful attention must be given when designing an exercise program for an older adult with cognitive impairment. An older adult's ability to anticipate and adapt to movement or environmental changes may be adversely affected by reductions in cognition. What precautions will you take and guidelines will you follow to ensure a safe environment and effective exercise routine for older clients who may have cognitive declines?

General Psychological Well-being

Although psychological health consists of both positive and negative components, previous research in the exercise sciences has focused predominantly on the effects of physical activity on negative components of psychological health, such as depression, anxiety, and other stress-related disorders. However, a more recent focus of study in this area centers on examining the relationship between physical activity and more positive elements of psychological functioning. One component of positive psychological health is well-being, which is a composite of relatively low levels of negative emotion, relatively high levels of positive emotion, and life satisfaction.

It has been suggested that a high level of cardiorespiratory fitness is associated with better psychological well-being. Moreover, cardiorespiratory fitness is one of the strongest predictors of all-cause mortality in healthy and unhealthy men and women (Mandsager et al., 2018). Accordingly, researchers have theorized that a high level of cardiorespiratory fitness buffers the adverse effects of negative emotion or enhances positive emotion, which results in a positive association with survival. Indeed, it has been shown that low levels of negative emotion and high levels of cardiorespiratory fitness are independent predictors of long-term survival in men and women. Investigators in one study that looked at approximately 5,000 men and women between the ages of 20 and 81 found that those subjects with both a low level of negative emotion and a high level of cardiorespiratory fitness had a 63% lower risk of death than those with higher levels of negative emotion and a low level of cardiorespiratory fitness (Ortega et al., 2010).

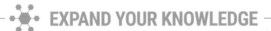

EXPAND YOUR KNOWLEDGE

Exercise and Depressive Symptoms in Older Adults

While the effects of exercise on mental health, including depression, are well established, it remains unclear which exercise-related variables produce these beneficial effects. Miller et al. (2019) examined the extent to which four exercise variables—exercise behavior, exercise-induced mood, exercise self-efficacy, and social support—can predict depression symptoms in older adults.

The research team surveyed nearly 600 community-dwelling older adults between the ages of 65 and 96 using five different questionnaires. What they found was that all four variables were negatively associated with depressive symptoms. In other words, the more exercise people performed, the better their mood and self-efficacy related to exercise, and the better their support system, the more improvement they saw in their symptoms (Miller et al., 2019).

Further, according to Mintzer and colleagues (2019), cognitive decline and depression have been linked and it is essential that exercise professionals examine multiple areas of wellness that can affect both cognition and emotional health. As such, the following behaviors should be encouraged among older adults:

- Partaking in regular physical activity
- Pursuing intellectually stimulating activities
- Staying socially active
- Practicing positive attitudes
- Managing stress
- Eating healthy
- Sleeping well

Exercise professionals working with community-dwelling older adults should create exercise programs that focus on the development of social support among participants, as well as that bring participants enjoyment and improve their self-efficacy.

SOCIAL IMPLICATIONS OF REGULAR PHYSICAL ACTIVITY

Social engagement encompasses contact with others in the context of living situations (cohabitation) and out-of-home activities (social and work activities with friends, colleagues, and family), as well as the level of satisfaction a person derives from these social encounters. Social encounters place a high demand on several cognitive-function areas, especially memory (e.g., social interaction requires individuals to remember names and elements of others' personal lives, families, and activities for the purposes of discussion).

Empowering older individuals and assisting them in playing a more active role in society are among the social benefits attributed to physical activity. The following lists present a number of significant short- and long-term effects of physical activity on sociocultural variables (WHO, 1997):

- Immediate benefits
  - *Empowering older individuals:* A large proportion of the older adult population voluntarily adopts a sedentary lifestyle, which eventually threatens to reduce independence and self-sufficiency. Participation in appropriate physical activity can help empower older individuals and assist them in playing a more active role in society.
  - *Enhanced social and cultural integration:* Physical-activity programs, particularly when carried out in small groups and/or in social environments, enhance social and intercultural interactions for many older adults.
- Long-term effects
  - *Enhanced integration:* Regularly active individuals are less likely to withdraw from society and more likely to actively contribute to the social milieu.
  - *Formation of new friendships:* Participation in physical activity, particularly in small groups and other social environments, stimulates new friendships and acquaintances.
  - *Widened social and cultural networks:* Physical activity frequently provides individuals with an opportunity to widen available social networks.

- *Role maintenance and new role acquisition:* A physically active lifestyle helps foster the stimulating environments necessary for maintaining an active role in society, as well as for acquiring positive new roles.

- *Enhanced intergenerational activity:* In many societies, physical activity is a shared activity that provides opportunities for intergenerational contact, thereby diminishing stereotypical perceptions about aging and the elderly.

Aging is associated with a need to adjust to changing roles and life transition. Factors such as the completion of caring for children, bereavement, retirement, financial hardship, ill health, and isolation force many older people to systematically relinquish more and more of the roles that are a meaningful part of their identity (Morgan et al., 2019). Physical activity can help older persons better adjust to these changing roles. Activity programs provide seniors with the opportunity to improve self-esteem, self-belief, and self-identity, and bolster feelings of togetherness and belonging (Morgan et al., 2019).

SUMMARY

Advancing age is characterized by a progressive and insidious decline in the functional capacity of most physiological systems. While these declines in functional capacity are, to a large extent, inevitable and inescapable, considerable differences exist among individuals in the rate and magnitude of this decline. Several lines of research suggest that individuals who engage in healthful behaviors, such as participating in regular physical activity, can often postpone or reduce these adverse consequences and, thereby deviate from expected patterns of aging. As the psychological and physiological advantages of physical activity for older adults become more widely accepted and appreciated, it is likely that a growing proportion of the population, regardless of age, will begin to include exercise as an integral component of their everyday routines.

REFERENCES

Academy of Nutrition and Dietetics (2012). Position of the Academy of Nutrition and Dietetics: Food and nutrition for older adults: Promoting health and wellness. *Journal of the Academy of Nutrition & Dietetics*, 112, 1255–1277.

American College of Sports Medicine (2018). *ACMS's Guidelines for Exercise Testing and Prescription* (10th ed.). Philadelphia: Wolters Kluwer.

American College of Sports Medicine (2009). American College of Sports Medicine position stand: Exercise and physical activity for older adults. *Medicine & Science in Sports & Exercise*, 41, 1510–1530.

Andrews, R.M. et al. (2017). Positive aging expectations are associated with physical activity among urban-dwelling older adults. *The Gerontologist*, 57, Suppl. 2, S178–186.

Anker, D. et al. (2018). Screening and treatment of hypertension in older adults: Less is more? *Public Health Reviews*, 39, 26.

Arsenis, N.C. et al. (2017). Physical activity and telomere length: Impact of aging and potential mechanisms of action. *Oncotarget*, 8, 27, 45008–45019.

Bamidis, P.D. et al. (2014). A review of physical and cognitive interventions in aging. *Neuroscience and Biobehavioral Reviews*, 44, 206–220.

Baumgart, M. et al. (2015). Summary of the evidence on modifiable risk factors for cognitive decline and dementia: A population-based perspective. *Alzheimer's & Dementia*, 11, 6, 718–726.

Bernadotte, A., Mikhelson, V.M., & Spivak, I.M. (2016). Markers of cellular senescence: Telomere shortening as a marker of cellular senescence. *Open-Access Impact Journal on Aging*, 8, 1, 3–11.

Bosnes, I. et al. (2019). Lifestyle predictors of successful aging: A 20-year prospective HUNT study. *PLoS ONE*, 14, 7: e0219200.

Bouaziz, W. et al. (2018). Effect of aerobic training on peak oxygen uptake among seniors aged 70 or older: A meta-analysis of randomized controlled trials. *Rejuvenation Research*, 21, 4, 341–349.

Breda, A.I. & Watts, A.S. (2017). Expectations regarding aging, physical activity, and physical function in older adults. *Gerontology & Geriatric Medicine*, 3, 1–8.

Bwiza, C.P., Son, J.M., & Lee, C. (2019). Integrated theories of biological aging. *Oxford Research Encyclopedia of Psychology*, DOI: 10.1093/acrefore/9780190236557.013.334.

Byrne, C. et al. (2016). Ageing, muscle power and physical function: A systematic review and implications for pragmatic training interventions. *Sports Medicine*, 46, 1311–1332.

Chen, H.T. et al. (2017). Effects of difference types of exercise on body composition, muscle strength, and IGF-1 in the elderly with sarcopenic obesity. *Journal of the American Geriatrics Society*, 65, 827–832.

Colberg, S.R. et al. (2016). Physical activity/exercise and diabetes: A position statement of the American Diabetes Association. *Diabetes Care*, 39, 2065–2079.

Crevenna, R. & Dorner, T.E. (2019). Association between fulfilling the recommendations for health-enhancing physical activity with (instrumental) activities of daily living in older Austrians. *The Central European Journal of Medicine*, 131, 265–272.

Crooke, S.N. et al. (2019). Immunosenescence and human vaccine immune responses. *Immunity & Aging*, 16, 25.

Cruz-Jentoft, A.J. et al. (2019). Sarcopenia: Revised European consensus on definition and diagnosis. *Age and Ageing*, 48, 1, 16–31.

Cruz-Jimenez, M. (2017). Normal changes in gait and mobility problems in the elderly. *Physical Medicine and Rehabilitations Clinics of North America*, 28, 4, 713–725.

Dhillon, R.J.S. & Hasni, S. (2017). Pathogenesis and management of sarcopenia. *Clinics in Geriatric Medicine*, 33, 1, 17–26.

Diamond, A. & Ling, D.S. (2016). Conclusions about interventions, programs, and approaches for improving executive functions that appear justified and those that, despite much hype, do not. *Developmental Cognitive Neuroscience*, 18, 34–48.

Dogra, S. & Stathokostas, L. (2012). Sedentary behavior and physical activity are independent predictors of successful aging in middle-aged and older adults. *Journal of Aging Research*, DOI: 10.1155/2012/190654.

Duggal, N.A. et al. (2018). Major features of immunesenscence, including reduced thymic output, are ameliorated by high levels of physical activity in adulthood. *Aging Cell*, 17, 2, 1–13.

Dunsky, A. (2019). The effect of balance and coordination exercises on quality of life in older adults: A mini-review. *Frontiers in Aging and Neuroscience*, DOI: 10.3389/fnagi.2019.00318.

Faselis, C. et al. (2012). Exercise capacity and progression from prehypertension to hypertension. *Hypertension*, 60, 333–338.

Fielding, R.A. et al. (2017). Dose of physical activity, physical functioning and disability risk in mobility-limited older adults: Results from the LIFE study randomized trial. *PLoS One*, e0182155.

Fragala, M.S. et al. (2019). Resistance training for older adults: Position statement from the National Strength and Conditioning Association. *Journal of Strength and Conditioning Research*, 33, 8, 2019–2052.

Gallaway, P.J. et al. (2017). Physical activity: A viable way to reduce the risks of mild cognitive impairment, Alzheimer's disease, and vascular dementia in older adults. *Brain Sciences*, 7, 22.

Gambardella, J. et al. (2020). Pathophysiology mechanisms underlying the beneficial effects of physical activity in hypertension. *Journal of Clinical Hypertension*, 22, 291–295.

Garatachea, N. et al. (2015). Exercise attenuates the major hallmarks of aging. *Rejuvenation Research*, 18, 1, 57–89.

Gent, D.N. & Norton, K. (2013). Aging has greater impact on anaerobic versus aerobic power in trained masters athletes. *Journal of Sports Sciences*, 31, 97–103.

Harridge, S.D.R. & Lazarus, N.R. (2017). Physical activity, aging, and physiological function. *Physiology*, 32, 152–161.

Hayflick, L. (1985). Theories of biological aging. *Experimental Gerontology*, 20, 145–159.

Inami, T. & Shimizu, T. (2014). Long-term stretching program in older active adults increases muscle strength. *Journal of Exercise, Sports & Orthopedics*, 1, 2, 1–8.

Jakovljevic, D.G. (2018). Physical activity and cardiovascular aging: Physiological and molecular insights. *Experimental Gerontology*, 109, 67–74.

Kao, C. et al. (2018). Effect of interactive cognitive motor training on gait and balance among older adults: A randomized controlled trial. *International Journal of Nursing Studies*, 82, 121–128.

Khan, S.S., Singer, B.D., & Vaughan, D.E. (2017). Molecular and physiological manifestations and measurement of aging in humans. *Aging Cell*, 16, 4, 624–633.

Lange, P. et al. (2015). Lung-function trajectories leading to chronic obstructive pulmonary disease. *New England Journal of Medicine*, 373, 111–122.

Laughlin, M.H., Bowles, D.K., & Duncker, D.J. (2012). The coronary circulation in exercise training. *American Journal of Physiology Heart & Circulatory Physiology*, 302, H10–23.

Lavie, C.J. et al. (2019). Sedentary behavior, exercise, and cardiovascular health. *Circulation Research*, 124, 5, 799–815.

Law, E. et al. (2016). Telomeres and stress: Promising avenues for research in psycho-oncology. *Asia-Pacific Journal of Oncology Nursing*, 3, 137–147.

Levy, S.S. et al. (2020). Effects of a community-based exercise program on older adults' physical function, activities of daily living, and exercise self-efficacy: Feeling Fit Club. *Journal of Applied Gerontology*, 39, 1, 40–49.

Luo, M. et al. (2020). Social engagement pattern, health behaviors and subjective well-being of older adults: An international perspective using WHO-SAGE survey data. *BMC Public Health*, 20, 99.

Mandsager, K. et al. (2018). Association of cardiorespiratory fitness with long-term mortality among adults undergoing exercise treadmill testing. *JAMA Network Open*, 1, 6, e183605.

Melton, L.J. et al. (2000). Epidemiology of sarcopenia. *Journal of the American Geriatric Society*, 48, 625–630.

Miller, K.J. et al. (2019). Exercise, mood, self-efficacy, and social support as predictors of depressive symptoms in older adults: Direct and interaction effects. *Frontiers in Psychology*, 10, 2145.

Mintzer, J. et al. (2019). Lifestyle choices and brain health. *Frontiers in Medicine*, 6, 204.

Morente-Oria, H. et al. (2020). Effects of 8-weeks concurrent strength and aerobic training on body composition, physiological and cognitive performance in older adult women. *Sustainability*, 12, 1–14.

Morgan, G.S. et al. (2019). A life fulfilled: Positively influencing physical activity in older adults—A systematic review and meta-ethnography. *BMC Public Health*, 19, 362.

Mozaffarian, D. et al. (2015). Heart disease and stroke statistics—2015 update: A report from the American Heart Association. *Circulation*, 131, e29–322.

Murphy, M.H. et al. (2019). The effects of continuous compared to accumulated exercise on health: A meta-analytic review. *Sports Medicine*, 49, 1585–1607.

Nomikos, N.N. et al. (2018). Exercise, telomeres, and cancer: "The Exercise-Telomere Hypothesis." *Frontiers in Physiology*, 9, 1978.

Ortega, F.B. et al. (2010). Psychological well-being, cardiorespiratory fitness, and long-term survival. *American Journal of Preventive Medicine, 39,* 440–448.

Pae, M., Meydani, S.N., & Wu, D. (2012). The role of nutrition in enhancing immunity in aging. *Aging & Disease, 3,* 91–129.

Passarino, G., De Rango, F., & Montesanto, A. (2016). Human longevity: Genetics or lifestyle? It takes two to tango. *Immunity & Ageing, 13,* 12.

Paterson, D.H. & Warburton, D.ER. (2010). Physical activity and functional limitations in older adults: A systematic review related to Canada's Physical Activity Guidelines. *International Journal of Behavioral Nutrition and Physical Activity, 7,* 38.

Peterson, M.D., Sen, A., & Gordon, P.M. (2011). Influence of resistance exercise on lean body mass in aging adults: A meta-analysis. *Medicine & Science in Sports & Exercise, 43,* 249–258.

Pollock, R.D. et al. (2015). An investigation into the relationship between age and physiological function in highly active older adults. *The Journal of Physiology, 593,* 3, 657–680.

Rahman, N.N.A.A., Singh, D.K.A., & Lee, R. (2017). Correlation between thoracolumbar curvatures and respiratory function in older adults. *Clinical Interventions in Aging, 12,* 523–529.

Reid, K.F. & Fielding, R.A. (2012). Skeletal muscle power: A critical determinant of physical functioning in older adults. *Exercise and Sport Sciences Reviews, 40,* 1, 4–12.

Rikli, R.E. & Jones, J.C. (2013). *Senior Fitness Test Manual* (2nd ed.). Champaign, Ill.: Human Kinetics.

Roman, M.A., Rossiter, H.B., & Casaburi, R. (2016). Exercise, ageing and the lung. *European Respiratory Journal, 48,* 1471–1486.

Saldmann, F. et al. (2019). The naked mole rat: A unique example of positive oxidative stress. *Oxidative Medicine and Cellular Longevity,* Article ID: 4502819.

Sanders, L.M.J. et al. (2019). Dose-response relationship between exercise and cognitive function in older adults with and without cognitive impairment: A systematic review and meta-analysis. *PLoS One, 14,* 1, e0210036.

Sgarbieri, V.C. & Pacheco, M.T.B. (2017). Healthy human aging: Intrinsic and environmental factors. *Brazilian Journal of Food Technology, 20.*

Sillanpää, E. et al. (2014). Associations between muscle length, spirometric pulmonary function and mobility in healthy older adults. *Age, 36,* 4, 9967.

Suzuki, T. et al. (2012). Effects of multicomponent exercise on cognitive function in older adults with amnestic mild cognitive impairment: A randomized controlled trial. *BMC Neurology, 12,* 128.

Tsai, C-L. et al. (2015). The effects of long-term resistance exercise on the relationship between neurocognitive performance and GH, IGF-1, and homocysteine levels in the elderly. *Frontiers in Behavioral Neuroscience, 9,* 23.

Tucker, L.A. (2017). Physical activity and telomere length in U.S. men and women: An NHANES investigation. *Preventive Medicine, 100,* 145–151.

Tun, B.C. et al. (2017). Exercise, blood pressure and mortality: Finding of eight years of follow-up. *Brazilian Journal of Sports Medicine, 23,* 2, 133–136.

United Nations, Department of Economic and Social Affairs, Population Division (2019). *World Population Ageing 2019: Highlights* (ST/ESA/SER.A/430).

United Nations, Department of Economic and Social Affairs, Population Division (2017). *World Population Ageing 2017: Highlights* (ST/ESA/SER.A/397).

U.S. Department of Health & Human Services (2018). *Physical Activity Guidelines for Americans* (2nd ed.). https://health.gov/paguidelines/second-edition/pdf/Physical_Activity_Guidelines_2nd_edition.pdf

Wackerage, H. (2017). Sarcopenia: Causes and treatments. *Dutch Journal of Sports Medicine, 68,* 178–184.

Wang, F. & Boros, S. (2019). The effect of physical activity on sleep quality: A systematic review. *European Journal of Physiotherapy,* DOI: 10.1080/21679169.2019.1623314.

Wang, Y. & Xu, D. (2017). Effects of aerobic exercise on lipids and lipoproteins. *Lipids in Health and Disease, 16,* 132.

Wilkinson, D.J., Piasecki, M., & Atherton, P.J. (2018). The age-related loss of skeletal muscle mass and function: Measurement and physiology of muscle fibre atrophy and muscle fibre loss in humans. *Ageing Research Reviews, 47,* 123–132.

World Health Organization (2018). *The Global Action Plan on Physical Activity 2018-2030: More Active People for a Healthier World.* https://www.who.int/ncds/prevention/physical-activity/global-action-plan-2018-2030/en/

World Health Organization (2011). *Global Recommendations for Physical Activity for Health.* https://www.who.int/dietphysicalactivity/leaflet-physical-activity-recommendations.pdf?ua=1

World Health Organization (1997). The Heidelberg guidelines for promoting physical activity among older persons. *Journal of Aging and Physical Activity,* 5, 1, 2–8.

SUGGESTED READINGS

American College of Sports Medicine (2009). American College of Sports Medicine position stand: Exercise and physical activity for older adults. *Medicine & Science in Sports & Exercise,* 41, 1510–1530.

Chodzko-Zajko, W.J., Kramer, A.F., & Poon, L.W. (2009). *Enhancing Cognitive Functioning and Brain Plasticity.* Champaign, Ill.: Human Kinetics.

Poon, L.W., Chodzko-Zajko, W., & Tomporowski, P.D. (2006). *Active Living, Cognitive Functioning, and Aging.* Champaign, Ill.: Human Kinetics.

Rikli, R.E. & Jones, J.C. (2013). *Senior Fitness Test Manual* (2nd ed.). Champaign, Ill.: Human Kinetics.

Spirduso, W.W., Poon, L.W., & Chodzko-Zajko, W. (2008). *Exercise and Its Mediating Effects on Cognition.* Champaign, Ill.: Human Kinetics.

U.S. Department of Health & Human Services (2018). *Physical Activity Guidelines for Americans* (2nd ed.). https://health.gov/paguidelines/second-edition/pdf/Physical_Activity_Guidelines_2nd_edition.pdf

World Health Organization (2018). *The Global Action Plan on Physical Activity 2018-2030: More Active People for a Healthier World.* https://www.who.int/ncds/prevention/physical-activity/global-action-plan-2018-2030/en/

CHAPTER 4
Senior Nutrition

LEARNING OBJECTIVES

After reading this chapter, you will be able to:

▸ Describe several physiological changes that occur with advanced age and dramatically affect nutrition choices and nutritional intake

▸ Explain how chronic diseases such as osteoporosis, sarcopenia, and sarcopenic obesity affect nutrition in older adulthood

▸ Describe how factors such as polypharmacy, access to food, and social isolation relate to older adult nutritional status

▸ Explain the caloric, macronutrient, micronutrient, and hydration needs unique to older adults

▸ Provide general nutrition guidelines for older adults

Nearly 80% of older adults have at least one chronic disease and it is estimated that 67% of community-dwelling older adults have two or more concurrent chronic conditions, with each additional chronic condition being associated with an increase in the number of functional limitations presented. There is a strong association between multimorbidity and functional limitations (National Council on Aging, 2018; Jindai et al., 2016). Practicing healthy lifestyle behaviors plays an important role in staving off illness and disease and keeping older adults healthy, independent, and in their homes. In fact, older adults who eat higher quality diets, such as the **Healthy Mediterranean-Style Eating Pattern,** which includes vegetables, fruits, whole grains, poultry, fish, and low-fat dairy products, have increased quality and quantity of life (Govindaraju et al., 2018; Mendez & Newman, 2018; U.S. Department of Agriculture, 2015; Anderson et al., 2011). Older adults face unique barriers when striving to eat a healthful diet, including:

▸ Age-related physiological changes in smell, taste, chewing, swallowing, **digestion,** and **absorption**

▸ Changes to physical-activity patterns and body composition

▸ Compromised dentition (i.e., arrangement and number of teeth) and dental health

▶ The use of multiple medications, each with varying food-medication interactions and restrictions and diet-altering side effects

▶ Economic hardships

▶ Changes in mental functioning

▶ Social isolation

Prior to delving into a discussion of the nutrition recommendations and ideal eating patterns of older adults, it is first important to understand the issues they face when making nutrition choices.

Physiological Changes Affecting Nutrition Choices

A large number of physiological changes occur with advanced age. For many older adults, these changes dramatically affect nutrition choices and nutritional intake.

SENSORY CHANGES

It should not be assumed that all older adults will experience age-related sensory loss, but the reality is that many older adults will be challenged with a decline in one or more of the five classical senses. In fact, one study looking at data collected from over 3,000 community-dwelling older adults suggests that 67% of older adults in the United States have two or more sensory deficits, while 27% suffer from just one and only 6% have no impairment (Correia et al., 2016). These sensory losses not only play an important role in disease but are also linked with unfavorable clinical and functional outcomes. In addition, sensory loss commonly affects how older adults live and interact with other people and their environments (National Institute on Aging, 2015). Global sensory impairment, or deficits in all five senses, predicts decreased mobility and function, weight loss, lower physical activity, decreased cognitive function, lower self-reported physical and mental health, and increased mortality at five years from baseline measurements (National Institute on Aging, 2015). Deficits in sensory function may predict major health outcomes and may signal general physiological decline (National Institute on Aging, 2015).

For many people, food selection is primarily determined not by **nutrient density,** but rather by a host of other factors, not the least of which is smell and taste, two sensations that are altered with increased age.

Alterations in Smell

Many adults (approximately 23% of Americans over the age of 40 and 32% of adults 80 and older) experience a self-reported decrease in **olfaction** (smell) (National Institute on Deafness and Other Communication Disorders, 2019). Age-related diminished olfaction is referred to as **presbyosmia,** while a complete loss of olfaction is called **anosmia. Dysosmia** is a distortion in olfaction such that one either experiences a smell incongruent with the actual smell (typically a pleasant smell is perceived as an unpleasant smell) or experiences a smell that does not exist (phantom odor perception). Decreased olfaction is thought to be due to both aging and a lifetime of environmental insults such as respiratory infections, exposure to toxic chemicals, and certain types of head injuries.

A diminished sense of smell can have dire consequences for an older adult. For example, an older adult may not notice the rancid smell of rotting leftover food in the refrigerator and may still opt to eat it, increasing the risk of foodborne illness. A person with a diminished sense of smell may also get less pleasure from eating, which may combine with decreased appetite to increase the risk of nutritional deficiency. **Depression** and a decrease in self-care, including proper nutrition, may also be amplified when one's diminished smell leads to poor hygiene, which may cause less socialization and more isolation.

✦ EXPAND YOUR KNOWLEDGE

Food Safety Considerations for Older Adults

An important but often underestimated key to healthy eating is to avoid foods contaminated with harmful bacteria, viruses, parasites, and other microorganisms. About one in six Americans, or 48 million people, become sick each year from foodborne illness, 128,000 are hospitalized, and approximately 3,000 die [Centers for Disease Control and Prevention (CDC), 2018]. Older adults are at particularly high risk for foodborne illness due to a weakened immune system, decreased ability to rid the body of harmful bacteria, and an impaired ability to recognize the smell of spoiled food. The majority of foodborne illnesses are preventable with a few simple precautions (Table 4-1). Refer to www.fightbac.org, www.foodsafety.gov, or www.cdc.gov/foodsafety for more information.

Advise older adults to follow these tips while grocery shopping to reduce the risk of foodborne illnesses:

▸ Check produce for bruises and feel and smell for ripeness (given these senses are reliable for the individual).

▸ Look for a sell-by date for breads and baked goods, a use-by date on some packaged foods, and an expiration date on yeast and baking powder. For more information on the shelf life of thousands of foods, visit www.stilltasty.com.

▸ Make sure packaged goods are not torn and cans are not dented, cracked, or bulging.

▸ Separate fish and poultry from other purchases by wrapping them separately in plastic bags.

▸ Pick up refrigerated and frozen foods last. Try to make sure all perishable items are refrigerated within one hour of purchase.

TABLE 4-1
Steps to Safe Food Handling

To avoid microbial foodborne illness:

▸ Clean hands, food contact surfaces, and fruits and vegetables. Meat and poultry should not be washed or rinsed.

▸ Separate raw, cooked, and ready-to-eat foods while shopping, preparing, or storing foods.

▸ Cook foods to a safe temperature to kill microorganisms [bacteria grow most rapidly between the temperatures of 40 and 140° F (4 and 60° C)]. Pregnant women should only eat certain deli meats and frankfurters that have been reheated to steaming hot.

▸ Refrigerate perishable food promptly (within two hours) and defrost foods properly. Eat refrigerated leftovers within three or four days.

▸ Avoid raw (unpasteurized) milk or any products made from unpasteurized milk, raw or partially cooked eggs, or foods containing raw eggs, raw or undercooked meat and poultry, unpasteurized juice, and raw sprouts. This is especially important for infants and young children, pregnant women, older adults, and those who are immunocompromised.

Reprinted from the United States Department of Agriculture (2015). *2015–2020 Dietary Guidelines for Americans* (8th ed.). www.health.gov/dietaryguidelines

Alterations in Taste

Diminished taste (**hypogeusia**), which affects 19% of Americans over the age of 40 and 27% of those over 80 (National Institute on Deafness and Other Communication Disorders, 2019), and absent taste (**ageusia**) also affects older adults, though the complete lack of taste is exceedingly rare. Taste perception can be altered in older adults due to mouth infections such as a fungal infection (thrush) that often occurs in response to conditions that compromise the immune system, such as **diabetes,** or as a side effect of medications. Older adults may also report decreased taste in foods for nonsensory reasons such as decreased pleasure from eating and decreased appetite. Any client who reports decreased sense of smell or taste should be referred to their primary care physician for further evaluation and intervention.

📖 APPLY WHAT YOU KNOW

Improving Nutritional Intake for Older Adults with Impaired Olfaction or Taste

Health coaches and exercise professionals should share the following tips with clients with impaired senses of smell or taste (National Institute on Aging, 2015).

▸ Mask the bitterness of vegetables and fruits with a small amount of salt or sugar (for example, add a teaspoon of sugar to grapefruit or top broccoli or Brussels sprouts with a small amount of melted cheese) (if appropriate, depending on client's other health considerations).

▸ Vary the texture and temperature of foods.

▸ Add an "irritant" such as black pepper, chili pepper, or ginger to maintain interest in eating.

▸ Increase visual appeal of meals by incorporating a wide range of colors and garnishes so that the individual "eats with the eyes" to stimulate appetite and food enjoyment.

STRUCTURAL CHANGES

Many structural changes occur in the functioning of the human body with increased age. Some of the most significant, when it comes to nutritional status, include the changes in the gastrointestinal tract, cardiovascular system, excretory system, and muscle composition.

Gastrointestinal System: Alterations in Digestion and Absorption

Age-related changes to the many organs of the gastrointestinal system do occur; however, most organs of the gastrointestinal system have such large reserves that these changes are inconsequential for most healthy older adults. However, those older adults who suffer from any of a number of gastrointestinal disorders (such as gallstones, **diverticular disease,** ulcers, constipation, **inflammatory bowel syndrome, lactose intolerance, gastroesophageal reflux disease,** and various cancers) may suffer from dramatic changes in digestion, absorption, and consequently nutritional intake and nutritional status.

The most obvious of the age- and disease-related alterations of the gastrointestinal system include chewing and swallowing, especially for the oldest adults (>85 years). These problems are often exacerbated by medication side effects, which include altered taste sensation, nausea, and altered attention and mood.

A pronounced age-related change affecting an individual's nutrition may be a loss of appetite. Referred to as "anorexia of aging," this condition is primarily due to a reduction in key **nutrients** (e.g., protein, fiber, fruits, vegetables, and whole grains) and poor oral intake as a result of changes to peripheral hormone signaling, gut motility, sensory perception due to aging, and environmental and social factors (Cox et al., 2019).

As described earlier, loss of the sense of taste is common among older people and has been associated with an age-related decline in the density of the taste buds and **papillae** (cone-shaped protuberances on the top of the tongue that contain the taste buds). Consequently, sensitivity to the four basic taste qualities (i.e., sweet, salty, bitter, and sour) can become impaired in older adults. Distorted ability to taste in old age may also be influenced by disease, functional and cognitive impairment, depression, or **polypharmacy.** These changes can have several clinical consequences, such as diminished appreciation of food and beverages, and a declining appetite, which may increase the risk of **anorexia,** weight loss, and **malnutrition.**

Cardiovascular System: Alterations in Cardiovascular Function

Cardiovascular disease is a leading cause of death and disability among older adults. Decline in cardiovascular function occurs with increased age, most notably in middle age onward. Older adults experience a decline in cardiovascular reserve for primarily three reasons: (1) age-associated changes, (2) physical deconditioning associated with low levels of physical activity, and (3) progressive **atherosclerosis.** While many cardiovascular changes that occur with aging may be natural, normal, and inevitable, they are at least to some extent affected by environmental factors, including a lifetime of nutrition choices. Older adults may consider adopting a **Dietary Approaches to Stop Hypertension (DASH) eating plan,** Healthy Mediterranean-Style Eating Pattern, **Healthy U.S.-Style Eating Pattern,** or **Healthy Vegetarian Eating Pattern** to optimize heart health and reduce the risk for a cardiovascular event (U.S. Department of Agriculture, 2015). These eating plans are described in more detail later in this chapter.

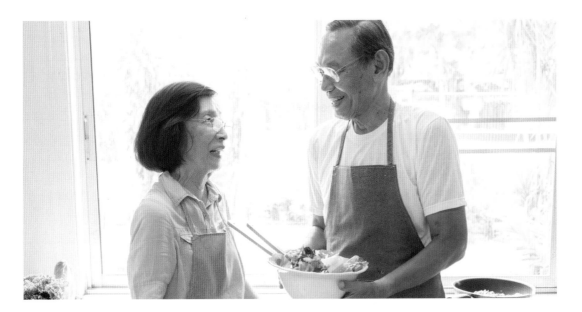

ACE→ M⊙VER METHOD▮

Empowering a Client to Make Dietary Changes

During the cool-down portion of an exercise session with your client Dave, he lets you know that he received a pamphlet of information about the DASH eating plan after a recent medical appointment. Dave has been your client for six months and has primarily been interested in increasing his physical-activity levels. This is the first time he has mentioned dietary changes. Dave is interested in incorporating the DASH eating plan and wants to know how he should go about it.

ACE→ ABC APPROACH

Following is an example of how the ACE Mover Method™ and the ACE ABC Approach™ can be utilized to explore the topic of making dietary changes while remaining within the scope of practice and honoring the client's resourcefulness and ability to change.

Ask: Use powerful open-ended questions to better understand the client's expectations and what he is hoping to achieve by implementing the DASH eating plan.

Exercise Professional: Thank you for letting me know about the information you received about the DASH eating plan. What is it about this eating plan that interests you?

Client: As you know, my blood pressure has been elevated for most of my adult life and recently my doctor let me know that my blood pressure is now considered high. The doctor says I should keep working with you to find ways to increase my physical-activity levels but also recommended dietary changes that might help. She knows I am not keen on the idea of taking medications and let me know that lifestyle changes can help. The information I received about the DASH plan is appealing to me because it looks like it can help with my blood pressure and it does not seem like a fad diet.

Exercise Professional: Taking medications to control your blood pressure is not something you want to do and eating more healthfully in addition to your increased physical activity is something you are considering. What do you already know about the DASH eating plan?

Client: That's correct. I don't want to be bothered with taking medications and having to fill prescriptions, especially if I can do things on my own to take control of my health. The pamphlet I received was informative and I did some research to see what is involved with this diet. I found some resources online that were recommended in the information my doctor gave me and they lay out an easy-to-follow plan. If I remember correctly, it looks like I need to eat more whole grains, fruits, and vegetables and less meat than I do now. Does that sound about right to you?

Exercise Professional: That does sound right. What else would you like to know about DASH?

Client: I think I have all the information I need for now, but one thing that struck me is the recommendation for sodium. I believe the literature said to eat 2,500 mg, or something like that. I don't even know what a mg is and I don't want to have to measure or weigh my food. If this gets complicated, I probably won't do it.

Exercise Professional: Keeping it simple is important to your success. The recommendation from your doctor is to consume no more than 2,300 mg of sodium per day. To keep things simple, you can think of it as having no more than one teaspoon of salt per day. Remember, sodium is found in many foods and I would be happy to give you a list of foods with their sodium amount to help you easily navigate through your daily consumption. In addition, I can educate you on label reading to help you make better choices and answer any of your other nutritional questions as they arise to help you meet your goals. Would that help?

Client: That would help and makes me feel less anxious about starting this journey because I feel supported. I would like to know more about the foods I am eating and how they help or hinder my health.

Break down barriers: Ask more open-ended questions to find out what is getting in the way of implementing this goal.

Exercise Professional: What, if anything, is stopping you from making dietary changes right now?

Client: I have been thinking about this for a while and it does not seem that complicated. My biggest hesitation at this point involves my wife. When I shared this information with her, she was not very excited about it. Don't get me wrong. She wants me to be healthy and supports me, but this plan seems like more work for her since she does most of the cooking.

Exercise Professional: Your wife cares for you and wants you to be healthy, but if the changes you have to make are too cumbersome for her, she will lack excitement about these healthy modifications and this will be a barrier to your success.

Client: Exactly. If she is not on board with me, it will make this change very challenging. Because this is important to me, I have been thinking of some strategies for gradually introducing this plan. I came up with some ideas that will move me toward full integration of DASH and make my wife happy or at least more open to the idea. I think if I sit down with her to discuss how important these changes are to me, that will resonate with her and show that I am serious. After that, I plan to add one **serving** of fruit to my daily routine and to cook one vegetable as part of dinner, which is quite a simple change for both of us.

Collaborate: Partner with your client to determine next steps for overcoming obstacles now that some potential options have been identified for moving forward.

Exercise Professional: You have already been thinking of ways to get started. That's great! What else would you like to do that will help move you closer to your goal?

Client: Not only am I going to increase my fruit and vegetable intake, but I am also going to decrease the burden on my wife by being the one to purchase the fruits and vegetables each week and I will prepare the vegetables at dinner time so I don't add to her workload at home.

Exercise Professional: What thoughtful ideas! Being as specific as possible, how will you get started this week?

Client: This week, I will go to the local farmers market on Sunday and select seven pieces of fruit so that I have one to eat each day. If my wife would like to start with me, I will get some for her as well. Also, I will pick out vegetables to add to each night's dinner this week, which I will prepare. The literature from the doctor had some recommendations, but I will ask the vendors at the market for suggestions on easy ways to prepare vegetables. I will eat one serving of fruit each day and one serving of vegetables with dinner every day for one week.

Exercise Professional: These goals seem realistic and meaningful to you! In addition to your new nutritional goals, you did a great job with your workout today. I look forward to seeing you next week and hearing about how you are doing with these new goals.

In this scenario, the topic of nutrition came up after the client received information about a specific eating pattern from his doctor. The client expressed an interest in pursuing a more healthful way of eating and the exercise professional engaged the client to find out more. Using the ACE Mover Method philosophy and the ACE ABC Approach, the exercise professional was able to find out what the client is hoping to achieve, what barriers might get in the way of the plan, and respected the client's autonomy by letting him decide what his next steps should be.

Renal System: Alterations in Fluid Balance

The kidneys are responsible for many important and complex functions, which include maintenance of body pH and fluid balance. The kidneys naturally decrease in size and function in old age. The **glomerular filtration rate,** the rate at which fluid is filtered by the kidney per minute, and **renal plasma flow,** the volume of plasma that flows through the kidney over a specified period of time, decrease with age and impact diluting and concentrating capacity, the secretion of potassium, and the ability to excrete an acid load, which affects the ability to maintain **homeostasis** under stressful conditions. Age-related changes to the kidneys culminate in a decreased ability to concentrate urine and, consequently an impairment of serum sodium levels, resulting in either **hyponatremia** or **hypernatremia,** depending upon other factors such as fluid intake and medications. Further, individuals with **hypertension** and diabetes (both increasingly common conditions in older adults) have a significantly higher risk for developing chronic kidney disease.

Musculoskeletal System: Alterations in Body Composition and Metabolism

Energy needs decrease with age. The decline is probably due in large part to decreased physical activity and subsequent decreased muscle mass (which is highly metabolically active) and increased fat mass (which is relatively metabolically inactive), although reduced **growth hormone** secretion, decreased sex hormones, and other unknown factors may also play a role. Though declining muscle mass is expected with advancing age, older adults who maintain a strenuous physical-activity regimen that includes some muscular training may be able to maintain muscle mass and minimize the decrease in metabolic rate. Therefore, physical activity and specificity training become even more important as body composition and metabolic changes occur with age.

CHANGES TO DENTITION AND DENTAL HEALTH

The oral cavity undergoes dramatic changes with aging, not the least of which include changes to the strength and integrity of the teeth. Any of a number of dental ailments can impair an older adult's ability to properly chew and swallow food, including decayed teeth; periodontal disease; poorly fitting dentures; poor oral hygiene; and pain, inflammation, or infection of the oral cavity. Attention to oral health is one of the first areas to become neglected as older adults develop chronic diseases, more difficulty completing activities of daily living, and decreased access to dental care.

Consequently, poor oral health afflicts a large percentage of older adults. Approximately 20% of older adults have untreated tooth decay, 68% of those 65 and older have gum disease, and 20% of older adults have lost all of their teeth (CDC, 2019). Other older adults suffer from dry mouth due to side effects of prescription medications. The decreased production of saliva that naturally contains bacteria-fighting substances and minerals that help to build tooth enamel increases the risk for oral disease (CDC, 2019). Those older adults with the poorest dental health tend to be of low socioeconomic status, reliant on Medicare (which does not cover dental services), from a minority population, and possibly disabled, homebound, or institutionalized (CDC, 2019).

Oral health is a crucial factor for overall well-being and its decline is associated with dry mouth, infection, pain, and problems with swallowing, chewing, smiling, speaking, socializing, and communicating (Kossioni, 2018). In addition, because the oral cavity is an important part of the digestive process responsible for biting, chewing, preparing food for transport, and moving it to the stomach, deterioration in any of these functions may lead to nutritional impairment. Dysfunctional mastication, or chewing, for example, may lead to a reduced consumption of fibrous foods and **micronutrients** such as thiamine and vitamin B12, which are associated with cognitive impairment, and an increase in consumption of easy-to-chew foods of poor nutritional quality, which may lead to unhealthy diets that are associated with an increased risk for **stroke** and **dementia** (Kossioni, 2018). Anyone identified as possibly suffering from a form of malnutrition should be immediately referred for evaluation by a physician and **registered dietitian (RD).**

Nutrition and Chronic Disease in Older Adulthood

Older adults are susceptible to a variety of chronic diseases and ailments. The implications of acquiring chronic diseases as an older adult extend beyond the challenges of managing a disease. In many cases, the treatments required have profound impacts on nutritional status. Moreover, the prevention of chronic diseases and reduction of their associated consequences is essential for keeping older adults healthy and independent. Healthy nutrition and physical activity are keys to a long and healthy life. Eating nutrient-dense foods and balancing energy intake with the necessary physical activity to maintain a healthy weight is essential at all stages of life. Unbalanced consumption of foods high in calories and low in essential nutrients contributes to caloric excess, **overweight,** and **obesity.** The amount of the calories consumed in relation to physical activity and the quality of food is a key determinant of nutrition-related chronic disease.

OSTEOPOROSIS

Osteoporosis is the most common bone disease and is defined as a weakening of the bones, which can lead to fracture of the hip, spine, and other skeletal sites. In America, 54% of people over the age of 50 have low bone mineral density (BMD), with an estimated 10.2 million people having osteoporosis. When combined with rates of **osteopenia,** or a below-average BMD that puts someone at risk for developing osteoporosis, the total prevalence in the U.S. is 35.5 million women and 18.2 million men. Fractures related to bone fragility are a worldwide concern and are expected to increase as the older adult population grows. In fact, by the year 2030, the number of fragility fractures is expected to increase by 32% (Goode, Wright, & Lynch, 2020). The disease most often affects elderly women, although it can occur in men and younger women as well (refer to Chapter 9 for more in-depth coverage of osteoporosis and **menopause**).

Some of the nutrients involved in the prevention and treatment of osteoporosis include calcium and vitamin D. Vitamin D deficiency is associated with bone softening (**osteomalacia**), reduced calcium absorption, and demineralization of bone, which can lead to thin, brittle, and misshaped bones [National Institutes of Health (NIH), 2020]. Older adults are at risk for vitamin D deficiency because of decreased dietary intake, more time spent indoors, and the fact that aged skin is less efficient at synthesizing vitamin D from sun exposure (NIH, 2020). Smoking and a lack of physical activity also increase the risk of osteoporosis, while engaging in weight-bearing physical activity decreases the risk (NIH, 2018; McMillan et al., 2017).

Exercise professionals should share the following strategies for preventing osteoporosis with senior clients.

▸ Consume a healthy diet with recommended amounts of calcium (1,000 mg/day for women ages 19 to 50; 1,200 mg/day for women over 50; 1,000 mg/day for men 51 to 70; and 1,200 mg/day for men over 70) and vitamin D [15 mcg/day (600 IU/day) for all adults up to 70 years, and 20 mcg/day (800 IU/day) for individuals over 70] (U.S. Department of Agriculture, 2015).

▸ Maintain a healthful body weight (**body mass index** of 18.5 to 24.9 kg/m^2).

▸ Engage in regular physical activity that includes weight-bearing cardiorespiratory exercise and muscular-strengthening exercise.

▸ Avoid heavy drinking and smoking.

In addition, exercise professionals can help clients minimize the risk of falls by encouraging them to:

▸ Evaluate the home environment for tripping hazards and lighting deficiencies.

▸ Get a medical check-up to evaluate health issues related to falling.

▸ Wear sensible shoes.

▸ Perform strength training and neuromuscular exercise to promote increased balance.

▸ Use assistive devices such as handrails.

SARCOPENIA AND SARCOPENIC OBESITY

Sarcopenic obesity is defined as having both **sarcopenia** (the age-related loss of muscle mass and either low muscular strength or low physical performance) and obesity (see Chapter 9). Sarcopenia has been hypothesized to be related to a combination of factors occurring over time. Nutrition-related factors include reduced dietary intake of protein and vitamin D deficiency, while other possible contributors include reduced physical activity, cumulative inflammatory responses, oxidative stress, and resistance to anabolic stimuli. Nutritional interventions have been trialed in chronic sarcopenia and there is increasing evidence that older adults have higher protein requirements than younger adults, with further increased requirements during acute illness. There are clear health benefits for promotion of physical activity and healthy nutrition. However, further research is needed to identify the characteristics of an optimal physical activity and nutrition approach (Welch et al., 2018).

·:·: EXPAND YOUR KNOWLEDGE

Are Age-related Loss of Muscle Mass and Weight Gain Inevitable?

It is well recognized that muscle mass declines with age. Consequently, many older adults suffer from sarcopenia, a notable risk factor for osteoporosis and other related negative health consequences. While muscular training plays some role in helping to preserve muscle mass with age, researchers have wondered whether certain nutritional factors may also play a role in protection from sarcopenia. To answer this question, researchers set out to conduct a review to understand the impact of nutrition on muscle mass, strength, and performance in older adults (Mithal et al., 2012). Their findings are summarized in Table 4-2.

TABLE 4-2

Impact of Specific Nutrients on Muscle Mass, Strength, and Performance in Older Adults

Nutrient	Likely Benefit	Recommendation
Protein	Protein stimulates a hormone called insulin-like growth factor 1 (IGF-1), which increases muscle synthesis. Most effective when consumed following resistance exercise	Combine high protein load (such as 15 g bolus of essential amino acids) with resistance training to boost muscle protein synthesis.
Vitamin D	Mechanism unknown Supplementation seems to increase the number and size of fast-twitch (type II) muscle fibers.	Many older adults do not meet vitamin D needs through sunshine and diet and may require supplementation. This should be discussed with a physician.
Alkaline diet	A high-acid diet likely contributes to the age-related decline in muscle function and possibly muscle mass.	Eat more alkaline foods like fruits and vegetables and less acid-producing foods like meat and cereal grains.
Vitamin B12/ folic acid	By correcting for high levels of the inflammatory marker homocysteine, vitamin B12 and/or folic acid may help improve postural stability and/or muscle function and strength.	Many older adults do not readily absorb vitamin B12 from foods. Whether supplementation is indicated should be discussed with a physician.
Antioxidants and anti-inflammatory compounds	Inflammation is thought to play a role in the development of sarcopenia. Antioxidants may help to buffer inflammation and its effects.	Eat naturally occurring antioxidants, such as those found in fruits and vegetables.

Source: Mithal, A. et al. (2012). Impact of nutrition on muscle mass, strength, and performance in older adults. *Osteoporosis International.* DOI: 10.1007/s00198-012-2236-y.

Sarcopenic obesity is common during older adulthood (Batsis & Villareal, 2018). Caloric intake and appetite decrease with age; however, many older adults have overweight or obesity because the age-related decrease in physical activity and metabolic rate is often more pronounced than reduced caloric intake. This scenario leads to a **positive energy balance** and weight gain. In addition, older adults are faced with age-related increases in body fat until the seventh decade of life and declining muscle mass beginning after peak levels are achieved in the fourth decade.

Exercise professionals working with older adults should develop programs to improve muscle mass, strength, performance, and weight status. The Academy of Nutrition and Dietetics (AND) and the Society for Nutrition Education and Behavior state that it is essential to first determine the health risk versus benefit for intentional weight loss in older adults. This determination is made by looking at the impact of weight loss on functionality, life expectancy, and disease prevention (Academy of Nutrition and Dietetics and Society for Nutrition Education and Behavior, 2019). A multidisciplinary team of allied health professionals including, at minimum, a nutrition specialist, exercise professional, and physician should work closely when developing a weight-management program for an older adult.

Other Factors Affecting Nutrition in Older Adults

In addition to age-related changes in body functioning and increased prevalence of chronic disease, other health, economic, and social factors can greatly affect the nutritional status of older adults.

POLYPHARMACY AND NUTRITION CONSIDERATIONS

While an individual takes medications to alleviate the symptoms or consequences of a disease, the medications themselves can cause dramatic side effects, not the least of which can include impaired sense of taste, digestion, and absorption; alterations in metabolism; disruption in normal voiding and defecation patterns; and increased frailty, falls, and mortality. Table 4-3 highlights several commonly prescribed medications in older adults and their potential nutritional interactions and common side effects. Older adults are two to three times more likely to experience adverse drug reactions as compared to younger people and are encouraged to discuss their medication regimen with their physicians and identify any options or alternatives that may have a less harmful effect on nutritional status and quality of life (Little, 2018).

FOOD ACCESS

Poverty status is determined by measuring a family's resources against a measure of its needs. In 2017, nearly 10% of people aged 65 and older had an income below federal poverty thresholds and the median income was $32,654 for men and $19,180 for women (Administration for Community Living, 2019; Congressional Research Service, 2019). With many factors such as housing, transportation, healthcare, and food competing for spending with a limited budget, many older adults suffer from **food insecurity,** which is defined as a lack of access to sufficient, safe, and nutritious food. In fact, it is estimated that about 8% of U.S. households with at least one adult aged 65 or older and nearly 9% of older adults living alone face food insecurity (Pooler et al., 2019). Risk factors for food insecurity include older age, living in poverty, having a low education level, being a minority, being divorced or separated, living with a grandchild, being a renter, having a

TABLE 4-3

Drug–Nutrient Interactions

Medication Class	Drug–Nutrient Interaction/Effect
Antihypertensives*	Zinc deficiency Effect: May cause dysgeusia†, anorexia, impotence, poor appetite, lethargy, and poor wound healing
Acetylcholinesterase inhibitors	Unknown drug–nutrient interaction Effect: May cause nausea, vomiting, diarrhea, and anorexia
Proton pump inhibitors	B12 deficiency Effect: May cause diarrhea, pneumonia, and hip fracture
Statins (HMG-Co reductase inhibitors)	Reductions in CoQ10, α-tocopheral, ß-carotene, and lycopene Effect: May cause myopathy
Long-term, high-dose aspirin	Vitamin C deficiency Effect: May cause thinning of gastric mucosa, with subsequent gastritis, peptic ulcer disease, nausea, anorexia, and malnutrition
Metformin	B12 deficiency Effect: May cause anemia, fatigue, and cognitive impairment

* Thiazide diuretics, angiotensin receptor blockers, angiotensin-converting enzyme inhibitors, and potassium-sparing diuretics

† Distortion of the sense of taste

Source: Little, M.O. (2018). Updates in nutrition and polypharmacy. *Current Opinion in Clinical Nutrition and Metabolic Care, 21,* 4–9.

chronic disease, and living alone (Jih et al., 2018; Bowman, 2007). There are many factors that contribute to poor health and wellness as individuals age. It is vital that exercise professionals look at the bigger picture and all the variables that could be contributing to poor health and wellness, particularly for individuals who live alone and have limited income and resources.

Food Assistance Programs for Seniors

Many older adults face the threat of hunger. To ensure that seniors receive adequate nutrition, there are a number of government and private food-assistance programs available that provide financial assistance for those in need as well as food delivery for the homebound. One such organization is Meals on Wheels America, which provides more than 1 million meals to community-residing older adults each day. The organization is comprised of 5,000 senior nutrition programs from all 50 states and the U.S. territories. The meals are served in community centers and/or delivered to the homes of seniors with limited mobility. Each chapter is an independent organization with varying programs and services, though most programs provide at least two meals per day, five days per week, with large-scale efforts underway to expand those offerings.

Find a Meals on Wheels chapter in your local area by entering your ZIP code at www.mealsonwheelsamerica.org.

SOCIAL ISOLATION

In 2018, Nearly 28% of noninstitutionalized older adults lived alone (9.5 million women and 4.8 million men) (Administration for Community Living, 2019). Older adults who do not have relationships or contact with others to help them are at high risk of nutritional deficiencies due to their inability to shop, prepare, and cook meals because of low income status and the distance from markets or inability to find transportation to the markets (Baugreet et al., 2017).

Social isolation can also influence dietary practices, as cooking a proper meal for oneself may feel burdensome because of the amount of time required (Leslie & Hankey, 2015). In fact, one of the most important suggestions that an exercise professional may make to an older adult to improve nutritional status is to increase the enjoyment level of mealtimes and eat more often with others. It is also important to consider that, in many cases, the nutritional habits of older adults—especially those who are not able to independently care for themselves—are greatly influenced by the shopping, meal preparation, and feeding practices of the caretaker. When providing information to an older adult about quality nutrition, it is also important to include the caregiver, considering the role they may play in determining what types of foods are available in the home.

The following tips can help older adults who eat most meals alone to increase the enjoyment level of mealtimes and help to protect against malnutrition:

▸ Start an eating club that meets regularly for a fun social time set around a good meal.

▸ Eat by a window and use your best dishes.

▸ Eat a lunch in the park.

▸ Invite friends to a potluck dinner or host cooking parties.

▸ Attend a nutrition program for older adults and enjoy meals in the community.

▸ During an illness, arrange for home-delivered meals from a community nutrition program for seniors.

▸ Turn leftovers into "planned leftovers."

▸ Prepare a new recipe each week and invite friends over for a tasting party.

▸ Use frozen prepared dinners for added variety and convenience.

▸ Add flavor to foods with seasoning and experiment with new recipes.

▸ Purchase produce that is in-season for the best flavor and sweetness.

▸ Add a special touch to your table, like a colorful tablecloth or placemats, a plant, flowers, candle, or decorative vase.

▸ Eat smaller meals more often throughout the day.

Caloric, Macronutrient, and Micronutrient Needs for Older Adults

Health status, physical-activity level, sex, and the presence or absence of disease help to determine an older adult's nutrient needs. The *Dietary Guidelines for Americans* provide daily nutritional goals based on age and sex. Table 4-4 provides dietary guidelines for adults 51 years and older.

TABLE 4-4

Nutritional Goals for Adults 51 and Over Based on Dietary Reference Intakes and *Dietary Guidelines* Recommendations

	Females 51+	Males 51+
Calorie Level	1,600	2,000
Macronutrients		
Protein (g)	46	56
Protein (% kcal)	10–35%	10–35%
Carbohydrate (g)	130	130
Carbohydrate (% kcal)	45–65%	45–65%
Dietary Fiber (g)	22.4	28
Added Sugars (% kcal)	<10%	<10%
Total Fat (% kcal)	20–35%	20–35%
Saturated Fat (% kcal)	<10%	<10%
Linoleic Acid (g)	11	14
Linolenic Acid (g)	1.1	1.6
Minerals		
Calcium (mg)	1,200	1,000*
Iron (mg)	8	8
Magnesium (mg)	320	420
Phosphorous (mg)	700	700
Potassium (mg)	4,700	4,700
Sodium (mg)	2,300	2,300
Zinc (mg)	8	11
Copper (mcg)	900	900
Manganese (mg)	1.8	2.3
Selenium (mcg)	55	55
Vitamins		
Vitamin A (mg) RAE	700	900
Vitamin E (mg) AT	15	15
Vitamin D (IU)	600[†]	600[†]
Vitamin C (mg)	75	90
Thiamin (mg)	1.1	1.2
Riboflavin (mg)	1.1	1.3
Niacin (mg)	14	16
Vitamin B6 (mg)	1.5	1.7
Vitamin B12 (mcg)	2.4	2.4
Choline (mg)	425	550
Vitamin K (mcg)	90	120
Folate (mcg) DFE	400	400

* Calcium Recommended Daily Allowance for males 71+ years is 1,200 mg.

† Vitamin D RDA for males and females ages 71+ years is 800 IU.

U.S. Department of Agriculture (2015). *2015–2020 Dietary Guidelines for Americans* (8th ed.). www.health.gov/dietaryguidelines

Sources: Institute of Medicine (2006). *Dietary Reference Intakes: The Essential Guide to Nutrient Requirements.* Washington, D.C.: The National Academies Press; Institute of Medicine (2010). *Dietary Reference Intakes for Calcium and Vitamin D.* Washington, D.C.: The National Academies Press.

CALORIC NEEDS

Energy requirements decrease with age, mostly due to an age-associated decline in physical activity. Despite a decline in energy needs with age, in many cases people do not change energy intake, leading to weight gain and an accumulation of fat mass. In fact, over 78% of men aged 60 and older have overweight as well 68% of women in this same age range. Also, obesity rates for older adults parallel the age-adjusted prevalence in the U.S., with 37% of men and nearly 34% of women 60 years of age and older having obesity (Malenfant & Batsis, 2019). Importantly, though energy needs decrease, micronutrient needs do not. Consequently, many older adults struggle to meet calorie, macronutrient, and micronutrient needs.

If a client over the age of 50 wants to maintain their current weight, the caloric needs are as follows (U.S. Department of Agriculture, 2015):

- ▶ Women:
  - Not physically active: 1,600 calories per day
  - Moderately active: 1,800 calories per day
  - Active lifestyle: 2,000 to 2,200 calories per day
- ▶ Men:
  - Not physically active: 2,000 to 2,200 calories per day
  - Moderately active: 2,200 to 2,400 calories per day
  - Active lifestyle: 2,400 to 2,800 calories per day

MACRONUTRIENT NEEDS

The typical older adult requires about 130 grams per day of **carbohydrate,** while active older adults may have higher needs (U.S. Department of Agriculture, 2015). High-fiber fruits, vegetables, and whole grains are excellent sources of carbohydrate for older adults. These foods are high in nutrients and the fiber provides additional benefits of improved glycemic control, gastric motility, and reduced **low-density lipoprotein (LDL)** cholesterol. However, a diet too high in fiber could be a detriment to very frail older adults and older adults with a

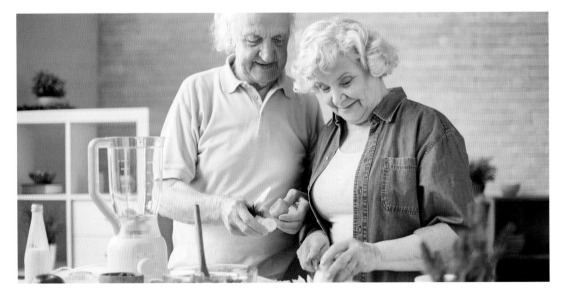

poor appetite, as the high fiber may contribute to early **satiety** and decreased intake of other nutrient-dense foods. For the typical older adult, the recommended fiber intake is 28 grams for men and 22.4 grams for women over age 50 (U.S. Department of Agriculture, 2015).

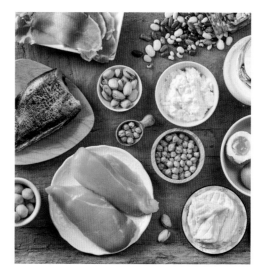

Protein needs for most older adults are similar to that of the general population—about 46 grams per day for women and 56 grams per day for men (U.S. Department of Agriculture, 2015). Very active older adults probably have increased needs to enhance muscle protein **anabolism** and reduce the loss of muscle mass that occurs with aging. While protein intake may play some role in attenuating sarcopenia, the research to date is inconclusive.

While the exact amount of protein needed is dependent on many variables and a clear consensus on daily values is yet to be elucidated, many authorities on this topic suggest amounts greater than the **Recommended Dietary Allowance (RDA)** for the prevention of sarcopenia, **cachexia,** and frailty. These recommendations range from 0.8 to 2.0 g/kg per day for healthy older adults (Franzke et al., 2018; Baum, Kim, & Wolfe, 2016).

Recommended total **fat** intake needs for older adults mirror those of younger adults. Daily nutritional goals for fat include 20 to 35% of total calories coming from fat with less than 10% coming from **saturated fat, trans fats** limited to as low as possible, and an intake of 1.1 grams of linolenic acid (**omega-3 fatty acid**) per day for women and 1.6 grams per day for men, and 11 grams of linoleic acid (**omega-6 fatty acid**) per day for women and 14 grams per day for men (U.S. Department of Agriculture, 2015). Otherwise, fat intake should be based on individual needs and weight-management goals.

Another way to look at macronutrient recommendations is in the context of a complete diet. This can be done using the **Acceptable Macronutrient Distribution Range (AMDR),** which provides target macronutrient values for a complete diet, represents an intake range associated with a decreased risk of chronic disease, and provides essential nutrients. The AMDR for older adults is the same as those for younger adults and suggests that an overall eating pattern should be comprised of 45 to 65% calories from carbohydrate, 10 to 35% calories from protein, and 20 to 35% of calories from fat (U.S. Department of Agriculture, 2015).

MICRONUTRIENT NEEDS

Though caloric needs decrease with age, many nutrient needs stay the same or increase. Thus, in order to consume appropriate amounts of needed nutrients without exceeding caloric needs, older adults need to increase the nutrient density of their diets, eating more lower-calorie nutrient-packed foods like fruits and vegetables and eating fewer **empty calories,** or foods that contain very little nutrition and a large number of calories, such as many desserts and snacks. Older adults suffer from nutritional insufficiencies of many vitamins and minerals such as calcium; zinc; iron; vitamins A, D, E, and K; potassium; B vitamins, especially vitamin B12; and fiber.

Hydration Needs for Older Adults

The risk of **dehydration** is pronounced in older adults, especially those older than 85 years or living in institutionalized settings (Bernstein & Munoz, 2012). An **Adequate Intake (AI)** of 2.7 liters per day for older women and 3.7 liters per day for older men is included in the DRIs (Jimoh et al., 2019; Food and Nutrition Board, 2005). This is the amount of fluid needed to replace normal daily losses and prevent dehydration. Many older adults do not meet these recommendations for a variety of reasons. The sensation of thirst decreases with age. The kidneys become less effective at concentrating urine, leading to excess water loss in urine. Medication side effects and interactions with other drugs may interfere with appropriate hydration. Consequently, unless prompted, many older adults may not achieve the AI for fluids, an amount intended to replace normal daily losses and prevent dehydration. Provision of sufficient fluids is especially critical for exercising older adults who have additional exercise-related fluid losses.

📖 APPLY WHAT YOU KNOW

Strategies to Help Older Adults Meet Fluid Needs

Exercise professionals can share the following tips to encourage clients to meet their fluid needs:

- Take sips from a glass of water, milk, or juice between bites during meals.
- Have a cup of low-fat soup as an afternoon snack.
- Drink a full glass of water if you need to take a pill.
- Have a glass of water before and after you exercise or go outside to garden or walk, especially on a hot day.
- Have small glasses or bottles of water at strategic locations in the house or at work for convenience and as reminders to hydrate.
- Set a timer to remind you to drink periodically throughout the day.
- Drink water first thing in the morning to help the hydration process and start a habit to be continued throughout the day.

General Nutrition Guidelines for Older Adults

An ideal eating pattern for older adults closely resembles an ideal eating pattern for the general adult population, with a few notable exceptions and considerations, which are depicted in the My Plate for Older Adults icon developed by Tuft University's Jean Mayer USDA Human Nutrition Research Center on Aging (Figure 4-1). As presented in the icon, older adults need to pay particular attention to fluid intake, affordable and easy-to-prepare food, and physical activity.

An optimal eating plan for an older adult should incorporate cultural norms and taste preferences, religious and personal beliefs, and food cost and availability. Many eating plans have not been adequately studied to draw firm conclusions on their health benefits. However,

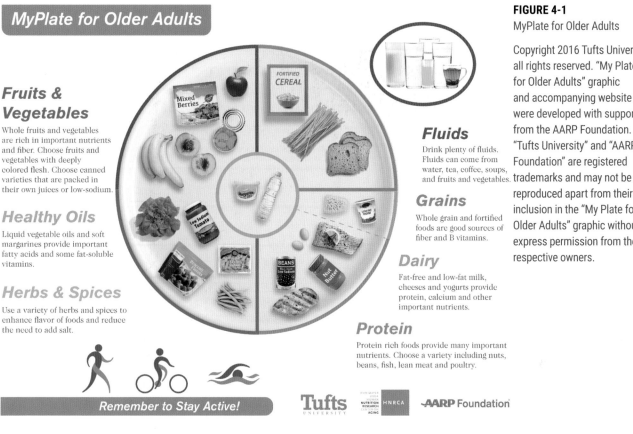

MyPlate for Older Adults

Fruits & Vegetables

Whole fruits and vegetables are rich in important nutrients and fiber. Choose fruits and vegetables with deeply colored flesh. Choose canned varieties that are packed in their own juices or low-sodium.

Healthy Oils

Liquid vegetable oils and soft margarines provide important fatty acids and some fat-soluble vitamins.

Herbs & Spices

Use a variety of herbs and spices to enhance flavor of foods and reduce the need to add salt.

Remember to Stay Active!

Fluids

Drink plenty of fluids. Fluids can come from water, tea, coffee, soups, and fruits and vegetables.

Grains

Whole grain and fortified foods are good sources of fiber and B vitamins.

Dairy

Fat-free and low-fat milk, cheeses and yogurts provide protein, calcium and other important nutrients.

Protein

Protein rich foods provide many important nutrients. Choose a variety including nuts, beans, fish, lean meat and poultry.

FIGURE 4-1
MyPlate for Older Adults

several popular and well-researched eating plans such as the Healthy U.S.-Style Eating Pattern, DASH eating plan, Healthy Mediterranean-Style Eating Pattern, and **vegetarian** and **vegan** eating plans offer health benefits and appeal to certain clients.

HEALTHY U.S.-STYLE EATING PATTERN

The 2015–2020 *Dietary Guidelines for Americans* make a point to emphasize overall eating patterns more so than individual nutrients, recognizing that the overall nutritional value of a person's diet is more than "the sum of its parts" (U.S. Department of Agriculture, 2015). The main components of a healthy eating pattern include:

▸ A variety of vegetables from five different groups—dark green, red and orange, legumes (beans and peas), starchy, and other

▸ Fruit

▸ Grains, primarily whole grains

▸ Fat-free or low-fat dairy, including milk yogurt, cheese, and/or fortified soy products

▸ A variety of foods rich in protein, including seafood, lean meats and poultry, eggs, legumes (beans and peas), nuts, seeds, and soy products

▸ Limited amounts of saturated fats (less than 10% of calories), trans fat (as low as possible) added sugars (less than 10% of calories), and sodium (less than 2,300 mg per day). If alcohol is consumed, it should be consumed in moderation, defined as up to one drink per day for women and two drinks per day for men. One drink is equivalent to 12 ounces of beer, 5 ounces of wine, or 1.5 ounces of hard liquor.

The Healthy U.S.-Style Eating Pattern is based on the types and proportions of foods Americans typically consume, but in nutrient-dense forms and appropriate amounts. It is designed to meet nutrient needs while not exceeding calorie requirements and while staying within limits for overconsumed dietary components.

DASH EATING PLAN

The DASH eating plan was initially developed to manage hypertension. This plan emphasizes the consumption of vegetables, fruits, and low-fat milk and milk products. It is higher in whole grains, poultry, seafood, and nuts and lower in sodium, red and processed meats, sweets, and sugar-containing beverages than the typical American diet. Studies of the DASH eating plan have found that it lowers blood pressure, improves cholesterol levels, and decreases cardiovascular disease risk (U.S. Department of Agriculture, 2015). A very-low-sodium DASH eating plan further reduces blood pressure for individuals with hypertension or elevated blood pressure.

HEALTHY MEDITERRANEAN-STYLE EATING PATTERN

The Healthy Mediterranean-Style Eating Pattern is adapted from the Healthy U.S.-Style Eating Pattern and models the traditional eating patterns of the countries bordering the Mediterranean Sea. While the U.S. Department of Agriculture (2015) offers a specific version of a Mediterranean eating plan, each country consumes a slightly different traditional diet based on culture and agricultural patterns, so there are several variations that share a few underlying features. Overall, it is an eating pattern that emphasizes vegetables, fruit, nuts, olive oil, and whole grains. Limited amounts of meat and milk products are included. Wine is typically included with a meal. People who follow an eating plan that resembles a Mediterranean diet have decreased cardiovascular disease risk factors, cardiovascular disease, and total mortality (Martínez-González, Gea, & Ruiz-Canela, 2019).

EXPAND YOUR KNOWLEDGE

Does the Mediterranean Diet Increase Longevity?

The Greek island of Crete is famous for more than its stunning scenery and ancient roots. Fifty years ago, American scientist Ancel Keys, who himself lived to 100, attributed the exceptional longevity and miniscule rates of cardiovascular disease and cancer on the island to the "Cretan" Mediterranean diet—a diet rich in fruits, vegetables, legumes, whole grains, fish, and olive oil and moderate in red wine. Since then, a large body of research on the Mediterranean diet has accumulated, suggesting that adhering to a Mediterranean diet offers numerous benefits such as enhanced weight loss, heart health, and mental health and reduced **Alzheimer's disease,** cancer, and **Parkinson's disease** (Tosti, Bertozzi, & Fontana, 2017). But is there enough evidence to support the assertion that adopting a Mediterranean diet may add years to your life?

What does the evidence say?
Greek researchers from the University of Athens medical school set out to rigorously evaluate the assertion that adherence to a Mediterranean diet may improve longevity. They enrolled 22,043 adults in Greece who completed a comprehensive survey that included a food-frequency questionnaire aimed to evaluate how closely the diet resembled the traditional Mediterranean diet. The researchers rated adherence to the Mediterranean diet on a nine-point scale that incorporated the diet's major features. They then followed up on the study participants 44 months later, during which 275 participants had died. A higher degree

of adherence to the Mediterranean diet was associated with a lower likelihood of death from any cause, as well as death from cardiovascular disease or cancer. Interestingly, associations between individual food groups within the Mediterranean diet and mortality were not significant. The authors concluded that adherence to the traditional Mediterranean diet is associated with a significant reduction in mortality and that greater adherence to a Mediterranean diet may be related to the increased longevity.

The authors evaluated adherence to a Mediterranean diet with a scale very similar to the one presented here. Exercise professionals can use this scale to assess how closely a client's typical diet resembles a Mediterranean diet. Clients get one point for each "yes." If they score 6 or higher, they are eating like they live in the Mediterranean.

	YES	NO
Vegetables (other than potatoes), 4 or more servings per day	☐	☐
Fruits, 4 or more servings per day	☐	☐
Whole grains, 2 or more servings per day	☐	☐
Beans (legumes), 2 or more servings per week	☐	☐
Nuts, 2 or more servings per week	☐	☐
Fish, 2 or more servings per week	☐	☐
Red and processed meat, 1 or fewer servings per day	☐	☐
Dairy foods, 1 or fewer servings per day	☐	☐
Alcohol, ½ to 1 drink per day for women, 1 to 2 for men	☐	☐

Source: Trichopoulou, A. et al. (2003). Adherence to a Mediterranean diet and survival in a Greek population. *New England Journal of Medicine,* 348, 2599–2608.

HEALTHY VEGETARIAN EATING PATTERN

Vegetarian eating patterns can range from a casual vegetarian who infrequently eats meat to a vegan who consumes no animal products. Vegetarians tend to consume fewer overall calories and calories from fat and more fiber, potassium, and vitamin C than nonvegetarians. Research suggests that vegetarian eating patterns contribute to improved health outcomes, including reduced rates of obesity, cardiovascular disease, hypertension, and mortality. The *Dietary Guidelines* endorse the Healthy Vegetarian Eating Pattern as a healthful alternative to the Healthy U.S-Style Eating Pattern. This pattern can be vegan if all dairy choices are replaced with fortified soy beverages (e.g., soy milk) or other plant-based dairy substitutes.

COMMON FEATURES OF HEALTHY EATING PATTERNS

While healthy eating patterns can exist in many different forms, they tend to share some common features, including the following:

▸ High in vegetables and fruits

▸ High in whole grains

▸ Moderate amounts of foods high in protein, including seafood, beans and peas, nuts, seeds, soy products, meat, poultry, and eggs

> ‣ Small amounts of added sugars

> ‣ More oils, especially olive, canola, and coconut oils, than solid fats

> ‣ Low in full-fat (whole) milk and milk products (though some include high amounts of low-fat and fat-free milk and milk products)

Unfortunately, many potential barriers may impede an older adult's ability to achieve dietary goals. Table 4-5 highlights several of these barriers and offers tips an exercise professional may provide to help clients overcome them.

TABLE 4-5
Barriers and Strategies for Achieving Healthy Dietary Goals

Barrier	Strategy
Food insecurity (disruption of food intake because of a lack of money or other resources)	‣ Stay informed: Find out about benefit programs in your area to help pay for food and other expenses at www.benefitscheckup.org ‣ Utilize grocery store reward programs ‣ Find and use coupons for foods you enjoy ‣ Transfer prescriptions to grocery stores that offer a discount ‣ Shop on days when grocery stores offer a discount for older adults ‣ Join or start a community garden ‣ Shop for discounted items marked down for quick sale ‣ Make a shopping list and meal plan ‣ Research options for free and reduced-cost food and meals in your area ‣ Sign up for a group meal program such as Meals on Wheels America ‣ Do not overlook store brand food items
Mobility issues, lack of transportation, and proximity of food	‣ Sign up for home-delivered food and meals (check to see if this is included with your insurance) ‣ Recruit a family member or friend to take you to the grocery store or shop for you ‣ Carpool with neighbors ‣ Sign up for the LyftUp grocery access program (www.lyft.com)
Cannot cook	‣ Sign up for an in-home cooking service ‣ Take a cooking class ‣ Purchase premade meals when shopping or have them delivered to your home ‣ Invite a friend or family member over to cook together ‣ Research simple recipes that you feel comfortable attempting
Difficulty eating and loss of appetite	‣ Talk to your doctor about the impact of medications on appetite (e.g., lack of saliva, nausea or reduced sense of smell and taste) ‣ Eat with others to increase pleasure ‣ Talk to your doctor about your decreased appetite, which could be caused by depression or other health conditions ‣ Use spices, herbs, and sauces to enhance flavor ‣ Improve ambience ‣ Use chopped, ground, or pureed foods to ease chewing and avoid sticky, hard, and tough to chew foods

Reading a Nutrition Label

For those older adults who are living independently and who select and purchase their own foods, another important skill to learn is how to read nutrition labels to make healthier choices. This can prove to be exceedingly difficult for even the most sophisticated younger and older adults alike.

It is one thing to understand in theory what foods are healthier than others, but it is quite another for many older adults to identify and choose the healthier items when purchasing foods. One important skill to teach clients who shop for themselves is how to use a nutrition label to help make healthier choices (Figure 4-2). An exercise professional can help clients dissect the food label by taking a stepwise approach.

▸ Start from the top with the number of servings per container and serving size. In general, serving sizes are not a recommendation of how much to eat but are standardized so that consumers can compare similar products. All of the nutrient amounts listed on the food label are for one serving, so it is important to determine how many servings are actually being consumed to accurately assess nutrient intake.

▸ Next, consumers should look at the total calories per serving. The calories indicate how much energy a person gets from a single serving of a particular food. To determine the total calories for the entire food, simply multiply the number of calories per serving by the number of servings per container. Americans tend to consume too many calories, and too many calories from fat, without meeting daily nutrient requirements. This part of the nutrition label is the most important factor for weight control. In general, 40 calories per serving is considered low, 100 calories is moderate, and 400 or more calories is considered high.

▸ The next two sections of the label note the nutrient content of the food product. Consumers should try to minimize intake of fat (especially saturated and trans fat), sugars, and sodium—and aim to consume adequate amounts of fiber, vitamins, and minerals, especially vitamin A, vitamin C, calcium, and iron. The food label includes the total amount of sugars and specifies the amount of added sugars.

The **percent daily value (PDV)** is listed for key nutrients to make it easier to compare products (just make sure that the serving sizes are similar), evaluate nutrient content claims (does 1/3 reduced sugar cereal really contain less carbohydrate than a similar cereal of a different brand?), observe contributions to total daily diet, and make informed dietary trade-offs (e.g., balance consumption of a high-fat product for lunch with lower-fat products throughout the rest of the day). In general, 5% daily value or less is considered low, while 20% daily value or more is considered high.

▸ The footnote at the bottom of the label reminds consumers that all PDVs are based on a 2,000-calorie diet. Individuals who need more or fewer calories should adjust recommendations accordingly. For example, 3 grams of fat provides 4% of the recommended amount for someone on a 2,000-calorie diet, but 5% for someone on a 1,500-calorie diet.

▸ Carefully review the ingredients list. Note that the ingredients list is in decreasing order of substance weight in the product. That is, the ingredients that are listed first are the most abundant ingredients in the product. The ingredient list is useful to help identify whether or not the product contains trans fat, solid fats, added sugars, whole grains, and refined grains.

FIGURE 4-2

Nutrition facts label

① Serving Size

The label presents serving sizes as the amount that most people actually consume in a sitting. This is not necessarily the same as how much one should eat per serving. All of the nutrition information on the label is based on one serving. If you eat twice the serving size shown here, multiply the nutrient and calorie values by two.

② Calories

The number of calories listed represents the total calories from fat, carbohydrate, and protein (manufacturers are allowed to round this value to the nearest 5- or 10-calorie increment). 100 calories per serving is considered moderate, while 400 calories or more per serving is considered high. A 5'4", 138-lb active woman needs about 2,200 calories each day. A 5'10", 174-lb active man needs about 2,900 calories.

③ Total Fat

Fat is calorie-dense and, if consumed in large portions, can increase the risk of weight problems. While once vilified, most fat, in and of itself, is not bad. Adults should consume 20 to 35% of total calories from fat.

④ Saturated Fat

Saturated fat is part of the total fat in food. It is listed separately because it plays an important role in raising blood cholesterol and your risk of heart disease. Eat less than 10% of total calories from saturated fat.

⑤ Trans Fat

Trans fat works a lot like saturated fat, except it is worse. This fat starts out as a liquid unsaturated fat, but then food manufacturers add some hydrogen to it, turning it into a solid saturated fat (that is what "partially hydrogenated" means when you see it in the food ingredients). They do this to increase the shelf-life of the product, but in the body the trans fat damages the blood vessels and contributes to increasing blood cholesterol and the risk of heart disease. Individuals should consume as little trans fat as possible.

⑥ Cholesterol

Many foods that are high in cholesterol are also high in saturated fat, which can contribute to heart disease. Dietary cholesterol itself likely does not cause health problems.

Nutrition Facts

8 Servings Per Container

Serving Size   2/3 cup (55g)

Amount Per Serving

Calories   230

% Daily Value*

Total Fat 8g	**10%**
Saturated Fat 1g	**5%**
Trans Fat 0g	**0%**
Cholesterol 0mg	**0%**
Sodium 160mg	**7%**
Total Carbohydrate 37g	**13%**
Dietary Fiber 4g	**14%**
Total Sugars 12g	
Includes 10g Added Sugars	**20%**
Protein 3g	
Vitamin D 2mcg	10%
Calcium 260mg	20%
Iron 8mg	45%
Potassium 235mg	6%

* The % Daily Value (DV) tells you how much a nutrient in a serving of food contributes to a daily diet. 2,000 calories a day is used for general nutrition advice.

Daily Value

Daily Values are listed based on a 2,000-calorie daily eating plan. Your calorie and nutrient needs may be a little bit more or less based on your age, sex, and activity level (see https://fnic.nal.usda.gov/fnic/interactiveDRI/). For saturated fat, trans fat, sodium, and added sugars, choose foods with a low % (5% or less) Daily Value. For dietary fiber, vitamins, and minerals, your Daily Value goal is to reach 100% of each.

Ingredients: *This portion of the label lists all of the foods and additives contained in a product, in descending order by weight.*

Allergens: *This portion of the label identifies which of the most common allergens may be present in the product.*

(More nutrients may be listed on some labels)

mcg = micrograms (1,000 mcg = 1 mg)
mg = milligrams (1,000 mg = 1 g)
g = grams (about 28 g = 1 ounce)

⑦ Sodium

You call it "salt," the label calls it "sodium." Either way, it may add up to high blood pressure in some people. So, keep your sodium intake low—less than 2,300 mg each day.

⑧ Total Carbohydrate

Carbohydrates are in foods like bread, potatoes, fruits, and vegetables, as well as processed foods. Carbohydrate is further broken down into dietary fiber and sugars. Consume foods high in fiber often and those high in sugars, especially added sugars, less often. Adults should consume 45 to 65% of total calories from carbohydrates.

⑨ Dietary Fiber

There are two kinds of dietary fiber: soluble and insoluble. Fruits, vegetables, whole-grain foods, beans, and peas are all good sources and can help reduce the risk of heart disease and cancer. Individuals should try to eat 14 grams of dietary fiber for every 1,000 calories consumed.

⑩ Sugars

Too much sugar contributes to weight gain and increased risk of diseases like diabetes and fatty liver disease. Foods like fruits and dairy products contain natural sugars (fructose and lactose), but also may contain added sugars. It is recommended to consume no more than 10% of total calories from added sugar, or a total of 50 g per day based on a 2,000-calorie eating plan.

⑪ Protein

To limit saturated fat, eat small servings of lean meat, fish, and poultry. Use skim or low-fat milk, yogurt, and cheese. Try vegetable proteins like beans, grains, and cereals. Adults should consume 10 to 35% of total calories from protein.

⑫ Vitamins and Minerals

Your goal here is 100% of each for the day. Don't count on one food to do it all. Let a combination of foods add up to a winning score.

- *Trans fat:* Although trans fat is included in the "fat" section of the nutrition label, if the product contains <0.5 g per serving, the manufacturer does not need to claim it. However, if a product contains "partially hydrogenated oils," then the product contains trans fat.

- *Solid fats:* If the ingredient list contains beef fat, butter, chicken fat, coconut oil, cream, hydrogenated oils, palm kernel oils, pork fat (lard), shortening, or stick margarine, then the product contains solid fats.

- *Added sugars:* Ingredients signifying added sugars include anhydrous dextrose, brown sugar, confectioner's powdered sugar, corn syrup, corn syrup solids, dextrin, fructose, high-fructose corn syrup, honey, invert sugar, lactose, malt syrup, maltose, maple syrup, molasses, nectar, pancake syrup, raw sugar, sucrose, sugar, white granulated sugar, cane juice, evaporated corn sweetener, fruit juice concentrate, crystal dextrose, glucose, liquid fructose, sugar cane juice, and fruit nectar. In many cases, products contain multiple forms of sugar.

- *Whole grains:* If whole grains are the primary food listed, then the product is considered 100% whole grain. The whole grain should be the first or second ingredient. Examples of whole grains include brown rice, buckwheat, bulgur (cracked wheat), millet, oatmeal, popcorn, quinoa, rolled oats, whole-grain sorghum, whole-grain triticale, whole-grain barley, whole-grain corn, whole oats/oatmeal, whole rye, whole wheat, and wild rice.

- *Refined grains:* Refined grains should be "enriched." Enrichment is the process of adding nutrients back to a food that were removed during processing. If the first ingredient is an enriched grain, then the product is *not* a whole grain. This is one way to be sure whether a "wheat bread" is actually whole wheat or a refined product.

▸ Legislation also requires food manufacturers to list all potential food **allergens** on food packaging. The most common food allergens are fish, shellfish, soybean, wheat, egg, milk, peanuts, and tree nuts. This information usually is included near the list of ingredients on the package. Clearly, this information is especially important to clients with food allergies. For clients who follow a gluten-free diet, this is also an easy way to identify if wheat is a product ingredient.

While the food label is found on the side or the back of products, other health and nutrition claims are often visibly displayed on the front of the package. Though the Food and Drug Administration (FDA) regulates these claims, they frequently are a source of confusion. Consumers should be skeptical of front-of-package claims and evaluate them on a case-by-case basis. A loophole allowing "qualified health claims" has paved the way for manufacturers to claim unproven benefits to products, as long as the label states the claim is supported by very little scientific evidence.

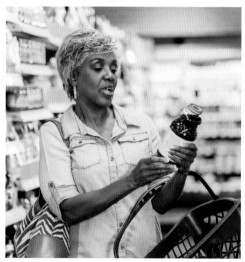

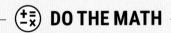 **DO THE MATH**

Nutrition Label Sample Problem

Using the nutrition label from Figure 4-2, determine (1) the number of calories per container; (2) the calories from carbohydrate, protein, and fat per serving; and (3) the percentage of calories from carbohydrate, protein, and fat.

1. 230 calories per serving x 8 servings per container = 1,840 calories per container

2. *Carbohydrate:* 37 grams carbohydrate per serving x 4 calories per gram = 148 calories per serving from carbohydrate

   Protein: 3 grams protein per serving x 4 calories per gram = 12 calories per serving from protein

   Fat: 8 grams fat per serving x 9 calories per gram = 72 calories per serving from fat

   Note that the label rounds the 232 calories calculated in question 2 to 230 calories.

3. *Carbohydrate:* 148 calories from carbohydrate/230 calories = 64% carbohydrate

   Protein: 12 calories from protein/230 calories = 5% protein

   Fat: 72 calories from fat/230 calories = 31% fat

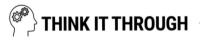 **THINK IT THROUGH**

Delivering Nutrition Education

While each client is unique in their needs and goals, providing sound nutrition education is typically part of helping a client reach health- and fitness-related goals. How much time will you devote during your sessions to nutrition? What resources will you use to provide clients with the best information for their needs? Will you develop handouts with nutrition facts or will you provide nutrition-related website addresses? Think about how you can consistently deliver this content to your clientele so that it becomes a built-in part of the services you offer.

SUMMARY

Ultimately, an exercise professional who helps an older adult improve nutritional intake must take many factors into consideration when providing information and making recommendations. Pertinent educational information and patience, coupled with skills in building rapport and collaborating to build self-efficacy, are essential skills for exercise professionals. To best meet the needs of older adults, the exercise professional should function as part of a multidisciplinary team of professionals including, at the very least, a physician and ideally a registered dietitian with expertise in working with older adults.

REFERENCES

Academy of Nutrition and Dietetics and Society for Nutrition Education and Behavior (2019). Position of the Academy of Nutrition and Dietetics and Society for Nutrition Education and Behavior: Food and nutrition program for community-residing older adults. *Journal of Academy of Nutrition and Dietetics*, 119, 7, 1188–1204.

Administration for Community Living (2019). *2018 Profiles of Older Americans.* https://acl.gov/sites/default/files/Aging%20and%20Disability%20in%20America/2018OlderAmericansProfile.pdf

Anderson, A.L. et al. (2011). Dietary patterns and survival of older adults. *Journal of the American Dietetic Association*, 111, 1, 840–891.

Batsis, J.A. & Villareal, D.T. (2018). Sarcopenic obesity in older adults: Aetiology, epidemiology and treatment strategies. *Nature Reviews Endocrinology*, 14, 9, 513–537.

Baugreet, S. et al. (2017). Mitigating nutrition and health deficiencies in older adults: A role for food innovation? *Journal of Food Science*, 82, 4, 848–855.

Baum, J.I., Kim, I-Y., Wolfe, R.R. (2016). Protein consumption and the elderly: What is the optimal level of intake? *Nutrients*, 8, 6, 359.

Bernstein, M. & Munoz, N. (2012). Position of the Academy of Nutrition and Dietetics: Food and nutrition for older adults: Promoting health and wellness. *Journal of the Academy of Nutrition and Dietetics*, 112, 8, 1255–1277.

Bowman, S. (2007). Low economic status is associated with suboptimal intakes of nutritious foods by adults in National Health and Nutrition Examination Survey 1999–2002. *Nutrition Research*, 27, 515–523.

Centers for Disease Control and Prevention (2019). *Oral Health for Older Americans.* https://www.cdc.gov/oralhealth/basics/adult-oral-health/adult_older.htm

Centers for Disease Control and Prevention (2018). *CDC Estimates of Foodborne Illness in the United States.* www.cdc.gov/foodborneburden/2011-foodborne-estimates.html

Congressional Research Service (2019). *Poverty among Americans Aged 65 and Older.* https://fas.org/sgp/crs/misc/R45791.pdf

Correia, C. et al. (2016). Global sensory impairment among older adults in the United States. *Journal of the American Geriatrics Society*, 64, 2, 306–313.

Cox, N.J. et al. (2019). Assessment and treatment of the anorexia of aging: A systematic review. *Nutrients*, 11, 1, 144.

Food and Nutrition Board (2005). *Dietary Reference Intakes for Energy, Carbohydrate, Fiber, Fat, Fatty Acids, Cholesterol, Protein, and Amino Acids.* Washington, D.C.: Institute of Medicine.

Franzke, B. et al. (2018). Dietary protein, muscle and physical function in the very old. *Nutrients*, 10, 7, 935.

Goode, S.C., Wright, T.F., & Lynch, C. (2020). Osteoporosis screening and treatment: A collaborative approach. *The Journal for Nurse Practitioners*, 16, 60–63.

Govindaraju, T. et al. (2018). Dietary patterns and quality of life in older adults: A systematic review. *Nutrients*, 10, 8, 971.

Institute of Medicine (2010). *Dietary Reference Intakes for Calcium and Vitamin D.* Washington, D.C.: The National Academies Press.

Institute of Medicine (2006). *Dietary Reference Intakes: The Essential Guide to Nutrient Requirements.* Washington, D.C.: The National Academies Press.

Jih, J. et al. (2018). Chronic disease burden predicts food insecurity among older adults. *Public Health Nutrition*, 21, 9, 1737–1742.

Jimoh, O.F. et al. (2019). Beverage intake and drinking patterns—Clues to support older people living in long-term care to drink well: DRIE and FISE studies. *Nutrients*, 11, 2, 447.

Jindai, K. et al. (2016). Multimorbidity and functional limitations among adults 65 or older, NHANES 2005–2012. *Preventing Chronic Disease*, 13, E151.

Kossioni, A.E. (2018). The association of poor oral health parameters with malnutrition in older adults: A review considering the potential implications for cognitive impairment. *Nutrients*, 10, 1709.

Leslie, W. & Hankey, C. (2015). Aging, nutritional status and health. *Healthcare*, 3, 3, 648–658.

Little, M.O. (2018). Updates in nutrition and polypharmacy. *Current Opinion in Clinical Nutrition and Metabolic Care*, 21, 4–9.

Malenfant, J.H. & Batsis, J.A. (2019). Obesity in the geriatric population: A global health perspective. *Journal of Global Health Reports*, 3, e2019045.

Martínez-González, M.A., Gea, A., & Ruiz-Canela, M. (2019). The Mediterranean diet and cardiovascular health: A critical review. *Circulation Research*, 124, 5, 779–798.

McMillan, L.B. et al. (2017). Prescribing activity for the prevention and treatment of osteoporosis in older adults. *Healthcare*, 5, 4, 85.

Mendez, M.A. & Newman, A.B. (2018). Can a Mediterranean diet pattern slow aging? *The Journal of Gerontology*, 73, 3, 315–317.

Mithal, A. et al. (2012). Impact of nutrition on muscle mass, strength, and performance in older adults. *Osteoporosis International*. DOI: 10.1007/ s00198-012-2236-y.

National Council on Aging (2018). *Fact Sheet: Healthy Aging.* https://d2mkcg26uvg1cz.cloudfront. net/wp-content/uploads/2018-Healthy-Aging-Fact-Sheet-7.10.18-1.pdf

National Institute on Aging (2015). *How Smell and Taste Change as You Age.* https://www.nia.nih.gov/ health/smell-and-taste

National Institute on Deafness and Other Communication Disorders (2019). *Quick Statistics about Taste and Smell.* https://www.nidcd.nih.gov/ health/statistics/quick-statistics-taste-smell

National Institutes of Health (2020). *Vitamin D: Fact Sheet for Health Professionals.* https://ods.od.nih.gov/ factsheets/VitaminD-HealthProfessional/

National Institutes of Health; Osteoporosis and Related Bone Diseases National Resource Center (2018). *Smoking and Bone Health.* https://www. bones.nih.gov/health-info/bone/osteoporosis/conditions-behaviors/bone-smoking

Pooler, J.A. et al. (2019). Food insecurity: A key social determinant of health for older adults. *Journal of the American Geriatrics Society*, 67, 3, 421–424.

Tosti, V., Bertozzi, B., & Fontana, L. (2018). Health benefits of the Mediterranean diet: Metabolic and Molecular Mechanisms. *The Journal of Gerontology*, 73, 3, 318–326.

Trichopoulou, A. et al. (2003). Adherence to a Mediterranean diet and survival in a Greek population. *New England Journal of Medicine*, 348, 2599–2608.

U.S. Department of Agriculture (2015). *2015–2020 Dietary Guidelines for Americans* (8th ed.). www.health.gov/dietaryguidelines

Welch, C. et al. (2018). Acute sarcopenia secondary to hospitalisation: An emerging condition affecting older adults. *Aging and Disease*, 9, 1, 151–164.

SUGGESTED READINGS

American Dietetic Association (2010). Position of the American Dietetic Association, American Society for Nutrition, and Society for Nutrition Education: Food and nutrition programs for community-residing older adults. *Journal of the American Dietetic Association*, 110, 463–472.

Eggersdorfer, M. et al. (2018). Hidden hunger: Solutions for America's aging populations. *Nutrients*, 10, 9, 1210.

U.S. Department of Agriculture (2015). *2015–2020 Dietary Guidelines for Americans* (8th ed.). www.health.gov/dietaryguidelines

CHAPTER 5

Preparticipation Health Screening and Interview

LEARNING OBJECTIVES

After reading this chapter, you will be able to:

▸ Identify characteristics of an older adult based on chronological age, biological age, and the ability to perform various levels of activities of daily living

▸ Implement a preparticipation health screening and interview that assesses an older client's readiness for exercise based on their current level of physical activity, diagnosed cardiovascular, metabolic, or renal disease and/or the presence of signs or symptoms of such disease, and the desired exercise intensity

▸ Utilize various preparticipation forms to record important client information

▸ Briefly describe the aging process and pharmacokinetics in older adults

The main purposes of fitness assessments for older adults are the same as those for all adults: to define the degree of risk associated with varying workloads and to establish appropriate intensities for an exercise program [American College of Sports Medicine (ACSM), 2018]. An exercise program should be developed and used only if it is based on sound information obtained from a reliable screening and assessment protocol. However, not all older people can or should be given assessments to determine their fitness levels, which is why conducting a pre-exercise screening is critically important.

Understanding Aging

Chapter 3 of this textbook provides information about the physiological effects of aging. Because the aging process is complex, physiology must be the first consideration when working with an older client, before proceeding with the assessment protocol. Likewise, it is imperative to ascertain both the general characteristics and the specific needs of older adults.

CHRONOLOGICAL AGE

No existing single model or paradigm clearly defines the older adult population; rather, a variety of approaches are blended according to individual differences. Because of the relationship between time and the aging process, **chronological age** is used as an initial identification. The following is an example of age categories that are commonly used in research to define the older adult population: young-old (65–74 years), middle-old (75–84 years), and oldest-old (85+ years). The oldest-old category constitutes the fastest growing segment of the U.S. population (U.S. Administration on Aging, 2018). The span of the older adult population is greater than in any other age group, and to label a person as an older adult based solely on age does not give many clues about their fitness level.

BIOLOGICAL AGE

As described in Chapter 3, scientists have theorized that **biological age** is a better construct than chronology when defining the older adult. Biological aging results from the accumulation of molecular and cellular damage over time, which leads to an increase risk of disease, gradual deterioration in physical and mental capacity, and eventually death (World Health Organization, 2018). It is common to hear someone refer to a person as "young for their age," suggesting that the person apparently has not suffered the decremental effects of biological aging that often accompany chronological age. However, simple observation of a person's appearance does not provide much more information about their **functional capacity** than chronology.

ACTIVITIES OF DAILY LIVING

Activities of daily living (ADL) are the basic tasks of everyday life and independent living, such as eating, bathing, and going to the bathroom. General measures of health status (e.g., diagnoses or medical conditions) are limited indicators of an individual's independence and functional capabilities.

ADL are classified into three levels of function as basic (BADL), instrumental or independent (IADL), and advanced (AADL). BADL include the elemental items of self-care (e.g., feeding, toileting, dressing, and bathing), IADL include tasks essential to maintaining independence (e.g., cooking, housework, handling medication and finances, doing laundry, and shopping), and AADL are functions well beyond the status necessary for living alone and tend to be specific to each individual. These include recreational, occupational, and community-service functions. ADL measurements are often used to determine whether an older adult is capable of living independently (Table 5-1). ADL can be simple or complex, depending on the lifestyle history of the individual. For example, stair climbing may or may not be considered a lifestyle activity, depending on the person's need to negotiate stairs. Ultimately, as a matter of lifestyle normalcy, it would be beneficial to train individuals to climb stairs. However, in terms of

TABLE 5-1

Hierarchy of Physical Function

Level of Function	Description
Physically elite	Engage in high-risk and power sports (e.g., hang gliding and weightlifting), including sports competition and the Senior Olympics
Physically fit	Engage in regular physical activity such as cardiovascular, resistance, and flexibility training
Physically independent	Can perform some AADL and all IADL, but are generally quite sedentary
	May engage in sedentary hobbies such as handcrafts, cards, and reading
	Borderline frail and are close to losing the ability to function independently
Physically frail	Can perform all BADL and some IADL
	Cannot perform household activities such as preparing meals, shopping, or housekeeping
	If still living at home, typically require outside services such as home nursing care
Physically dependent	Cannot perform BADL and are dependent upon others for daily functioning
	Require institutionalized care or full-time care at home

Note: AADL = Advanced activities of daily living; IADL = Independent activities of daily living; BADL = Basic activities of daily living

assessment, determining the person's immediate needs and abilities is the primary objective. Measurement of the ADL is an informative strategy for answering the question, "What can the older adult actually do?"

Pre-exercise Interview

The pre-exercise interview provides an opportunity for rapport building and gathering pertinent information to be used in determining if initial assessments are needed and conceptualizing exercise program design when working with older adults. For every individual who desires to begin an exercise program, there is a myriad of potential roadblocks that must first be identified and discussed. The very reason to conduct an initial interview and determine if assessments are needed is to establish a rationale for developing an effective and personalized training program that supports client goal attainment. What is learned from the interview and the results from any assessments should directly transfer to the sets, repetitions, duration, frequency, intensity, and load of each exercise recommended and honor client goals.

Begin the pre-exercise interview by addressing the client's present level of daily activity. Use questions of frequency, duration, and perceived intensity to identify ADL and the extent to which they are carried out. One person's ceiling may be another person's floor, but everyone is at some level of activity. Discover each individual's true level before proceeding with further investigation.

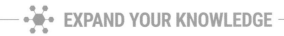

EXPAND YOUR KNOWLEDGE

Asking the Right Pre-exercise Interview Questions

Finding out as much information as possible about each client's lifestyle, habits, and physical-activity history will facilitate the program-design process. Begin with a simple statement that can open a treasure chest of information about the individual's ADL, and then ask for specifics:

▶ Tell me about a typical week in your life.

▶ Are you still working or are you retired? If you're working, is any part of your work physical?

▶ Do you consistently face stairs, lifting, or walking? If so, are any of these tasks difficult for you?

▶ Do you participate in consistent business activities, such as travel or entertaining, that extend the hours of your workday or week?

▶ How do you spend your time away from work?

▶ Do you participate in any regular physical activity, recreational travel, or physical play?

▶ Who maintains the upkeep of the home, both inside and out? What is the extent of the upkeep?

▶ Do you experience any pain during movement?

If the person is retired, ask what their occupation was. Depending on the answer, the same line of questioning detailed above may be appropriate. Based on how long ago the individual was employed, they may maintain a certain level of fitness due to on-the-job physical demands. The opposite also is true regarding the potential for deconditioning if the individual spent most of their time sitting at a desk. Ask if the retirement was by choice or disability. Further questioning after an answer of "disability" may lead to relevant information specific to the physical assessment:

▶ Have you ever fallen? If so, what were the circumstances?

▶ Have you had any other injuries?

▶ Did you ever undergo rehabilitation?

Health coaches and exercise professionals must decipher clues about the client's lifestyle to determine ability and conditioning, whether it is associated with work, social activities, or recreational activities. For example, if a person reports that the extent of their housecleaning is vacuuming and dusting, this suggests a particular level of ability. If another client reports that their housecleaning involves more ambitious chores, such as mopping floors, cleaning tubs and tile, and washing the windows both inside and out, it is reasonable to assume a higher level of ability. An exercise professional can assume that a person who can maneuver up and down from the floor to mop or clean a tub is likely to have conditioned leg muscles and **connective tissue.** From a strength standpoint, they also are likely to have greater strength during the **eccentric** phase of a movement and may be less likely to fall.

Seeking information about recreational activity can be helpful because it transfers directly to the activities of the physical assessment. Try these questions:

▶ When was the last time you went for a walk? Was it a brisk walk or a stroll?

▶ How often do you walk? How far and for how long do you typically walk?

▶ Do you ever experience pain while walking? If so, where and how long has it been occurring? How long does it take for the pain to subside?

In addition to the pre-exercise screening forms and evaluations, the answers to these questions can provide valuable information for individualizing an older client's physical-activity program. In this section, note the interplay between the use of closed questions (requiring a simple "yes," "no," or another single-word answer) and open-ended questions (inviting the client to talk in detail about a topic). When asking questions, consider what you are wanting to achieve. If you are wanting to find out more about a client's overall lifestyle, open-ended questioning encouraging thought and discussion would be best. However, if the reason for your question is to find out about a specific health condition, more direct, closed questioning may be more helpful for gathering the information you need. Here is an example to reinforce this point when the presence of a cardiovascular, metabolic, or renal disease needs to be determined:

Scenario 1: Use of Open-ended Questioning

Exercise Professional: How has your health changed over the years and what makes you think you may have a health condition?

Client: Well, over the years I have become less physically active and it sometimes feels harder to do things that once felt easy. I notice that it takes me longer to recover from activities and that I have to be more mindful of planning activities to make sure I have the energy to do physical things on multiple days. For example, if I know I am going to spend the day at the local zoo with my family, it will probably mean that I will not feel up to walking much the next day. Over the years, I have gradually started to eat less and have less of an appetite, but I do make sure to drink plenty of water.

In this first example, there is much to be learned about the client's lifestyle, social support, possible signs and symptoms, and maybe even motivation, but we still don't know if the client has a cardiovascular, metabolic, or renal disease.

Scenario 2: Use of Direct, Closed Questioning

Exercise Professional: Have you ever been diagnosed as having a cardiovascular, metabolic, or renal disease?

Client: Yes.

In this example, the exercise professional is looking for a "yes" or "no" answer and the client provided an appropriate response. However, this closed question did not open the door for more communication and thought-provoking discussion.

During the initial interview and in all client-centered interactions, the use of both closed and open-ended questioning may be appropriate and some efficient combination of the two allows exercise professionals to gather both direct information when needed, as well as insights into client's values, perspectives, and goals. Used together, important information is gathered for facilitating a safe and effective exercise program.

Preparticipation Health Screening

The preparticipation health screening is the best way to continue gathering information about an older adult's individual needs. A self-reported medical history and an interview enable the exercise professional to discern the most appropriate exercise-testing protocol. As described in the previous section, the interview process often is the most comfortable way to begin gathering information and establishing a relationship. A seemingly casual conversation can reveal philosophical and attitudinal biases about exercise. Using a variety of evaluation forms can help guide the information-gathering process. In addition, the initial interview is an appropriate time to have the client sign any required documentation prior to the initial session.

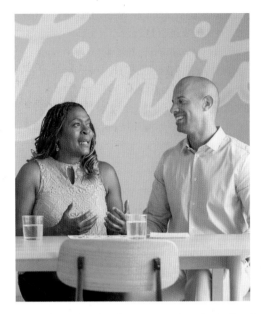

The ACSM preparticipation guidelines are designed to remove any unnecessary barriers to becoming more physically active (ACSM, 2018). Risk-factor profiling or classification is not part of the exercise preparticipation health-screening process because supporting evidence is lacking for the presence of risk factors without underlying disease increasing the risk for activity-related cardiovascular events, and screening must not become a barrier to participation. Further, the guidelines note that when an individual becomes more physically active, their risks decline. The health-screening process is based on three factors that have been identified as important risk modulators of exercise-related cardiovascular events:

▸ The individual's current level of physical activity

▸ Diagnosed cardiovascular, metabolic, or renal disease and/or the presence of signs or symptoms of cardiovascular, metabolic, or renal disease

▸ The desired exercise intensity

This screening protocol makes general recommendations for medical clearance, leaving the specifics—such as the need for medical exams or exercise tests—up to the discretion of the healthcare provider.

The goal of this process is to identify individuals:

▸ Who should receive medical clearance before initiating an exercise program or increasing the frequency, intensity, and/or volume of their current program

▸ With clinically significant disease(s) who may benefit from participating in a medically supervised exercise program

▸ With medical conditions that may require exclusion from exercise programs until those conditions are resolved or better controlled

Figure 5-1 presents the preparticipation health-screening algorithm, while an exercise preparticipation checklist is presented in Figure 5-2. This algorithm shows that medical clearance is advised only under the following circumstances, with regular exercise defined as performing planned, structured physical activity for at least 30 minutes at moderate intensity on at least three days/week for at least the past three months:

▸ **For those who do not exercise regularly:** If a client has cardiovascular, metabolic, or renal disease, or signs or symptoms that suggest they do, then medical clearance is recommended.

▸ **For regular exercisers:** If a client has signs or symptoms suggestive of cardiovascular, metabolic, or renal disease, they should discontinue exercise and seek medical clearance. If a client has a known history of cardiovascular, metabolic, or renal disease and has a desire to progress to vigorous-intensity aerobic exercise, medical clearance is recommended.

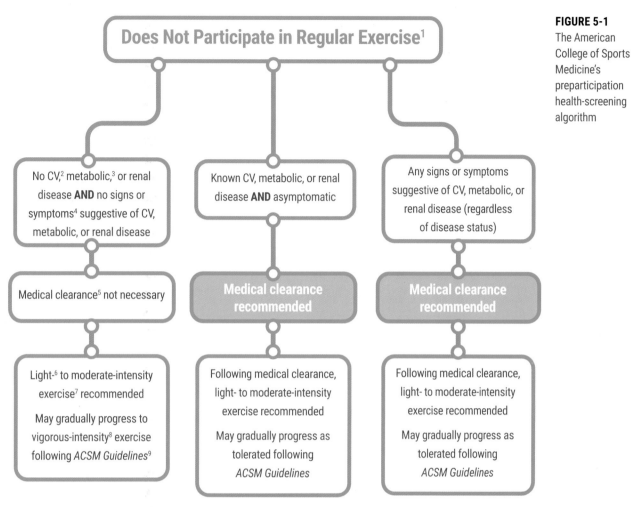

FIGURE 5-1

The American College of Sports Medicine's prepartipation health-screening algorithm

[1] **Exercise participation** Performing planned, structured physical activity for at least 30 minutes at moderate intensity on at least 3 days/week for at least the past 3 months

[2] **Cardiovascular disease** Cardiac, peripheral vascular, or cerebrovascular disease

[3] **Metabolic disease** Type 1 and 2 diabetes mellitus

[4] **Sign and symptoms** At rest or during activity. Includes pain, discomfort in the chest, neck, jaw, arms, or other areas that may result from ischemia; shortness of breath at rest or with mild exertion; dizziness or syncope; orthopnea or paroxysmal nocturnal dyspnea; ankle edema; palpitations or tachycardia; intermittent claudication; known heart murmur; unusual fatigue or shortness of breath with usual activities

[5] **Medical clearance** Approval from a healthcare professional to engage in exercise

[6] **Light-intensity exercise** 30–39% HRR or $\dot{V}O_2R$, 2–2.9 METs, RPE 9–11, an intensity that causes slight increases in HR and breathing

[7] **Moderate-intensity exercise** 40–59% HRR or $\dot{V}O_2R$, 3–5.9 METs, RPE 12–13, an intensity that causes noticeable increases in HR and breathing

[8] **Vigorous-intensity exercise** ≥60% HRR or $\dot{V}O_2R$, ≥6 METs, RPE ≥14, an intensity that causes substantial increases in HR and breathing

[9] **ACSM Guidelines** *ACSM's Guidelines for Exercise Testing and Prescription,* 10th edition

Note: CV = Cardiovascular; HRR = Heart-rate reserve; $\dot{V}O_2R$ = Oxygen uptake reserve; METs = Metabolic equivalents; RPE = Rating of perceived exertion; HR = Heart rate; ACSM = American College of Sports Medicine

Reprinted with permission from American College of Sports Medicine (2018). *ACSM's Guidelines for Exercise Testing and Prescription* (10th ed.). Philadelphia: Wolters Kluwer.

Continued on the next page

FIGURE 5-1
(continued)

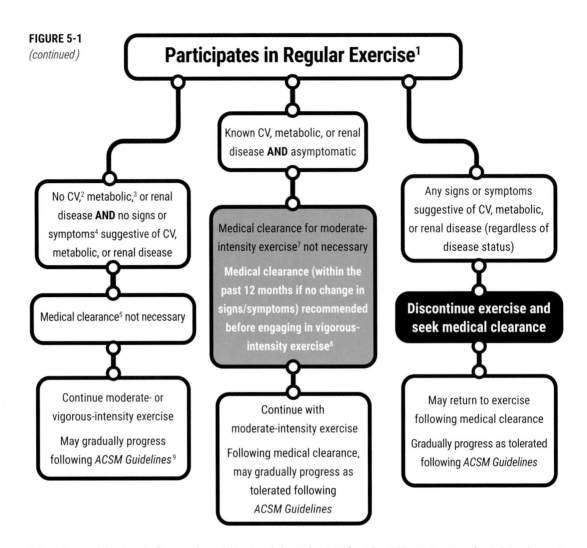

¹ **Exercise participation**   Performing planned, structured physical activity for at least 30 minutes at moderate intensity on at least 3 days/week for at least the past 3 months

² **Cardiovascular disease**   Cardiac, peripheral vascular, or cerebrovascular disease

³ **Metabolic disease**   Type 1 and 2 diabetes mellitus

⁴ **Sign and symptoms**   At rest or during activity. Includes pain, discomfort in the chest, neck, jaw, arms, or other areas that may result from ischemia; shortness of breath at rest or with mild exertion; dizziness or syncope; orthopnea or paroxysmal nocturnal dyspnea; ankle edema; palpitations or tachycardia; intermittent claudication; known heart murmur; unusual fatigue or shortness of breath with usual activities

⁵ **Medical clearance**   Approval from a healthcare professional to engage in exercise

⁶ **Light-intensity exercise**   30–39% HRR or $\dot{V}O_2R$, 2–2.9 METs, RPE 9–11, an intensity that causes slight increases in HR and breathing

⁷ **Moderate-intensity exercise**   40–59% HRR or $\dot{V}O_2R$, 3–5.9 METs, RPE 12–13, an intensity that causes noticeable increases in HR and breathing

⁸ **Vigorous-intensity exercise**   ≥60% HRR or $\dot{V}O_2R$, ≥6 METs, RPE ≥14, an intensity that causes substantial increases in HR and breathing

⁹ **ACSM Guidelines**   *ACSM's Guidelines for Exercise Testing and Prescription,* 10th edition

Note: CV = Cardiovascular; HRR = Heart-rate reserve; $\dot{V}O_2R$ = Oxygen uptake reserve; METs = Metabolic equivalents; RPE = Rating of perceived exertion; HR = Heart rate; ACSM = American College of Sports Medicine

Reprinted with permission from American College of Sports Medicine (2018). *ACSM's Guidelines for Exercise Testing and Prescription* (10th ed.). Philadelphia: Wolters Kluwer.

FIGURE 5-2
Exercise preparticipation health-screening questionnaire for exercise professionals

EXERCISE PREPARTICIPATION HEALTH-SCREENING QUESTIONNAIRE FOR EXERCISE PROFESSIONALS

Assess your client's health needs by marking all *true* statements.

Step 1

SYMPTOMS

Does your client experience:

☐ chest discomfort with exertion

☐ unreasonable breathlessness

☐ dizziness, fainting, blackouts

☐ ankle swelling

☐ unpleasant awareness of a forceful, rapid, or irregular heart rate

☐ burning or cramping sensations in your lower legs when walking short distances

If you **did** mark any of these statements under the symptoms, **STOP,** your client should seek medical clearance before engaging in or resuming exercise. Your client may need to use a facility with a **medically qualified staff**.

If you **did not** mark any symptoms, continue to steps 2 and 3.

Step 2

CURRENT ACTIVITY

Has your client performed planned, structured physical activity for at least 30 minutes at moderate intensity on at least 3 days per week for at least the past 3 months?

Yes ☐ No ☐

Continue to Step 3.

Step 3

MEDICAL CONDITIONS

Has your client had or does he or she currently have:

☐ a heart attack

☐ heart surgery, cardiac catheterization, or coronary angioplasty

☐ pacemaker/implantable cardiac defibrillator/rhythm disturbance

☐ heart valve disease

☐ heart failure

☐ heart transplantation

☐ congenital heart disease

☐ diabetes

☐ renal disease

Evaluating Steps 2 and 3:

• If you **did not mark any of the statements in Step 3,** medical clearance is not necessary.

• If you marked Step 2 **"yes"** and **marked any of the statements in Step 3,** your client may continue to exercise at light to moderate intensity without medical clearance. Medical clearance is recommended before engaging in vigorous exercise.

• If you marked Step 2 **"no"** and **marked any of the statements in Step 3,** medical clearance is recommended. Your client may need to use a facility with a **medically qualified staff.**

Reprinted with permission from American College of Sports Medicine (2018). *ACSM's Guidelines for Exercise Testing and Prescription* (10th ed.). Philadelphia: Wolters Kluwer.

While the identification of the signs and symptoms referenced in this algorithm may be within the scope of practice of most health coaches and exercise professionals, interpretation of those same signs and symptoms should be made only by qualified healthcare professionals within the context in which they appear (ACSM, 2018):

▸ Pain; discomfort (or other **angina** equivalent) in the chest, neck, jaw, arms, or other areas that may result from **myocardial ischemia**

▸ Shortness of breath or **dyspnea** at rest or with mild exertion

▸ **Orthopnea** (dyspnea in a reclined position) or **paroxysmal nocturnal dyspnea** (onset is usually two to five hours after the beginning of sleep)

▸ Dizziness, or **syncope,** most commonly caused by reduced perfusion to the brain

▸ Ankle **edema**

▸ **Palpitations** or **tachycardia**

▸ **Intermittent claudication** (pain sensations or cramping in the lower extremities during exercise that is associated with inadequate blood supply)

▸ Known heart murmur

▸ Unusual fatigue or shortness of breath with usual activities

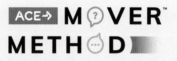

The Excited New Client in Need of Medical Clearance

During an initial meeting with your new client, Nathaniel, he lets you know that he is excited to begin a structured exercise program and that he has been looking forward to working with an exercise professional.

ACE→ ABC APPROACH

The following is an example of how using the ACE ABC Approach™ to coaching can facilitate the preparticipation health-screening process.

Ask: Asking powerful open-ended questions will help you learn more about Nathaniel's goals and what he would like to accomplish by working with an exercise professional.

Exercise Professional: Thank you for letting me know how excited you are to get started working together. How would you describe your health and fitness journey up to this point?

Client: Well, when I was in my 20s and 30s, I used to enjoy hiking, lifting weights, and even doing martial arts. I was very consistent when I was younger but once I was in my 40s, doing these activities became sporadic at best, but it's been over a decade since I did any of those things. Over the past two months, I started walking two days per week for 10 or 15 minutes to try to manage my **diabetes.**

Exercise Professional: Managing your diabetes is important to you. How do you envision me helping to support your goals?

Client: Yes, it is imperative that I manage my diabetes. I need help figuring out a structured physical-activity program that is consistent and includes different types of activities, so I don't get bored. I want to make sure that I keep my diabetes under control by improving my diet and moving more. If I could get back to a point where I felt like being active more than two days per week, that would be great!

Break down barriers: At this point in the conversation, asking more open-ended questions could help to uncover the potential barriers that might prevent Nathaniel from participating in a structured, consistent program.

Exercise Professional: Structure, consistency, and variety are important to you, and you also want to make sure your diabetes stays under control. You mentioned earlier that you enjoyed hiking, lifting weights, and martial arts. What changed? Why do you no longer do those activities?

Client: I'm not 100% sure why I stopped. It seems like I just started slowing down and finding reasons not to exercise. Then I started gaining weight, and the more I put on, the less I felt like doing.

Exercise Professional: You lost momentum. What did you learn from that experience? Are there any specific obstacles you think might disrupt your momentum this time?

Client: That's a nice way to put it. I think the main obstacles I'll face will be my work schedule, my "non-exercise"-related habits, and the difficulty of starting something new. Even finding the time to walk for 15 minutes twice per week is sometimes challenging, but I'm pretty motivated right now to get myself moving. I try to encourage myself by remembering how good I feel after my walks.

Exercise Professional: Reminding yourself of that fantastic post-walk feeling is a great strategy. What else?

Client: I think I need a plan that makes it easy to schedule activity as part of my day. It's easy to get wrapped up in my job, so I forget to get up and move. Maybe it will help if I put activity breaks in my calendar. Having regularly scheduled sessions with you before or after work will also help me to be accountable.

Exercise Professional: Adopting a consistent and varied exercise program is exciting for you, and you've come up with some great ideas for how to overcome potential obstacles. Part of my job is to make sure I do everything possible to create safe and effective programs for you, with exercises that you enjoy, so start thinking about what types of physical activity you'd like to incorporate. In addition, it is crucial to know if you are on any medications for your diabetes or if you have discussed your plans for increasing your physical activity with your doctor.

Client: No medications at the moment. I hope if I keep walking and get my diet figured out, I won't ever have to be on them. I haven't seen my doctor in a little over a year. The last time we talked, she told me about the benefits of being more active, but I was not ready to get started at that time. I think she would like the idea of me exercising. Do I need to ask her?

Collaborate: Working together on goals is the next step now that barriers and solutions for adopting healthier behaviors have been identified. Also, because this client is not currently physically active, and he presents with diabetes, it is vital to ensure that he has received clearance from his doctor before setting or working on any exercise-related goals.

Exercise Professional: The more your doctor knows about how you are managing your diabetes, the better equipped she is to help you. By discussing your plans with your doctor before we start working together, it allows her to communicate any limitations, restrictions, or guidelines. This will help to ensure that any plan we create for you will be safe and effective and that everyone on your healthcare team is on the same page. Are you open to the idea of contacting your doctor?

Client: I am, yes. Thank you. I like the idea of us all working together. It's probably a good idea for me to connect with my doctor anyway, since I have not seen her in over a year.

Exercise Professional: I want to be clear that asking you to see your doctor before we can work together is by no means a way of saying I don't want to help you. It is just the opposite. I want to see you get the right kind of help so that I can do what I do best when we work together: give you a great physical-activity experience that is enjoyable and helps you manage your diabetes. What can you do within the next week to get started?

Client: I will contact my doctor's office this week to make them aware of my plans to increase my physical activity. I am not sure if they will clear me for exercise over the phone or want me to come in for an appointment. Either way, I will work with my doctor to make sure she supports my goals and to see if she has any recommendations. Also, I want to make sure I am ready to start working with you once my doctor signs off, so I will keep walking twice a week. This way, I'll be set to go once I hear back from my doctor!

Exercise Professional: Great! I will provide you with a medical release form that your doctor can sign to make sure we have everything we need to get started. Please let me know when you have the form filled out and we will get our first training session scheduled. I look forward to hearing back from you and I will also plan to reach out to you to see if you need any assistance so we can begin as soon as possible.

The preparticipation health-screening process is an important initial step to take with clients, as it provides an opportunity to build rapport, get to know each other, learn about past exercise experience and health history, and determine if medical clearance is needed before beginning a formal exercise program. The ACE ABC Approach can be used throughout the screening process to gather all the pertinent information in a way that feels like a conversation and not an interview.

Addressing the need for medical clearance while also supporting the client's enthusiasm and readiness to get started is important, especially in the early stages of change. Staying in contact with the client and lending support is imperative, as you do not want the requirement for medical clearance to be a barrier to becoming more physically active.

RESISTANCE TRAINING

Current evidence is insufficient regarding cardiovascular complications during low-to-moderate intensity resistance training to warrant formal prescreening recommendations (ACSM, 2018). Limited data are available on the topic, but it appears that the risk of complications is low.

SELF-GUIDED SCREENING

Preparticipation health screening for individuals wanting to initiate an exercise program may be conducted using the **Physical Activity Readiness Questionnaire for Everyone (PAR-Q+)** form (Figure 5-3). This form is evidence-based and was developed with a goal of reducing unnecessary barriers to exercise. The PAR-Q+ can be used as either a self-guided screening tool or as an additional element of screening for use by exercise professionals seeking additional client information.

This important screening document is regularly updated and revised and there are different versions depending on the clientele with whom you are working. The PAR-Q+ and ePARmed-X+ (for clients who have had a positive response to the PAR-Q+ or have been referred to use this more comprehensive form by a healthcare professional) were created to reduce barriers for all individuals to become more physically active. These forms are publicly available at www.eparmedx.com.

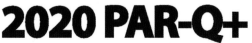

2020 PAR-Q+

The Physical Activity Readiness Questionnaire for Everyone

The health benefits of regular physical activity are clear; more people should engage in physical activity every day of the week. Participating in physical activity is very safe for MOST people. This questionnaire will tell you whether it is necessary for you to seek further advice from your doctor OR a qualified exercise professional before becoming more physically active.

GENERAL HEALTH QUESTIONS

Please read the 7 questions below carefully and answer each one honestly: check YES or NO.	YES	NO
1) Has your doctor ever said that you have a heart condition ☐ OR high blood pressure ☐?	☐	☐
2) Do you feel pain in your chest at rest, during your daily activities of living, OR when you do physical activity?	☐	☐
3) Do you lose balance because of dizziness OR have you lost consciousness in the last 12 months? Please answer NO if your dizziness was associated with over-breathing (including during vigorous exercise).	☐	☐
4) Have you ever been diagnosed with another chronic medical condition (other than heart disease or high blood pressure)? PLEASE LIST CONDITION(S) HERE: _____	☐	☐
5) Are you currently taking prescribed medications for a chronic medical condition? PLEASE LIST CONDITION(S) AND MEDICATIONS HERE: _____	☐	☐
6) Do you currently have (or have had within the past 12 months) a bone, joint, or soft tissue (muscle, ligament, or tendon) problem that could be made worse by becoming more physically active? Please answer NO if you had a problem in the past, but it does not limit your current ability to be physically active. PLEASE LIST CONDITION(S) HERE: _____	☐	☐
7) Has your doctor ever said that you should only do medically supervised physical activity?	☐	☐

☑ **If you answered NO to all of the questions above, you are cleared for physical activity.**
Please sign the PARTICIPANT DECLARATION. You do not need to complete Pages 2 and 3.

▶ Start becoming much more physically active – start slowly and build up gradually.

▶ Follow Global Physical Activity Guidelines for your age (https://apps.who.int/iris/handle/10665/44399).

▶ You may take part in a health and fitness appraisal.

▶ If you are over the age of 45 yr and NOT accustomed to regular vigorous to maximal effort exercise, consult a qualified exercise professional before engaging in this intensity of exercise.

▶ If you have any further questions, contact a qualified exercise professional.

PARTICIPANT DECLARATION
If you are less than the legal age required for consent or require the assent of a care provider, your parent, guardian or care provider must also sign this form.

I, the undersigned, have read, understood to my full satisfaction and completed this questionnaire. I acknowledge that this physical activity clearance is valid for a maximum of 12 months from the date it is completed and becomes invalid if my condition changes. I also acknowledge that the community/fitness center may retain a copy of this form for its records. In these instances, it will maintain the confidentiality of the same, complying with applicable law.

NAME _____ DATE _____

SIGNATURE _____ WITNESS _____

SIGNATURE OF PARENT/GUARDIAN/CARE PROVIDER _____

⬤ **If you answered YES to one or more of the questions above, COMPLETE PAGES 2 AND 3.**

⚠ **Delay becoming more active if:**

✓ You have a temporary illness such as a cold or fever; it is best to wait until you feel better.

✓ You are pregnant - talk to your health care practitioner, your physician, a qualified exercise professional, and/or complete the ePARmed-X+ at www.eparmedx.com before becoming more physically active.

✓ Your health changes - answer the questions on Pages 2 and 3 of this document and/or talk to your doctor or a qualified exercise professional before continuing with any physical activity program.

Copyright © 2020 PAR-Q+ Collaboration 1 / 4
01-11-2019

Continued on the next page

Continued on the next page

FIGURE 5-3
The Physical Activity Readiness Questionnaire for Everyone

FIGURE 5-3
(continued)

2020 PAR-Q+

FOLLOW-UP QUESTIONS ABOUT YOUR MEDICAL CONDITION(S)

1.	**Do you have Arthritis, Osteoporosis, or Back Problems?**	
	If the above condition(s) is/are present, answer questions 1a-1c **If NO ☐** go to question 2	
1a.	Do you have difficulty controlling your condition with medications or other physician-prescribed therapies? (Answer **NO** if you are not currently taking medications or other treatments)	YES ☐ NO ☐
1b.	Do you have joint problems causing pain, a recent fracture or fracture caused by osteoporosis or cancer, displaced vertebra (e.g., spondylolisthesis), and/or spondylolysis/pars defect (a crack in the bony ring on the back of the spinal column)?	YES ☐ NO ☐
1c.	Have you had steroid injections or taken steroid tablets regularly for more than 3 months?	YES ☐ NO ☐
2.	**Do you currently have Cancer of any kind?**	
	If the above condition(s) is/are present, answer questions 2a-2b **If NO ☐** go to question 3	
2a.	Does your cancer diagnosis include any of the following types: lung/bronchogenic, multiple myeloma (cancer of plasma cells), head, and/or neck?	YES ☐ NO ☐
2b.	Are you currently receiving cancer therapy (such as chemotheraphy or radiotherapy)?	YES ☐ NO ☐
3.	**Do you have a Heart or Cardiovascular Condition? This includes Coronary Artery Disease, Heart Failure, Diagnosed Abnormality of Heart Rhythm**	
	If the above condition(s) is/are present, answer questions 3a-3d **If NO ☐** go to question 4	
3a.	Do you have difficulty controlling your condition with medications or other physician-prescribed therapies? (Answer **NO** if you are not currently taking medications or other treatments)	YES ☐ NO ☐
3b.	Do you have an irregular heart beat that requires medical management? (e.g., atrial fibrillation, premature ventricular contraction)	YES ☐ NO ☐
3c.	Do you have chronic heart failure?	YES ☐ NO ☐
3d.	Do you have diagnosed coronary artery (cardiovascular) disease and have not participated in regular physical activity in the last 2 months?	YES ☐ NO ☐
4.	**Do you currently have High Blood Pressure?**	
	If the above condition(s) is/are present, answer questions 4a-4b **If NO ☐** go to question 5	
4a.	Do you have difficulty controlling your condition with medications or other physician-prescribed therapies? (Answer **NO** if you are not currently taking medications or other treatments)	YES ☐ NO ☐
4b.	Do you have a resting blood pressure equal to or greater than 160/90 mmHg with or without medication? (Answer **YES** if you do not know your resting blood pressure)	YES ☐ NO ☐
5.	**Do you have any Metabolic Conditions? This includes Type 1 Diabetes, Type 2 Diabetes, Pre-Diabetes**	
	If the above condition(s) is/are present, answer questions 5a-5e **If NO ☐** go to question 6	
5a.	Do you often have difficulty controlling your blood sugar levels with foods, medications, or other physician-prescribed therapies?	YES ☐ NO ☐
5b.	Do you often suffer from signs and symptoms of low blood sugar (hypoglycemia) following exercise and/or during activities of daily living? Signs of hypoglycemia may include shakiness, nervousness, unusual irritability, abnormal sweating, dizziness or light-headedness, mental confusion, difficulty speaking, weakness, or sleepiness.	YES ☐ NO ☐
5c.	Do you have any signs or symptoms of diabetes complications such as heart or vascular disease and/or complications affecting your eyes, kidneys, **OR** the sensation in your toes and feet?	YES ☐ NO ☐
5d.	Do you have other metabolic conditions (such as current pregnancy-related diabetes, chronic kidney disease, or liver problems)?	YES ☐ NO ☐
5e.	Are you planning to engage in what for you is unusually high (or vigorous) intensity exercise in the near future?	YES ☐ NO ☐

2020 PAR-Q+

FIGURE 5-3
(continued)

6.   Do you have any Mental Health Problems or Learning Difficulties? This includes Alzheimer's, Dementia, Depression, Anxiety Disorder, Eating Disorder, Psychotic Disorder, Intellectual Disability, Down Syndrome

If the above condition(s) is/are present, answer questions 6a-6b   If **NO** ☐ go to question 7

6a.	Do you have difficulty controlling your condition with medications or other physician-prescribed therapies? (Answer **NO** if you are not currently taking medications or other treatments)	YES ☐ NO ☐
6b.	Do you have Down Syndrome **AND** back problems affecting nerves or muscles?	YES ☐ NO ☐

7.   Do you have a Respiratory Disease? This includes Chronic Obstructive Pulmonary Disease, Asthma, Pulmonary High Blood Pressure

If the above condition(s) is/are present, answer questions 7a-7d   If **NO** ☐ go to question 8

7a.	Do you have difficulty controlling your condition with medications or other physician-prescribed therapies? (Answer **NO** if you are not currently taking medications or other treatments)	YES ☐ NO ☐
7b.	Has your doctor ever said your blood oxygen level is low at rest or during exercise and/or that you require supplemental oxygen therapy?	YES ☐ NO ☐
7c.	If asthmatic, do you currently have symptoms of chest tightness, wheezing, laboured breathing, consistent cough (more than 2 days/week), or have you used your rescue medication more than twice in the last week?	YES ☐ NO ☐
7d.	Has your doctor ever said you have high blood pressure in the blood vessels of your lungs?	YES ☐ NO ☐

8.   Do you have a Spinal Cord Injury? This includes Tetraplegia and Paraplegia

If the above condition(s) is/are present, answer questions 8a-8c   If **NO** ☐ go to question 9

8a.	Do you have difficulty controlling your condition with medications or other physician-prescribed therapies? (Answer **NO** if you are not currently taking medications or other treatments)	YES ☐ NO ☐
8b.	Do you commonly exhibit low resting blood pressure significant enough to cause dizziness, light-headedness, and/or fainting?	YES ☐ NO ☐
8c.	Has your physician indicated that you exhibit sudden bouts of high blood pressure (known as Autonomic Dysreflexia)?	YES ☐ NO ☐

9.   Have you had a Stroke? This includes Transient Ischemic Attack (TIA) or Cerebrovascular Event

If the above condition(s) is/are present, answer questions 9a-9c   If **NO** ☐ go to question 10

9a.	Do you have difficulty controlling your condition with medications or other physician-prescribed therapies? (Answer **NO** if you are not currently taking medications or other treatments)	YES ☐ NO ☐
9b.	Do you have any impairment in walking or mobility?	YES ☐ NO ☐
9c.	Have you experienced a stroke or impairment in nerves or muscles in the past 6 months?	YES ☐ NO ☐

10.   Do you have any other medical condition not listed above or do you have two or more medical conditions?

If you have other medical conditions, answer questions 10a-10c   If **NO** ☐ read the Page 4 recommendations

10a.	Have you experienced a blackout, fainted, or lost consciousness as a result of a head injury within the last 12 months **OR** have you had a diagnosed concussion within the last 12 months?	YES ☐ NO ☐
10b.	Do you have a medical condition that is not listed (such as epilepsy, neurological conditions, kidney problems)?	YES ☐ NO ☐
10c.	Do you currently live with two or more medical conditions?	YES ☐ NO ☐

PLEASE LIST YOUR MEDICAL CONDITION(S) AND ANY RELATED MEDICATIONS HERE: _____

_____

GO to Page 4 for recommendations about your current medical condition(s) and sign the PARTICIPANT DECLARATION.

Continued on the next page

FIGURE 5-3
(continued)

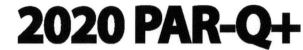

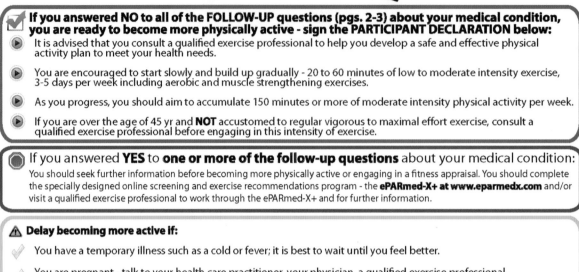

If you answered **NO** to all of the FOLLOW-UP questions (pgs. 2-3) about your medical condition, you are ready to become more physically active - sign the PARTICIPANT DECLARATION below:

▶ It is advised that you consult a qualified exercise professional to help you develop a safe and effective physical activity plan to meet your health needs.

▶ You are encouraged to start slowly and build up gradually - 20 to 60 minutes of low to moderate intensity exercise, 3-5 days per week including aerobic and muscle strengthening exercises.

▶ As you progress, you should aim to accumulate 150 minutes or more of moderate intensity physical activity per week.

▶ If you are over the age of 45 yr and **NOT** accustomed to regular vigorous to maximal effort exercise, consult a qualified exercise professional before engaging in this intensity of exercise.

If you answered **YES** to **one or more of the follow-up questions** about your medical condition:
You should seek further information before becoming more physically active or engaging in a fitness appraisal. You should complete the specially designed online screening and exercise recommendations program - the **ePARmed-X+ at www.eparmedx.com** and/or visit a qualified exercise professional to work through the ePARmed-X+ and for further information.

⚠ **Delay becoming more active if:**

✓ You have a temporary illness such as a cold or fever; it is best to wait until you feel better.

✓ You are pregnant - talk to your health care practitioner, your physician, a qualified exercise professional, and/or complete the ePARmed-X+ **at www.eparmedx.com** before becoming more physically active.

✓ Your health changes - talk to your doctor or qualified exercise professional before continuing with any physical activity program.

● You are encouraged to photocopy the PAR-Q+. You must use the entire questionnaire and NO changes are permitted.
● The authors, the PAR-Q+ Collaboration, partner organizations, and their agents assume no liability for persons who undertake physical activity and/or make use of the PAR-Q+ or ePARmed-X+. If in doubt after completing the questionnaire, consult your doctor prior to physical activity.

PARTICIPANT DECLARATION

● All persons who have completed the PAR-Q+ please read and sign the declaration below.

● If you are less than the legal age required for consent or require the assent of a care provider, your parent, guardian or care provider must also sign this form.

I, the undersigned, have read, understood to my full satisfaction and completed this questionnaire. I acknowledge that this physical activity clearance is valid for a maximum of 12 months from the date it is completed and becomes invalid if my condition changes. I also acknowledge that the community/fitness center may retain a copy of this form for records. In these instances, it will maintain the confidentiality of the same, complying with applicable law.

NAME _____   DATE _____

SIGNATURE _____   WITNESS _____

SIGNATURE OF PARENT/GUARDIAN/CARE PROVIDER _____

——— For more information, please contact ———
www.eparmedx.com
Email: eparmedx@gmail.com

Citation for PAR-Q+
Warburton DER, Jamnik VK, Bredin SSD, and Gledhill N on behalf of the PAR-Q+ Collaboration. The Physical Activity Readiness Questionnaire for Everyone (PAR-Q+) and Electronic Physical Activity Readiness Medical Examination (ePARmed-X+). Health & Fitness Journal of Canada 4(2):3-23, 2011.

The PAR-Q+ was created using the evidence-based AGREE process (1) by the PAR-Q+ Collaboration chaired by Dr. Darren E. R. Warburton with Dr. Norman Gledhill, Dr. Veronica Jamnik, and Dr. Donald C. McKenzie (2). Production of this document has been made possible through financial contributions from the Public Health Agency of Canada and the BC Ministry of Health Services. The views expressed herein do not necessarily represent the views of the Public Health Agency of Canada or the BC Ministry of Health Services.

Key References
1. Jamnik VK, Warburton DER, Makarski J, McKenzie DC, Shephard RJ, Stone J, and Gledhill N. Enhancing the effectiveness of clearance for physical activity participation; background and overall process. APNM 36(S1):S3-S13, 2011.
2. Warburton DER, Gledhill N, Jamnik VK, Bredin SSD, McKenzie DC, Stone J, Charlesworth S, and Shephard RJ. Evidence-based risk assessment and recommendations for physical activity clearance; Consensus Document. APNM 36(S1):S266-s298, 2011.
3. Chisholm DM, Collis ML, Kulak LL, Davenport W, and Gruber N. Physical activity readiness. British Columbia Medical Journal. 1975;17:375-378.
4. Thomas S, Reading J, and Shephard RJ. Revision of the Physical Activity Readiness Questionnaire (PAR-Q). Canadian Journal of Sport Science 1992;17:4 338-345.

Copyright © 2020 PAR-Q+ Collaboration   4/ 4
11-01-2019

PATIENTS IN CARDIAC REHABILITATION AND MEDICAL FITNESS FACILITIES

Health coaches and exercise professionals working with clients with known CVD in clinical settings, such as cardiac rehabilitation and medical fitness facilities, should use a more in-depth screening tool than the ones presented in the previous sections (ACSM, 2018). Specifically, it is recommended they use the risk-stratification criteria from the American Association of Cardiovascular and Pulmonary Rehabilitation, which can found on their website (www.aacvpr.org).

It is imperative that the client's personal physician be made aware of any signs or symptoms suggestive of **coronary artery disease** that may have been discovered as a result of the preparticipation health screening or during an ongoing exercise program.

Additional Forms

PREPARTICIPATION FORMS

Before a health coach or exercise professional begins using any of the documents presented in this chapter, it is critical that legal counsel specializing in health and exercise in the professional's state be consulted.

Informed Consent

An **informed consent** form can be utilized by an exercise professional to demonstrate that a client acknowledges that they have been specifically informed about the risks associated with the activity in which they are about to engage (Figure 5-4). It is primarily intended to communicate the potential benefits and dangers of the program or exercise-testing procedures to the client. Informed consent forms should detail the possible discomforts involved and potential alternatives. Exercise professionals should remember that many potential clients will be unaccustomed to straining their bodies through physical exertion. The informed consent form, combined with oral communication, prepares the client for the positive and negative effects of certain types of exercise.

FIGURE 5-4
Sample informed consent form

CARDIORESPIRATORY FITNESS TEST

Informed Consent for Exercise Testing of Apparently Healthy Adults
(without known heart disease)

Name _____

1. Purpose and Explanation of Test

I hereby consent to voluntarily engage in an exercise test to determine my cardiorespiratory fitness. It is my understanding that the information obtained will help me evaluate future physical activities and sports activities in which I may engage.

Initial: _____

Continued on the next page

FIGURE 5-4
(continued)

Before I undergo the test, I certify that I am in good health and have had a physical examination conducted by a licensed medical physician within the past _____ months. Further, I hereby represent and inform the facility that I have accurately completed the pre-test health-history questionnaire or interview presented to me by the facility staff and have provided correct responses to the questions as indicated on the health-history form or as supplied to the interviewer. It is my understanding that I will be interviewed by a physician or other person prior to my undergoing the test who will in the course of interviewing me determine if there are any reasons that would make it undesirable or unsafe for me to take the test. Consequently, I understand that it is important that I provide complete and accurate responses to the interviewer and recognize that my failure to do so could lead to possible unnecessary injury to myself during the test.

The test that I will undergo will be performed on a motor-driven treadmill or bicycle ergometer with the amount of effort gradually increasing. As I understand it, this increase in effort will continue until I feel and verbally report to the operator any symptoms such as fatigue, shortness of breath, or chest discomfort that I may experience. It is my understanding and I have been clearly advised that it is my right to request that a test be stopped at any point if I feel unusual discomfort or fatigue. I have been advised that I should, immediately upon experiencing any such symptoms or if I so choose, inform the operator that I wish to stop the test at that or any other point. My wishes in this regard shall be absolutely carried out.

During the test itself, it is my understanding that a trained observer will monitor my responses continuously and take frequent readings of blood pressure, the electrocardiogram, and my expressed feelings of effort. I realize that a true determination of my exercise capacity depends on progressing the test to the point of fatigue.

Once the test has been completed, but before I am released from the test area, I will be given special instructions about showering and recognition of certain symptoms that may appear within the first 24 hours after the test. I agree to follow these instructions and promptly contact the facility personnel or medical providers if such symptoms develop.

2. Risks

It is my understanding and I have been informed that there exists the possibility of adverse changes during the actual test. I have been informed that these changes could include abnormal blood pressure, fainting, disorders of heart rhythm, stroke, and very rare instances of heart attack or even death. Every effort, I have been told, will be made to minimize these occurrences by preliminary examination and by precautions and observations taken during the test. I have also been informed that emergency equipment and personnel are readily available to deal with these unusual situations should they occur. I understand that there is a risk of injury, heart attack, stroke, or even death as a result of my performance of this test, but knowing those risks, it is my desire to proceed to take the test as herein indicated.

Initial: _____

FIGURE 5-4
(continued)

3. Benefits to Be Expected and Alternatives Available to the Exercise Testing Procedure

The results of this test may or may not benefit me. Potential benefits relate mainly to my personal motives for taking the test (e.g., knowing my exercise capacity in relation to the general population, understanding my fitness for certain sports and recreational activities, planning my physical conditioning program, or evaluating the effects of my recent physical habits). Although my fitness might also be evaluated by alternative means (e.g., a bench step test or an outdoor running test), such tests do not provide as accurate a fitness assessment as the treadmill or bike test, nor do those options allow equally effective monitoring of my responses.

4. Confidentiality and Use of Information

I have been informed that the information that is obtained from this exercise test will be treated as privileged and confidential and will consequently not be released or revealed to any person without my express written consent or as required by law. I do, however, agree to the use of any information for research or statistical purposes so long as same does not provide facts that could lead to the identification of my person. Any other information obtained, however, will be used only by the facility staff to evaluate my exercise status or needs.

5. Inquiries and Freedom of Consent

I have been given an opportunity to ask questions about the procedure. Generally, these requests, which have been noted by the testing staff, and their responses are as follows:

_____

_____

I further understand that there are also other remote risks that may be associated with this procedure. Despite the fact that a complete accounting of all remote risks is not entirely possible, I am satisfied with the review of these risks, which was provided to me, and it is still my desire to proceed with the test.

I acknowledge that I have read this document in its entirety or that it has been read to me if I have been unable to read same.

I consent to the rendition of all services and procedures as explained herein by all facility personnel.

Date _____

Client's Signature _____

Witness' Signature _____

Test Supervisor's Signature _____

Modified with permission from Herbert, D.L. & Herbert, W.G. (2002). *Legal Aspects of Preventive, Rehabilitative, and Recreational Exercise Programs* (4th ed.). Canton, Oh.: PRC Publishing. Pages 467–470. All rights reserved. No form should be adopted without individualized legal advice.

Note: This document has been prepared to serve as a guide to improve understanding. Exercise professionals should not assume that this sample form will provide adequate protection in the event of a lawsuit. Please see an attorney before creating, distributing, and collecting any agreements to participate, informed consent forms, or waivers.

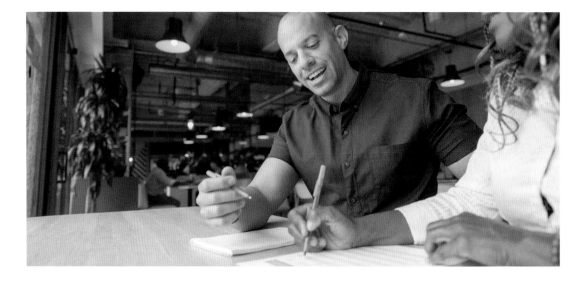

Agreements to Participate

An **agreement to participate** is designed to protect the exercise professional from a client claiming to be unaware of the potential risks of physical activity (Figure 5-5). An agreement to participate is not typically considered a formal contract, but rather serves to demonstrate that the client was made aware of the "normal" outcomes of certain types of physical activity and willingly assumed the risks of participation. Typically, the agreement to participate is utilized for "class" settings (e.g., bootcamp and group cycling) rather than for one-on-one situations. The agreement to participate should detail the nature of the activity, the potential risks to be encountered, and the expected behaviors of the participant (Cotten & Cotten, 2016). This last consideration is important, as the participant recognizes that they may need to follow instructions while participating.

Typically, agreements to participate are incorporated into other documents, such as informed consent forms and **waivers.** One potential consideration for each of these documents is a general request, or in some cases a requirement, that participants consult with a doctor prior to beginning any exercise routine. This practice is particularly important if vigorous-intensity exercise is to be performed. Though most exercise professionals know to "start slowly" with new clients, professionals cannot evaluate the overall health of a client in the same manner as a medical doctor. Some agreements to participate also ask that health insurance information be provided. This not only lets the exercise professional know that the client has coverage, but also enables the professional to provide that information if a client were in need of medical attention.

Waivers

Exercise professionals who hire employees need to understand the concept of **vicarious liability** (also known as **respondeat superior**). Employers are responsible for the employment actions of their employees. If an employee is negligent while working within the normal scope of employment, it is likely that the injured party will sue not only the employee who breached the duty to cause injury, but also the employer or employers. Since employees often do not have the financial resources of employers, courts have typically upheld the right of the injured party to seek damages from the employer's "deep pockets." In most cases, litigants name every possible entity linked to the employee when **negligence** occurs.

FIGURE 5-5
Sample agreement
to participate

"I, _____ , have enrolled in a program of strenuous physical activity including, but not limited to, high-intensity interval training, weight training, stationary bicycling, and the use of various aerobic-conditioning machinery offered by [name of personal trainer and/or business]. I am aware that participating in these types of activities, even when completed properly, can be dangerous. I agree to follow the verbal instructions issued by the personal trainer. I am aware that potential risks associated with these types of activities include, but are not limited to, death, serious neck and spinal injuries that may result in complete or partial paralysis or brain damage, serious injury to virtually all bones, joints, ligaments, muscles, tendons, and other aspects of the musculoskeletal system, and serious injury or impairment to other aspects of my body, general health, and well-being.

Because of the dangers of participating, I recognize the importance of following the personal trainer's instructions regarding proper techniques and training, as well as other organization rules.

I am in good health and have provided verification from a licensed physician that I am able to undertake a general fitness-training program. I hereby consent to first aid, emergency medical care, and admission to an accredited hospital or an emergency care center when necessary for executing such care and for treatment of injuries that I may sustain while participating in an exercise-training program.

I understand that I am responsible for my own medical insurance and will maintain that insurance throughout my entire period of participation with [name of personal trainer and/or business]. I will assume any additional expenses incurred that go beyond my health coverage. I will notify [name of personal trainer and/or business] of any significant injury or change in health status that requires medical attention (such as emergency care, hospitalization, etc.).

Signed _____

Printed Name _____

Phone Number _____

Address _____

Emergency Contact _____

Contact Phone Number _____

Insurance Company _____

Policy # _____

Effective Date _____

Name of Policy Holder _____

Note: This document has been prepared to serve as a guide to improve understanding. Exercise professionals should not assume that this sample form will provide adequate protection in the event of a lawsuit. Please see an attorney before creating, distributing, and collecting any agreements to participate, informed consent forms, or waivers.

The use of waivers is critical, as a properly worded **exculpatory clause** bars the injured party from potential recovery (Figure 5-6). There are some potential issues that every exercise professional must investigate with an attorney prior to crafting a waiver. Each state has slightly different rules regarding the validity of waivers, meaning that a waiver that is valid in one state may not be valid in another. In addition, confusion and litigation can arise when a facility utilizes exercise professionals who are not employees. Consider the following court case, which addressed the situation in which a member of a health club signed a supplemental contract for personal-training services in the club setting. When the client was injured in a session with the personal trainer, she contended that the waiver signed with her membership contract did not extend and cover the services of the personal trainer. The court disagreed and ruled that the services of the personal trainer were part of the activities and benefits offered at the club and were therefore covered by the original waiver (Cotten, 2000a). Despite the outcome of this case, exercise professionals should utilize their own waivers in addition to the ones potentially already signed when the client joined the fitness center or club.

FIGURE 5-6

Sample waiver

I, _____ , through the purchase of training sessions, have agreed to voluntarily participate in an exercise program, including, but not limited to, cardiorespiratory, muscular, and flexibility training under the guidance of [name of personal trainer and/or business]. I hereby stipulate and agree that I am physically and mentally sound and currently have no physical conditions that would be aggravated by my involvement in an exercise program. I have provided verification from a licensed physician that I am able to undertake a general fitness-training program.

I understand and am aware that physical-fitness activities, including the use of equipment, are potentially hazardous activities. I am aware that participating in these types of activities, even when performed properly, can be dangerous. I agree to follow the verbal instructions issued by the personal trainer. I am aware that potential risks associated with these types of activities include, but are not limited to: death, fainting, disorders in heartbeat, serious neck and spinal injuries that may result in complete or partial paralysis or brain damage, serious injury to virtually all bones, joints, ligaments, muscles, tendons, and other aspects of the musculoskeletal system, and serious injury or impairment to other aspects of my body, general health, and well-being.

I understand that I am responsible for my own medical insurance and will maintain that insurance throughout my entire period of participation with [name of personal trainer and/or business]. I will assume any additional expenses incurred that go beyond my health coverage. I will notify the [name of personal trainer and/or business] of any significant injury or change in health status that requires medical attention (such as emergency care, hospitalization, etc.).

[name of personal trainer or business] or I will provide the equipment to be used in connection with workouts, including, but not limited to, benches, dumbbells, barbells, and similar items. I represent and warrant any and all equipment I provide for training sessions is for personal

FIGURE 5-6
(continued)

use only. [name of personal trainer or business] has not inspected my equipment and has no knowledge of its condition. I understand that I take sole responsibility for my equipment. I acknowledge that although [name of personal trainer and/or business] takes precautions to maintain the equipment, any equipment may malfunction and/or cause potential injuries. I take sole responsibility to inspect any and all of my or [name of personal trainer and/or business]'s equipment prior to use.

Although [name of personal trainer and/or business] will take precautions to ensure my safety, I expressly assume and accept sole responsibility for my safety and for any and all injuries that may occur. In consideration of the acceptance of this entry, **I, for myself and for my executors, administrators, and assigns, waive and release any and all claims against [name of personal trainer and/or business] and any of their staffs, officers, officials, volunteers, sponsors, agents, representatives, successors, or assigns and agree to hold them harmless from any claims or losses, including but not limited to claims for negligence for any injuries or expenses that I may incur while exercising or while traveling to and from training sessions.** These exculpatory clauses are intended to apply to any and all activities occurring during the time for which I have contracted with [name of personal trainer and/or company].

I represent and warrant I am signing this agreement freely and willfully and not under fraud or duress.

HAVING READ THE ABOVE TERMS AND INTENDING TO BE LEGALLY BOUND HEREBY AND UNDERSTANDING THIS DOCUMENT TO BE A COMPLETE WAIVER AND DISCLAIMER IN FAVOR OF [name of personal trainer and/or business], I HEREBY AFFIX MY SIGNATURE HERETO.

_____

Client's name (please print clearly)

_____   Date: _____

Client's signature

_____

Client's address

_____   Date: _____

Parent/guardian signature (if applicable)

_____   Date: _____

Exercise Professional's signature

Note: This document has been prepared to serve as a guide to improve understanding. Exercise professionals should not assume that this sample form will provide adequate protection in the event of a lawsuit. Please see an attorney before creating, distributing, and collecting any agreements to participate, informed consent forms, or waivers.

Waivers also must detail the types of activities and potential risks of injury that would be barred from recovering remuneration in a court of law. A client must knowingly understand the nature of the activities and the potential risks before they can waive the right to potentially sue for injuries occurring during participation. Waivers also typically do not protect the exercise professional from injuries directly caused by **gross negligence**—an action that demonstrates recklessness or a willful disregard for the safety of others. As a general rule, gross negligence occurs when someone deliberately acts in a manner that extends beyond the scope of employment or fails to meet the accepted **standard of care.** For example, a correctly worded waiver would likely protect an exercise professional who did not properly spot a client completing an overhead press, as spotting would likely be considered part of the normal activities conducted during the course of an exercise session. However, if the exercise professional knowingly and intentionally used a piece of equipment after a safety screw was removed from the seat for use on another machine prior to the client's arrival, the waiver would likely not apply, because using a machine without the proper safety equipment in place is something that should *never* occur during the normal course of a professional's activities. Ultimately, the use of proper waivers protects the exercise professional from lawsuits that arise not only from injuries that typically occur during exercises, but also from injuries that might occur due to mistakes the exercise professional may make while interacting with clients. Hopefully, mistakes are mitigated, injuries are limited, and potential lawsuits are completely avoided.

Even if a waiver is not utilized properly, an exercise professional may successfully defend against a negligence lawsuit in certain situations, even if they are partially at fault. Courts will typically examine every aspect of the scenario to determine who was at fault. In some cases, the client may have contributed to the potential injury. In certain states, **contributory negligence** laws prevent a plaintiff in a lawsuit who has played some role in the injury from receiving *any* remuneration. For example, if a client failed to notify the exercise professional that the soles of one of their shoes had been slipping, they would be partially to blame if their foot slipped while conducting a squat exercise, even if the professional did not properly spot the client. The clients' improper actions bar them from recovering any money, even though the professional was partially at fault.

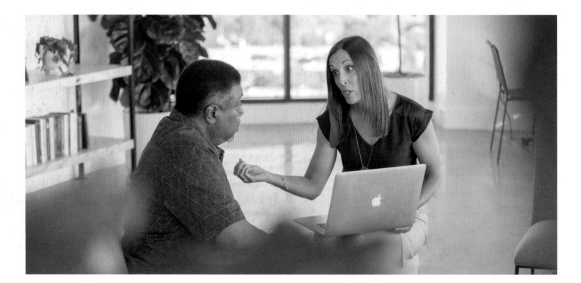

The majority of states do not use the contributory negligence standard, instead utilizing **comparative negligence** when deciding negligence cases. When multiple parties may have caused injuries, the court will apportion guilt and any subsequent award for damages. For instance, in the earlier example the client may be deemed to be 40% at fault for the injury (for failing to inform the exercise professional of the issue with their shoes) and the exercise professional 60% at fault (for failing to spot the client during the lift). If the court were to normally award $100,000 in damages, the award would be lowered to $60,000 (i.e., 60% of the damages). There are a variety of state standards regarding comparative negligence and its potential impact upon monetary awards.

Inherent Risks

Agreements to participate and informed consent forms, though potentially important in the defense against a lawsuit, primarily cover the **inherent risks** of participation in an activity. For instance, even if proper stretching and lifting techniques are utilized, injuries can occur to ligaments, tendons, muscles, and other parts of the body. An agreement to participate and an informed consent form would help to protect the exercise professional in the event that a lawsuit is filed by an injured client. However, it is often difficult to determine an inherent risk of participation and what might have been caused, in whole or in part, by the actions of the professional. A client may claim that an exercise professional did not provide proper spotting during an exercise and that this action specifically caused an injury. The exercise professional might counter that an injury was unfortunate, but part of the normal, safe lifting process, and that the spotting provided was well within the normal standard of care. This dispute would likely be settled in court. To potentially avoid this type of a scenario, professionals should have all clients sign a waiver prior to beginning any exercise routine. The waiver (sometimes called a release) will not only typically incorporate similar language included in an agreement to participate and an informed consent form, but will also include an exculpatory clause that bars the clients from seeking damages for injuries caused by the inherent risk of activities and by the ordinary negligence of exercise professionals and their employees and agents (see boldface text in Figure 5-6).

Procedures

Valid agreements to participate, informed consent forms, and waivers must be administered properly to clients. There should not be any underhanded attempt to hide the true nature of these agreements prior to a client signing the document. Though some states permit **group waivers** that have a list of spaces for multiple patrons to sign below the waiver, it is advisable to have a stand-alone document for each client. Often, exercise professionals properly insist that a new client sign a waiver prior to the first session, but then fail to allow sufficient time for the new client to read, understand, and ask questions about the document. Requiring a client to rush when reviewing a waiver can result in a court invalidating an otherwise properly crafted waiver. In addition, though courts have typically found that individuals who cannot read English retain the responsibility to have someone translate the waiver prior to signing, it is a good practice to have someone available to assist with the translation if needed (Cotten & Cotten, 2016). If the document is multiple pages, a space for the client to initial the bottom of each page should be provided (see Figure 5-4 as an example).

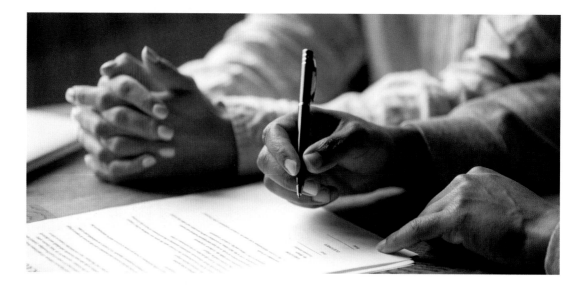

Minors cannot legally sign a contract, so in most cases a waiver signed by a child will be invalidated by the courts. However, some states do allow parents to sign paperwork that may provide limited protection for the exercise professional. An attorney specializing in this area should be consulted if children will be utilizing an exercise professional's services. A waiver signed by one spouse may not cover the other spouse (Cotten, 2000b). Once agreements to participate, informed consent forms, and waivers have been signed, the exercise professional should retain the paperwork on file at least until the **statute of limitations**—the time allotted to sue for damages—has elapsed. Some attorneys even recommend retaining records past the statute of limitations to ensure that a sudden change in the law does not negatively impact the ability of a service provider to defend against potential litigation.

Ultimately, the goal of any exercise professional should be to eliminate all client injuries. However, even in the safest conditions, physical activity may result in some physical injuries, even when proper care is provided. Professionals should utilize paperwork to notify new clients of *all* risks and potential dangers. This creates a situation in which the client knows and assumes the risks of participation. Exercise professionals should then also utilize waivers to protect against costly lawsuits that arise both from the normal physical injuries associated with physical activity and from mistakes that may occur during sessions.

Lifestyle and Health-history Questionnaire

This form collects more detailed medical and health information beyond the preparticipation health screening, including the following (Figure 5-7):

- ▶ Past and present exercise and physical-activity information
- ▶ Medications and supplements
- ▶ Recent or current illnesses or injuries, including chronic or acute pain
- ▶ Surgery and injury history
- ▶ Family medical history
- ▶ Lifestyle information (related to nutrition, stress, work, sleep, etc.)

FIGURE 5-7
Sample lifestyle
and health-history
questionnaire

Name: _____   Date: _____   Date of birth: _____

Medical Information

1. How would you describe your present state of health?
   ☐ Very well   ☐ Healthy   ☐ Unhealthy   ☐ Unwell   ☐ Other: _____

2. List current medications, how often you take them, and dosages (include prescriptions and over-the-counter medications). _____

   _____

   _____

3. Do you take all of your medications as they have been prescribed by your healthcare provider? ☐ Yes   ☐ No

   If not, please share why (e.g., cost, side effects, or feeling as though they are unnecessary). _____

   _____

   _____

4. Do you take any vitamin, mineral, or herbal supplements? ☐ Yes   ☐ No

   If yes, list type and amount per day: _____

5. When was the last time you visited your physician? _____

6. Have you ever had your cholesterol checked?   ☐ Yes   ☐ No

   Date of test: _____ What were the results? _____

   Total cholesterol: _____ High-density lipoprotein (HDL): _____ Low-density lipoprotein (LDL): _____

   Triglycerides: _____

7. Have you ever had your blood sugar checked?   ☐ Yes   ☐ No

   What were the results? _____

8. Please check any that apply to you and list any important information about your condition:

   ☐ Allergies (Specify: _____)

   ☐ Amenorrhea

   ☐ Anemia

   ☐ Anxiety

   ☐ Arthritis

   ☐ Asthma

   ☐ Celiac disease

   ☐ Chronic sinus condition

   ☐ Constipation

   ☐ Crohn's disease

   ☐ Depression

   ☐ Diabetes

   ☐ Diarrhea

   ☐ Disordered eating

   ☐ Gastroesophageal reflux disease (GERD)

   ☐ High blood pressure

   ☐ Hypoglycemia

   ☐ Hypo/hyperthyroidism

   ☐ Insomnia

   ☐ Intestinal problems

   ☐ Irritability

   ☐ Irritable bowel syndrome (IBS)

   ☐ Menopausal symptoms

   ☐ Osteoporosis

   ☐ Premenstrual syndrome (PMS)

   ☐ Polycystic ovary syndrome (PCOS)

   ☐ Pregnant

   ☐ Skin problems

   ☐ Ulcer

   ☐ Major surgeries: _____

   _____

   _____

   ☐ Past injuries: _____

   _____

   _____

   ☐ Describe any other health conditions that you have: _____

   _____

   _____

   _____

   _____

Continued on the next page

FIGURE 5-7
(continued)

Family History

1. Has anyone in your immediate family been diagnosed with the following?

☐ Heart disease   If yes, what is the relation? _____ Age of diagnosis: _____

☐ High cholesterol   If yes, what is the relation? _____ Age of diagnosis: _____

☐ High blood pressure   If yes, what is the relation? _____ Age of diagnosis: _____

☐ Cancer   If yes, what is the relation? _____ Age of diagnosis: _____

☐ Diabetes   If yes, what is the relation? _____ Age of diagnosis: _____

☐ Osteoporosis   If yes, what is the relation? _____ Age of diagnosis: _____

Nutrition

1. What are your dietary goals? _____

2. Have you ever followed a modified diet?   ☐ Yes   ☐ No

   If yes, describe: _____

3. Are you currently following a specialized eating plan (e.g., low-sodium or low-fat)?   ☐ Yes   ☐ No

   If yes, what type of eating plan? _____

4. Why did you choose this eating plan? _____

   Was the eating plan prescribed by a physician?   ☐ Yes   ☐ No

   How long have you been on the eating plan? _____

5. Have you ever met with a registered dietitian or attended diabetes education classes?   ☐ Yes   ☐ No

   If no, are you interested in doing so?   ☐ Yes   ☐ No

6. What do you consider to be the major issues with your nutritional choices or eating plan (e.g., eating late at night, snacking on high-fat foods, skipping meals, or lack of variety)? _____

   _____

   _____

7. How many glasses of water do you drink per day? _____ 8-ounce glasses

8. What do you drink other than water? List what and how much per day. _____

9. Do you have any food allergies or intolerance?   ☐ Yes   ☐ No

   If yes, what? _____

10. Who shops for and prepares your food?   ☐ Self   ☐ Spouse   ☐ Parent   ☐ Minimal preparation

11. How often do you dine out? _____ times per week

12. Please specify the type of restaurants for each meal:

    Breakfast: _____   Lunch: _____

    Dinner: _____   Snacks: _____

FIGURE 5-7
(continued)

13. Do you crave any foods?   ☐ Yes   ☐ No

    If yes, please specify: _____

Substance-related Habits

1. Do you drink alcohol?   ☐ Yes   ☐ No

    If yes, how often? _____ times per week   Average amount? _____

2. Do you drink caffeinated beverages?   ☐ Yes   ☐ No

    If yes, average number per day: _____

3. Do you use tobacco?   ☐ Yes   ☐ No

    If yes, how much (cigarettes, cigars, or chewing tobacco per day)? _____

Physical Activity

1. Do you currently participate in any structured physical activity?   ☐ Yes   ☐ No

    If so, please describe:

    _____ minutes of cardiorespiratory activity, _____ times per week

    _____ muscular-training sessions per week

    _____ flexibility-training sessions per week

    _____ minutes of sports or recreational activities per week

    List sports or activities you participate in: _____

2. Do you engage in any other forms of regular physical activity?   ☐ Yes   ☐ No

    If yes, describe: _____

3. Have you ever experienced any injuries that may limit your physical activity?   ☐ Yes   ☐ No

    If yes, describe: _____

4. Do you have any physical-activity restrictions? If so, please list:_____

    _____

    _____

5. What are your honest feelings about exercise/physical activity? _____

    _____

    _____

6. What are some of your favorite physical activities? _____

    _____

    _____

Continued on the next page

FIGURE 5-7
(continued)

Occupational

1. Do you work?   ☐ Yes   ☐ No

　　If yes, what is your occupation? _____

　　If you work, what is your work schedule? _____

2. Describe your activity level during the work day: _____

Sleep and Stress

1. How many hours of sleep do you get at night? _____

2. Rate your average stress level from 1 (no stress) to 10 (constant stress) _____

3. What is most stressful to you? _____

4. How is your appetite affected by stress?   ☐ Increased   ☐ Not affected   ☐ Decreased

Weight History

1. What is your present weight? _____   ☐ Don't know

2. What would you like to do with your weight?   ☐ Lose weight   ☐ Gain weight   ☐ Maintain weight

3. What was your lowest weight within the past 5 years? _____

4. What was your highest weight within the past 5 years? _____

5. What do you consider to be your ideal weight (the sustainable weight at which you feel best)? _____ ☐ Don't know

6. What are your current waist and hip circumferences? _____ Waist   _____ Hip   ☐ Don't know

7. What is your current body composition? _____% body fat   ☐ Don't know

Goals

1. On a scale of 1 to 10, how likely are you to adopt a healthier lifestyle (1 = very unlikely; 10 = very likely)? _____

2. Do you have any specific goals for improving your health? ☐ Yes ☐ No If yes, please list them in order of importance.

　　_____

　　_____

3. Do you have a weight-loss goal?   ☐ Yes   ☐ No

　　If yes, what is it? _____

4. If you want to lose weight, why is that important to you?

　　_____

　　_____

Fall Risk Questionnaire

The fear of falling is itself a risk factor for falling and can lead to a reduced quality of life and a decline in activity. Therefore, assessing fall risk can be helpful for identifying individuals with excessive fear that requires intervention and determining which activities are most feared and which could be targeted for training (Pena et al., 2019; Yardley et al., 2005).

The Falls Efficacy Scale-International (FES-I) can be used to assess concerns relating to basic and more demanding activities, both physical and social (Figure 5-8).

FIGURE 5-8
The Falls Efficacy Scale-International (FES-I)

I would like to ask some questions about how concerned you are about the possibility of falling. Please reply after thinking about how you usually do the activity. If you currently don't perform the activity (e.g., if someone does your shopping for you), please respond after considering whether you would be concerned about falling *if* you did the activity.

		Not at all concerned	Somewhat concerned	Fairly concerned	Very concerned
1	Cleaning the house (e.g., sweep, vacuum, or dust)	1 ☐	2 ☐	3 ☐	4 ☐
2	Getting dressed or undressed	1 ☐	2 ☐	3 ☐	4 ☐
3	Preparing simple meals	1 ☐	2 ☐	3 ☐	4 ☐
4	Taking a bath or shower	1 ☐	2 ☐	3 ☐	4 ☐
5	Going to the shop	1 ☐	2 ☐	3 ☐	4 ☐
6	Getting in or out of a chair	1 ☐	2 ☐	3 ☐	4 ☐
7	Going up or down stairs	1 ☐	2 ☐	3 ☐	4 ☐
8	Walking around in the neighborhood	1 ☐	2 ☐	3 ☐	4 ☐
9	Reaching for something above your head or on the ground	1 ☐	2 ☐	3 ☐	4 ☐
10	Going to answer the telephone before it stops ringing	1 ☐	2 ☐	3 ☐	4 ☐
11	Walking on a slippery surface (e.g., wet or icy)	1 ☐	2 ☐	3 ☐	4 ☐
12	Visiting a friend or relative	1 ☐	2 ☐	3 ☐	4 ☐
13	Walking in a place with crowds	1 ☐	2 ☐	3 ☐	4 ☐
14	Walking on an uneven surface (e.g., rocky ground or poorly maintained pavement)	1 ☐	2 ☐	3 ☐	4 ☐
15	Walking up or down a slope	1 ☐	2 ☐	3 ☐	4 ☐
16	Going out to a social event (e.g., religious service, family gathering, or club meeting)	1 ☐	2 ☐	3 ☐	4 ☐

Reprinted and modified with permission from Yardley, L. et al. (2005). Development and initial validation of the Falls Efficacy Scale-International (FES-I). *Age and Ageing*, 34, 614–619.

To score the FES-I, add up all the selected responses to determine the client's concern about falling. A score of 16 to 19 reflects a low level of concern, a score of 20 to 27 reflects a moderate level of concern, and a score above 27 reflects a high level of concern (Delbaere et al., 2010).

Medical Release

The medical release form provides the exercise professional with the client's medical information and explains physical-activity limitations and/or guidelines as outlined by their physician (Figure 5-9). *Deviation from these guidelines must be approved by the client's personal physician.*

FIGURE 5-9

Sample medical release form

Date _____

Dear Doctor:

Your patient, _____, wishes to start a personalized training program. The activity will involve the following:

(type, frequency, duration, and intensity of activities)

If your patient is taking medications that will affect their exercise capacity or heart-rate response to exercise, please indicate the manner of the effect (raises or lowers exercise capacity or heart-rate response):

Type of medication(s) _____

Effect(s) _____

Please identify any recommendations or restrictions that are appropriate for your patient in this exercise program:

_____

_____

_____

Thank you.
Sincerely,

Fred Fitness
Personalized Gym
Address
Phone

_____ has my approval to begin an exercise program with the recommendations or restrictions stated above.

Signed_____Date_____

Phone_____

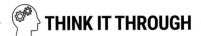

THINK IT THROUGH

Application of Legal Forms

Training or coaching clients requires carefully gathering information about lifestyle, goals, physical-activity history, and health history, conditions, or concerns. After reviewing all of the sample forms presented in this chapter, decide which ones you will use and how you will adapt them to your own practice. Be sure to have all of the forms you plan to use in your practice reviewed by a legal professional in your area. Protecting your clients and yourself from the risks associated with exercise is a prudent and necessary part of doing business as a health coach or exercise professional.

RECORD KEEPING

Keeping current and accurate records for every client is essential for an exercise professional. The important legal principle to remember is that if information is not written down, then from the perspective of the court system, it did not occur and does not exist.

Medical History

An exercise professional must maintain current records of each client's medical conditions and should document a client's condition prior to beginning any exercise. This will provide a baseline against which to compare in the future. It is advisable for the professional to update each client's records every time new information is provided or observed. Positive changes from the baseline can be used for motivation and goal development.

Exercise Record

A client's exercise record needs to stay current with specific notations for any changes, such as a new onset of pain. This will provide the exercise professional with an accurate record of any program changes and when the incident occurred. A good practice is to write down some important details of every single session.

Incident Report

If an injury does occur during a workout session, it needs to be recognized and addressed appropriately. The client's injury will need immediate medical attention. This may include

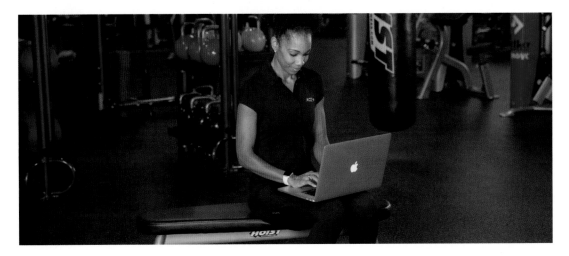

minor first aid or, potentially, something drastic like the activation of emergency medical services. Client safety is the number-one priority throughout the entire process. After the client is safe and stable, a formal written account of the incident needs to be documented. Most organizations will have a specific "incident" report that is completed after an injury has occurred. Copies of these reports are typically distributed to all pertinent parties. However, to protect their interests and to support their memory of the incident and the response, exercise professionals need to keep their own account of what occurred and maintain any pertinent documentation. This will help ensure that an accurate account of the incident is maintained.

Correspondence

Since the passage of the 1996 **Health Insurance Portability and Accountability Act (HIPAA),** maintaining the privacy of medical records has not only been a good ethical practice, but it has also been mandated by law. **Protected health information** includes any identifiable health information that is kept or communicated in any form. Like any other healthcare professional, health coaches and exercise professionals cannot print, email, or discuss a client's health information unless the client has granted written permission to do so. Though most professionals inherently know to protect the confidentiality of written health information, some have become lax in their approach to conversations with other professionals, facility employees, or even other clients. If there is any chance for someone to be able to determine which client's health information is being discussed, the professional should refrain from engaging in such conversations. If outside consultation is deemed by the professional to be necessary, they should obtain written permission from the client. In cases where permission has been granted, the professional should document all conversations and sharing of information. This will help ensure protection of the client's personal information. See Figure 5-10 for a sample HIPAA permission form.

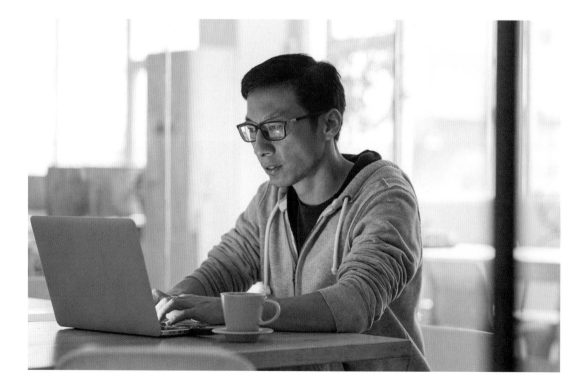

FIGURE 5-10

Sample HIPAA permission form for a medical doctor and personal trainer to disclose information

I, _____ , direct my healthcare and medical service provider
[client]

_____ to disclose and release my protected health
[healthcare provider]

information that is *pertinent* and *necessary* for _____ , acting
[personal trainer]

as my personal trainer, to design, implement, and supervise an exercise program. Further, I permit
my personal trainer and my healthcare provider to discuss my medical condition as it pertains to
my general health and my ongoing participation in said designed fitness program.

Health Information to be disclosed upon the request of the person named above (Check either A or B):

☐ A. Disclose my complete health record (including but not limited to diagnoses, lab tests,
prognosis, treatment, and billing, for all conditions) **OR**

☐ B. Disclose my health record, as above, BUT do not disclose the following
(check as appropriate):

  ☐ Mental health records

  ☐ Communicable diseases (including HIV and AIDS)

  ☐ Alcohol/drug abuse treatment

  ☐ Other (please specify): _____

This authorization shall be effective until (check one):

☐ All past, present, and future periods, **OR**

☐ Date or event: _____ unless I revoke it. (NOTE: You may revoke
this authorization at any time by notifying your healthcare provider and personal trainer,
preferably in writing.)

Printed Name of the Individual Granting this Authorization   Date of birth

_____   _____

Signature of the Individual Granting this Authorization

_____

Medical Personnel Name and Contact Information

_____

_____

Personal Trainer Name and Contact Information

_____

_____

Medications

Medication or substance (e.g., caffeine and nicotine) use is another important topic to review when discussing health history. These substances alter the biochemistry of the body and may affect a client's ability to perform or respond to exercise. The properties of these drugs must be understood by the exercise professional and discussed with the client. When designing and supervising an exercise program, it is important to realize that many substances, over-the-counter medications, and prescription drugs affect the heart's response to exercise. There are hundreds of thousands of different drugs on the market and each may be referred to by the manufacturer's brand name (e.g., Inderal) or by the scientific generic name (e.g., propranolol). Table 5-2 lists select medications and substances that may affect a person's response to exercise. To use the table, consult the client, the client's physician, or a medical reference to find the correct category for the medication. Then, refer to the general category under which each drug is grouped, such as **beta blockers, antihistamines,** or **bronchodilators.** The drugs in each group are thought to have a similar effect on most people, although individual responses will vary.

A particular response is usually dose dependent; the larger the dose, the greater the response. An important factor to consider in this dose-related response is the time when the medication is taken. As medications are metabolized, their effects diminish. If an exercise professional has any questions concerning a client's medications, it is essential that the professional discuss them with the client and their physician. If the professional or client is concerned about the effects of a medication and its impact on exercise, a medical clearance form can be utilized to seek clarification and recommendations (see Figure 5-9). The following are some of the most common categories of medications of which exercise professionals should be aware.

ANTIHYPERTENSIVES

High blood pressure, or **hypertension,** is common in modern society, and there are many medications used for its treatment. Most antihypertensives primarily affect one of four different sites: the heart, to reduce its force of contraction; the peripheral blood vessels, to open or dilate them to allow more room for the blood; the brain, to reduce the sympathetic nerve outflow; or the kidneys, to reduce blood volume by excreting more fluid. The site that the medication acts on helps to determine its effect on the individual as well as any potential side effects. The following are common antihypertensives.

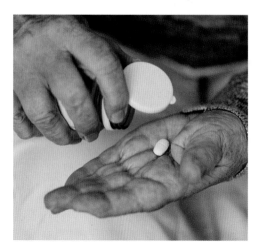

Beta Blockers

Beta-adrenergic blocking agents, or beta blockers, are commonly prescribed for a variety of cardiovascular and other disorders. These medications block beta-adrenergic receptors and limit **sympathetic nervous system** stimulation. In other words, they block the effects of **catecholamines (epinephrine** and **norepinephrine)** throughout the body, and reduce resting, exercise, and **maximal heart**

TABLE 5-2

Effects of Select Substances on Heart-rate Response

Medications	Resting HR	Exercise HR	Exercise Capacity	Comments
Beta blockers	↓	↓	↓ V̇O₂max with acute and ↑ with chronic administration	Dose-related response
Angiotensin II receptor blockers (ARBs) and calcium channel blockers (CCBs)	↓ or ↔	↓ or ↔	↔	
Other antihypertensives*	↑, ↔, or ↓	↑, ↔, or ↓	Usually ↔	Many antihypertensive medications are used. Some may decrease, a few may increase, and others do not affect HR. Some exhibit variable and dose-related responses.
Antihistamines	↑	↔	↔ performance and endurance	
Antidepressants and antianxiety medications	↑ or ↔	↑ or ↔		
Stimulants	↑	↑	↑ or ↔ endurance and performance	
Caffeine	↑	↑ or ↔	↑ endurance	
Bronchodilators	↔	↔	↔ V̇O₂max; ↑ or ↔ in individuals with COPD	
Alcohol	↔	↔	↓ performance and V̇O₂max	Exercise prohibited while under the influence; effects of alcohol on coordination increase possibility of injuries
Nicotine-replacement therapy	↑	↑	↔ or ↓	
Nonsteroidal anti-inflammatory drugs (NSAIDs)			↔ or ↑ performance	

Note: ↑ = increase; ↔ = no significant change; ↓ = decrease; HR = Heart rate; V̇O₂max = Maximal oxygen uptake; COPD = Chronic obstructive pulmonary disease

* Many antihypertensive medications can cause positional hypotension, meaning the blood pressure drops when changing positions (sitting to standing). Therefore, a client may become dizzy if they move too fast after performing abdominal work on the floor.

Note: Many medications are prescribed for conditions that do not require clearance. Do not forget other indicators of exercise intensity (e.g., client's appearance or rating of perceived exertion).

This table in not intended to be an exhaustive list of all medications and their effects on heart rate. For more information on this topic, refer to American College of Sports Medicine (2018). *ACSM's Guidelines for Exercise Testing and Prescription* (10th ed.). Philadelphia: Wolters Kluwer.

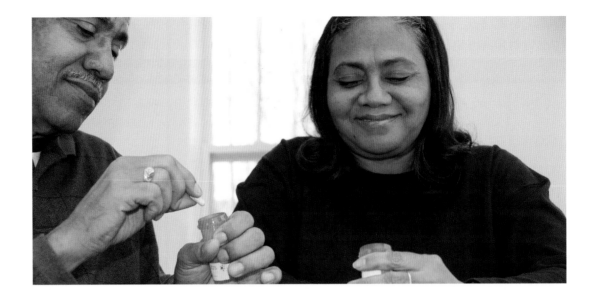

rates. This reduction in **heart rate (HR)** requires modifying the method used for determining exercise intensity. Using **rating of perceived exertion** or the **talk test** versus **target heart rate,** for example, would be appropriate for ensuring a safe and effective cardiorespiratory exercise intensity for someone on beta blockers.

Calcium Channel Blockers

Calcium channel blockers prevent calcium-dependent contraction of the smooth muscles in the arteries, causing them to dilate, which lowers blood pressure (BP). These agents also are used for angina and heart dysrhythmias (rapid or irregular HR). There are several types of calcium channel blockers on the market, and their effect on BP and HR depends on the specific agent. Notice in Table 5-2 that calcium channel blockers may decrease or have no effect on the HR. Therefore, while it is important to know the general effects of a category of medication, remember that individual responses can vary.

Angiotensin-converting Enzyme Inhibitors

Angiotensin-converting enzyme (ACE) inhibitors block an enzyme secreted by the kidneys, preventing the formation of a potent hormone (angiotensin II) that constricts blood vessels. If this enzyme is blocked, the vessels dilate and BP decreases. ACE inhibitors should not affect HR but will cause a decrease in BP at rest and during exercise.

Angiotensin II Receptor Antagonists

Angiotensin II receptor antagonists (or blockers) are a newer class of antihypertensive agents. These drugs are selective for angiotensin II (type 1 receptor). Angiotensin II receptor antagonists are well tolerated, and do not adversely affect blood lipid profiles or cause "rebound hypertension" after discontinuation.

Diuretics

Diuretics are medications that increase the excretion of water and **electrolytes** through the kidneys. They are usually prescribed for high BP, or when a person is accumulating too much fluid, as occurs with congestive heart failure. They have no primary effect on the

HR, but they can cause water and electrolyte imbalances, which may lead to dangerous cardiac **arrhythmias.** Because diuretics can compromise hydration status and decrease blood volume, they may predispose an exerciser to dehydration. A client taking diuretics needs to maintain adequate fluid intake before, during, and after exercise, especially in a warm, humid environment. Diuretics are sometimes used by athletes to try to lose weight for sport. This is a dangerous practice that should not be condoned by a responsible exercise professional.

BRONCHODILATORS

Asthma medications, also known as bronchodilators, relax or open the air passages in the lungs, allowing better air exchange. There are many different types, but the primary action of each is to stimulate the sympathetic nervous system. Bronchodilators increase exercise capacity in persons limited by **bronchoconstriction** but otherwise have minimal effect on resting and exercise HRs and BPs.

COLD MEDICATIONS

Sympathomimetic drugs are compounds that mimic the activity of the sympathetic nervous system (e.g., increase BP and HR) and are often found in medications that treat allergic rhinitis, nasal congestion, and asthma. For example, decongestants act directly on the smooth muscles of the blood vessels to stimulate **vasoconstriction.** In the upper airways, this constriction reduces the volume of the swollen tissues and results in more air space. Vasoconstriction in the peripheral vessels may raise BP and increase HR both at rest and possibly during exercise.

Antihistamines block the histamine receptor, which is involved with the mast cells and the allergic response. These medications do not have a direct effect on the HR or BP, but they do produce a drying effect in the upper airways and may cause drowsiness.

Most cold medications are a combination of decongestants and antihistamines and may have combined effects. However, they are normally taken in low doses and have minimal effect on exercise capacity.

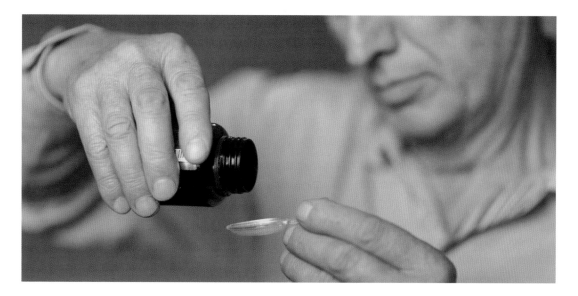

For additional information about medications and their impact on older adults, refer to *ACSM's Guidelines for Exercise Testing and Prescription* (ACSM, 2018) and *The Exercise Professional's Guide to Personal Training* (ACE, 2020).

THE AGING PROCESS AND PHARMACOKINETICS

Pharmacokinetics involves the absorption, distribution, metabolism, and excretion of drugs in the human body. Following are four physiological changes that affect the pharmacokinetics of medications in older adults:

▶ *Decrease in lean body mass as body fat increases:* A decrease in lean body tissue and an increase in body fat are due not only to the aging process, but also are partially dependent on lifestyle behaviors. Body weight typically increases between the ages of 40 and 60 due to an increase in fat tissue, then declines between the ages of 60 and 80 as lean muscle mass is lost. These changes profoundly affect the distribution and elimination of drugs outside the circulatory system (Shi & Klotz, 2011). If a drug must bind to protein tissues, such as acid-organic drugs (diazoxide, digitoxin, and penicillin), its distribution is adversely affected by the decrease in muscle mass. When body fat increases, liposoluble drugs, such as barbiturates and psychotropic agents, accumulate in fat tissue and increase the chance of prolonged and toxic effects.

▶ *Reduction in total body water:* The body consists of about 80% water at birth. This volume decreases gradually with age, and it is generally agreed that total body water drops by 10 to 15% between the ages of 30 and 80 (Beaufrère & Morio, 2000). Since body water helps dilute water-soluble medications (i.e., diuretics), this decrease in the amount of water in the body lessens the distribution and increases the concentration of these drugs, causing a higher susceptibility to the drugs' toxic effects in older adults.

▶ *Decreased efficiency of the gastrointestinal tract:* As people age, the efficiency of the gastrointestinal tract diminishes. Enzyme and glandular secretion, blood flow, gastric motility, and sphincter activity decrease, and the effective surface area available for drug absorption is reduced (Hurwitz et al, 2003). Thus, the absorption of oral medications in the gastrointestinal tract is slow and less complete. Differences in drug absorption are due to gastrointestinal diseases associated with the aging process, mixing various medications, drug/nutrient interactions, and the effects of exercise (Fischer & Fadda, 2016).

▶ *Decreased efficiency of the liver and kidneys:* The liver is the most predominant organ in drug metabolism. As humans age, liver mass diminishes, hepatic blood flow decreases, and fat tends to accumulate in the liver (Hunt et al., 2019). Combined with other lifestyle factors, these conditions cause a decline in liver function and a slower, less complete metabolism of drugs. This slower metabolism of drugs—particularly cardiac medications—increases an older adult's vulnerability to adverse effects.

Aging also induces changes in the structure and function of the kidneys. Evidence suggests that by age 85, kidney mass is about 25% less than that of a younger person and renal plasma flow is less than half. These and other changes, such as the build-up of fatty tissue, decrease the filtration rate and secretion in the kidneys and account for a slower removal of drugs (Denic, Glassock, & Rule, 2016). A study by Takahashi et al. (2018) found that individuals with reduced hepatic and renal function experienced an increased risk of adverse drug effects.

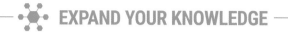
EXPAND YOUR KNOWLEDGE

Disease and Heterogeneity in the Older Adult Population

The high prevalence of disease in the elderly also results in a higher dependence on medications (polypharmacy) and the incidence of adverse drug effects with increasing age. It has been reported that approximately 9 to 15% of hospitalizations in the older adult are due to adverse effects of medications (Oscanoa, Lizaraso, & Carvajal, 2017; Chalmers et al., 2016), while up to 30% of those admitted for an adverse drug reaction result in death (Shepherd et al., 2012). Thus, an important consideration for medication use in older people is that there is greater heterogeneity in older populations, which means not only that there is significant variation in disease states, but also significant variations in responses to medications.

SUMMARY

The pre-exercise interview and health-screening process are the ideal time for beginning or continuing to build rapport; gathering information about values, goals, and health history; clarifying expectations; ensuring appropriate legal forms are reviewed and signed; ensuring clients have the opportunity to ask questions and express concerns; and to determine if it is safe and appropriate for clients to begin or increase the intensity of an exercise program. When it comes to effective exercise program design and supporting clients in health behavior change, it is essential for exercise professionals to gather relevant information for the creation of safe exercise programs and goals. The forms and screening tools covered in this chapter are options to be used when working with clients and, when used appropriately, can set the stage for an open, honest, meaningful, and effective professional relationship.

REFERENCES

American College of Sports Medicine (2018). *ACSM's Guidelines for Exercise Testing and Prescription* (10th ed.). Philadelphia: Wolters Kluwer.

American Council on Exercise (2020). *The Exercise Professional's Guide to Personal Training.* San Diego: American Council on Exercise.

Beaufrère, B. & Morio, B. (2000). Fat and protein redistribution with aging: Metabolic considerations. *European Journal of Clinical Nutrition,* 54, Suppl3, S48–S53.

Chalmers, L., et al. (2016). Prediction of hospitalization due to adverse drug reactions in elderly community-dwelling patients (The PADR-EC Score). *PLoS One,* 11,10, p.e0165757.

Cotten, D.J. (2000a). Carefully worded liability waiver protects Bally's from liability for personal trainer negligence. *Exercise Standards and Malpractice Reporter,* 14, 5, 65.

Cotten, D.J. (2000b). Non-signing spouses: Are they bound by a waiver signed by the other spouse? *Exercise Standards and Malpractice Reporter,* 14, 2, 18.

Cotten, D.J. & Cotten, M.B. (2016). *Waivers & Releases of Liability* (9th ed.). Scotts Valley, Calif.: CreateSpace Independent Publishing.

Delbaere, K. et al. (2010). The Falls Efficacy Scale International (FES-I): A comprehensive longitudinal validation study. *Age and Ageing,* 39, 210–216.

Denic, A., Glassock, R.J., & Rule, A.D. (2016). Structural and functional changes with the aging kidney. *Advanced in Chronic Kidney Disease,* 23, 1, 19–28.

Fischer, M. & Fadda, H.M. (2016). The effect of sex and age on small intestinal transit times in humans. *Journal of Pharmacological Science,* 105, 682–686.

Herbert, D.L. & Herbert, W.G. (2002). *Legal Aspects of Preventive and Rehabilitative Exercise Programs* (4th ed.). Canton, Ohio: PRC Publishing.

Hunt, N.J. et al. (2019). Hallmarks of aging in the liver. *Computational and Structural Biotechnology Journal,* 17, 1151–1161.

Hurwitz, C.E. et al. (2003). Gastric function in the elderly: Effects on absorption of ketoconazole. *Journal of Clinical Pharmacology,* 43, 996–1002.

Oscanoa, T.J., Lizaraso, F., & Carvajal, A. (2017). Hospital admissions due to adverse drug reactions in the elderly. A meta-analysis. *European Journal of Clinical Pharmacology,* 73, 6, 759–770.

Pena, S.B. et al. (2019). Fear of falling and risk of falling: A systematic review and meta-analysis. *Acta Paulista de Enfermagem,* 32, 4, 456–463.

Shepherd, G. et al. (2012). Adverse drug reaction deaths reported in United States vital statistics, 1999-2006. *Annals of Pharmacotherapy,* 46, 2, 169–175.

Shi, S. & Klotz, U. (2011). Age-related changes in pharmacokinetics. *Current Drug Metabolism,* 12, 7, 601–610.

Takahashi, Y. et al. (2018). Effect of baseline renal and hepatic function on the incidence of adverse drug events: The Japan Adverse Drug Events study. *Drug Metabolism and Personalized Therapy,* 33, 4, 165–173.

U.S. Administration on Aging (2018). *Profile of Older Americans.* Washington, D.C.: U.S. Department of Health and Human Services. https://acl.gov/sites/default/files/Aging%20and%20Disability%20in%20America/2018OlderAmericansProfile.pdf

World Health Organization (2018). *Ageing and Health.* https://www.who.int/news-room/fact-sheets/detail/ageing-and-health

Yardley, L. et al. (2005). Development and initial validation of the Falls Efficacy Scale-International (FES-I). *Age and Ageing,* 34, 614–619.

SUGGESTED READINGS

American College of Sports Medicine (2018). *ACSM's Guidelines for Exercise Testing and Prescription* (10th ed.). Philadelphia: Wolters Kluwer.

American Council on Exercise (2020). *The Exercise Professional's Guide to Personal Training.* San Diego: American Council on Exercise.

American Council on Exercise (2015). *ACE Medical Exercise Specialist Manual.* San Diego: American Council on Exercise.

CHAPTER 6

ACE Integrated Fitness Training Model

LEARNING OBJECTIVES

After reading this chapter, you will be able to:

▸ Describe the components of the ACE Integrated Fitness Training® (ACE IFT®) Model and how they apply to older adults of various levels of functional ability

▸ Explain the differences among individuals who are at different points along the function–health–fitness–performance continuum

▸ Describe important considerations for training older adults and provide general strategies for how to approach those considerations through exercise programming for the senior population

Safe and effective programming for older adults requires integrating knowledge of their unique needs with appropriate assessment procedures and exercise techniques, giving special attention to program implementation. This chapter facilitates this integration of concepts by first providing specific strategies for determining current levels of function, identifying and prioritizing specific needs at each functional level, and then providing general programming guidelines that effectively meet these needs without exposing participants to unnecessary risks.

This chapter also introduces the ACE Integrated Fitness Training (ACE IFT) Model, which provides health coaches and exercise professionals with a systematic and comprehensive approach to exercise programming. Special considerations and practical guidelines for the older client are discussed as well.

Exercise professionals are seeing an influx of clientele with an increasingly long list of special needs. Furthermore, the vast heterogeneous characteristics of older adults makes designing an appropriate exercise program for this clientele even more complex.

Both novice and veteran exercise professionals are well aware of the positive benefits exercise can yield in improving health, fitness, mood, cognition, weight management, stress management, quality of life, and other health-related parameters. The *Physical Activity Guidelines for Americans* reinforce these positive benefits by acknowledging that regular exercise is a critical component of good health for people of all ages and that individuals can reduce their risk of developing chronic disease by staying physically active and participating in structured exercise on a regular basis (U.S. Department of Health & Human Services, 2018). The guidelines specifically state that regular physical activity (any bodily movement caused by the contraction of skeletal muscle) and/or exercise (physical activity that is planned, repetitive, structured, and performed with a goal of improving fitness or health) will help prevent, slow, or delay many common diseases, such as **type 2 diabetes, cardiovascular disease** (including heart failure, **stroke,** and heart attack), **hypertension,** and the health risks associated with **obesity.**

The *Physical Activity Guidelines for Americans* suggest that adults participate in cardiorespiratory physical activity at a moderate intensity for at least 150 minutes per week or a vigorous intensity for at least 75 minutes per week, or an equivalent combination of both moderate and vigorous activity to experience substantial health benefits. In addition, it is recommended that adults incorporate muscle-strengthening activities at least two days a week. While this document endorses physical activity and exercise as a means to achieve good health, it does not provide specific instructions for how to exercise (U.S. Department of Health & Human Services, 2018). Table 6-1 provides examples of physical activities for older adults.

In addition, exercise guidelines exist for individuals with special considerations, including people who have cardiovascular disease, pulmonary disease, metabolic disease,

TABLE 6-1
Examples of Physical Activities for Older Adults

Aerobic Activities	Muscle-strengthening Activities
▸ Walking or hiking ▸ Dancing ▸ Swimming ▸ Water aerobics ▸ Jogging or running ▸ Aerobic exercise classes ▸ Some forms of yoga ▸ Bicycle riding (stationary or outdoors) ▸ Some yard work, such as raking and pushing a lawn mower ▸ Sports like tennis or basketball ▸ Walking as part of golf	▸ Strengthening exercises using exercise bands, weight machines, or hand-held weights ▸ Body-weight exercises (push-ups, pull-ups, planks, squats, lunges) ▸ Digging, lifting, and carrying as part of gardening ▸ Carrying groceries ▸ Some yoga postures ▸ Some forms of tai chi

Reprinted from U.S. Department of Health & Human Services (2018). *Physical Activity Guidelines for Americans* (2nd ed.). www.health.gov/paguidelines/

hypertension, **dyslipidemia, osteoporosis,** and a variety of other special needs. These guidelines are based on medical and scientific research, are published by the governing body of practitioners for each respective group, and provide specific exercise guidelines to help these individuals improve their health and quality of life. So how does an exercise professional pull it all together? How does a novice or even an experienced exercise professional know which assessments to perform, when to perform them, which guidelines are most important, when to address foundational imbalances in posture or movement, and how to progress or modify a program based on observed and reported feedback?

To address these questions and more, the American Council on Exercise developed the ACE IFT Model to provide exercise professionals with a systematic and comprehensive approach to exercise programming that integrates assessments and programming to facilitate behavioral change, while also improving posture, movement, flexibility, balance, core function, cardiorespiratory fitness, and **muscular fitness.**

Function–Health–Fitness–Performance Continuum

The function–health–fitness–performance continuum is based on the premise that human movement and fitness can progress and regress along a spectrum that starts with developing or reestablishing basic functional movements and extends to performing highly advanced and specialized movements and physical work seen in athletics (Figure 6-1). Each individual is at a unique point on this continuum based upon factors that include health status and physical limitations; frequency, intensity, and types of physical activities; and any participation in, and goals for, athletic performance. Both lifecycle and lifestyle factors can influence where an individual currently falls on the continuum.

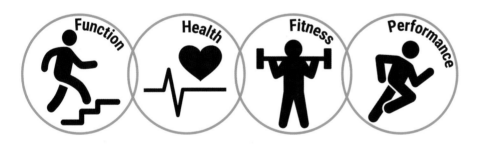

FIGURE 6-1
The function–health–fitness–performance continuum

Lifecycle factors include infant and child development, adolescent and pubescent growth spurts, adulthood, pregnancy, and aging. Early child development is focused primarily on gaining the strength, stability, and balance to perform basic human functional movements like holding one's head up, rolling over, sitting, crawling, standing, and eventually taking first steps. As children grow, their movements help them to build healthier bodies and develop the fitness to jump, climb, and run longer and faster. As adolescents and teens, human development includes considerable skeletal growth and muscular development. This developmental progression helps people progress from low-functioning infants to young adults who have good health, fitness, and even some performance-related skills and abilities. Unfortunately, far too often, lifestyle factors (e.g., smoking, excessive alcohol consumption, poor nutrition, and inadequate sleep and physical activity) disrupt natural human development, resulting in individuals regressing along the continuum to where they are less fit, are at risk for, or have, chronic disease and other health issues, and may even have impaired functional movement.

While the function–health–fitness–performance continuum is not a training method, exercise professionals can utilize this concept to understand that clients ebb and flow along this continuum based on the lifecycle and lifestyle factors that are impacting, positively or negatively, their opportunities for, and participation in, physical activity. Professionals can help clients progress along this continuum by meeting them where they are and providing personalized exercise programs and coaching based on each client's current health, fitness, and goals.

An exercise professional working with a client who has difficulties performing activities of daily living (ADL) should first establish goals aimed at helping the client improve basic functional movements. If a client has been insufficiently active for an extended period or is at risk for health issues, the professional should provide the client with personalized programming that improves both health and functional movements. Exercise professionals working with clients who have adequate functional movements and health can help them to improve fitness and, if appropriate, incorporate performance-related exercises.

Introduction to the ACE Integrated Fitness Training Model

Meeting each client's personalized needs can be a welcome challenge for an experienced exercise professional—and at the same time a potentially confusing and frustrating endeavor for a newly certified exercise professional. While the function–health–fitness–performance continuum provides a suggested sequence for training clients ranging from physically inactive to performance-oriented, it does not address the individual components of fitness and how they fit together.

The ACE IFT Model is a comprehensive system for exercise programming that pulls together the multifaceted training parameters required to be a successful exercise professional. It organizes the latest exercise science and health-behavior research into a systematic approach to designing, implementing, and modifying exercise programs based on the unique abilities, needs, and goals of each individual. Since its launch in 2010, the ACE IFT Model has evolved to incorporate new evidence-based practices in fitness assessments, exercise programming, and coaching skills. It has also evolved, based on user feedback, into a model that is just as robust in terms of science, content, and comprehensive programming, while being simplified in its presentation and terminology.

The ACE IFT Model has two training components:

- ▸ Cardiorespiratory Training
- ▸ Muscular Training

Each training component has three phases that are named to accurately reflect the training focus of each phase (Figure 6-2). The two training components of the ACE IFT Model feature evidence-based exercise programming and progressions, along with associated fitness and functional assessments, that produce physiological adaptations to exercise that improve function, health, fitness, and performance. The training components are independent of each other, allowing for the integration of any Cardiorespiratory Training phase with any Muscular Training phase to meet the personalized health and fitness goals and capabilities of each client. This adaptable programming allows the ACE IFT Model to be used with everyone from **previously physically inactive** clients who have limited exercise experience to high-performance endurance athletes who have poor postural stability and seasoned weight lifters who have low cardiorespiratory fitness.

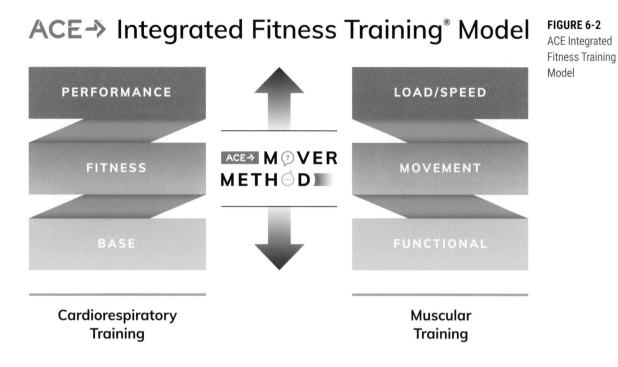

FIGURE 6-2
ACE Integrated Fitness Training Model

The ACE IFT Model also provides exercise professionals with tools and methods to help clients make fitness-related behavior changes that facilitate physical-activity participation and adherence to make lasting improvements in health and well-being. The ACE IFT Model is introduced here and detailed further in Chapter 8.

CARDIORESPIRATORY TRAINING

The ACE IFT Model provides a systematic approach to cardiorespiratory training that can help move a client all the way from being physically inactive to training for a personal record in an event like a half marathon. While this will not be a training goal of most previously physically inactive individuals, having an organized system of training that can allow for long-term progression is empowering for exercise professionals because it provides them with strategies for training the entire spectrum of clientele—from the physically inactive person to the competitive athlete.

The Cardiorespiratory Training component of the ACE IFT Model is divided into three phases, each with a title that defines its training focus (see Figure 6-2). An overview of the primary objectives of Base, Fitness, and Performance Training follows, with detailed information about cardiorespiratory assessments and programming associated with each training phase presented in Chapters 7 and 8.

Base Training

Base Training is focused on developing an initial aerobic base in clients who have been insufficiently active. This should not be confused with the "aerobic-base training" that

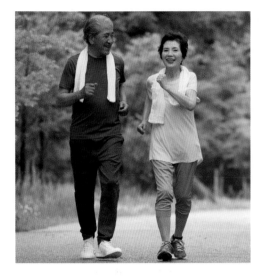

is performed by endurance athletes as the foundation of their offseason training. Instead, it is focused on getting people to move consistently to establish basic cardiorespiratory endurance to improve health, energy, mood, and caloric expenditure and to serve as a foundation for progressing to Fitness Training.

Any client who is not consistently performing moderate-intensity cardiorespiratory exercise for bouts of at least 20 minutes on at least three days per week should begin with Base Training. The initial cardiorespiratory exercise performed should be of an appropriate duration and intensity that the client can tolerate. Exercise professionals can learn about their clients' current cardiorespiratory exercise participation during the initial interview process. No cardiorespiratory assessments are recommended during the Base Training phase, since many of the clients who start in this phase will be unfit and may have difficulty completing an assessment of this nature.

A client who has been physically inactive for an extended period might only be able to initially perform five minutes of continuous cardiorespiratory exercise at a moderate or low-to-moderate intensity. In a scenario of this nature, the exercise professional should give the client positive feedback for completing the five-minute exercise bout, remind the client that bouts of physical activity of any length are beneficial in reducing health risks, and document the total time completed. This would serve as the client's baseline cardiorespiratory fitness data and the starting point for Cardiorespiratory Training progressions to build an aerobic base.

Regardless of the initial duration, the goal for all clients in Base Training is to create early positive exercise experiences to help clients become regular exercisers while gradually increasing exercise duration and frequency until the client is performing cardiorespiratory exercise three to five days per week for a duration of 20 minutes or more. The easiest method for monitoring intensity with clients during Base Training is to use the **talk test.** If the client can perform the exercise and talk comfortably, they are likely below the **first ventilatory threshold (VT1).** When exercising below VT1, clients should be exercising at a moderate intensity classified by a rating of perceived exertion (RPE) of 3 to 4 (0 to 10 scale) (see Chapter 8).

Fitness Training

Fitness Training is focused on enhancing the client's aerobic efficiency by progressing the program through increased duration of sessions, increased frequency of sessions when possible, and the integration of exercise performed at and above VT1. The inclusion of cardiorespiratory exercise performed at and above VT1 allows exercise professionals to blend moderate-intensity exercise (below VT1) with moderate- to vigorous-intensity exercise [at or above VT1 to just below the **second ventilatory threshold (VT2)**; RPE = 5 to 6 on the 0 to 10 scale] in a client's program to create variety and facilitate physiological adaptations leading to greater cardiorespiratory fitness levels. Both new and existing clients who can consistently perform moderate-intensity physical activity for bouts of 20 minutes or more on at least three days per week can perform Fitness Training. As with Base Training, the initial Fitness Training program should be performed at an appropriate duration, intensity, and frequency for the client based on their current level of exercise participation.

Exercise professionals can incorporate intervals into exercise programs for clients with Fitness Training goals to add variety to individual sessions and to introduce more intense training stimuli to elicit desired physiological adaptations to exercise. Professionals should keep in mind each client's current cardiorespiratory fitness level when selecting interval intensities and durations to ensure that the increased challenge is appropriate for the client. By providing clients with intervals that offer increased yet achievable challenges, exercise professionals can help their clients simultaneously increase fitness and self-efficacy.

Individual goals for Fitness Training will vary greatly among clients. Those looking to improve fitness and overall health can benefit from increased exercise frequency, duration, and the introduction of intervals. Clients with goals for longer endurance events, such as completing a 10K run or a half marathon, will need to include some exercise sessions of longer duration to reach the total exercise duration required to complete the event. Exercise professionals can help each client work toward their unique goals by manipulating training variables and then adjusting them regularly based on the client's progress, recovery, challenges, and timeline. Many clients will spend years focused on various cardiorespiratory goals within Fitness Training, while those with endurance performance–oriented goals should be progressed to Performance Training.

Performance Training

Individuals who progress to Performance Training will have goals that are focused on success in endurance sports and events. This may include achieving a personal record in a cycling, swimming, or rowing event, running a local marathon in a time that qualifies them for a national-level event, or finishing top-five at a state or national championship. In these examples, the training programs will progress beyond the parameters of fitness to focus on performance through increased **speed, power,** and endurance. Performance Training requires adequate training volume to prepare clients to comfortably complete their events. This is only the first step, as clients focused on Performance Training will have goals that go far beyond simply finishing an event. To help them achieve higher-level performance goals, professionals will want to continue building on the moderate- and vigorous-intensity exercise in their programs while integrating intervals that push clients up to and beyond VT2, where efforts are of very high intensity (RPE = 7 to 10 on the 0 to 10 scale) and short duration. Exercise professionals can help clients advance their endurance performance by designing programs that include periodized training plans, with each day's training focused on specific variables such as distance, recovery, increased speed, or improved power. Periodized training plans allow professionals to manipulate key training variables, including total training volume, as well as frequency and duration of intervals performed both between VT1 and just below VT2 and at or above VT2, to help each client reach their unique performance goals. As a client's total weekly training time increases, a greater percentage of their training time will typically be at moderate intensities to accommodate the increased training volume and to allow for recovery from higher-intensity interval-training sessions. Table 6-2 provides a summary of the three phases of Cardiorespiratory Training.

TABLE 6-2
Cardiorespiratory Training

Base Training	▶ Focus on moderate-intensity cardiorespiratory exercise (RPE = 3 to 4), while keeping an emphasis on enjoyment.
	▶ Keep intensities below the talk-test threshold (below VT1).
	▶ Increase duration and frequency of exercise bouts.
	▶ Progress to Fitness Training when the client can complete at least 20 minutes of cardiorespiratory exercise below the talk test threshold at least three times per week.
Fitness Training	▶ Progress cardiorespiratory exercise duration and frequency based on the client's goals and available time.
	▶ Integrate vigorous-intensity (RPE = 5 to 6) cardiorespiratory exercise intervals with segments performed at intensities below, at, and above VT1 to just below VT2.
Performance Training	▶ Progress moderate- and vigorous-intensity cardiorespiratory exercise.
	▶ Program sufficient volume for the client to achieve goals.
	▶ Integrate near-maximal and maximal intensity (RPE = 7 to 10) intervals performed at and above VT2 to increase aerobic capacity, speed, and performance.
	▶ Periodized training plans can be used to incorporate adequate training time below VT1, from VT1 to just below VT2, and at or above VT2.

Note: RPE = Rating of perceived exertion (0 to 10 scale); VT1 = First ventilatory threshold; VT2 = Second ventilatory threshold

MUSCULAR TRAINING

The Muscular Training component of the ACE IFT Model provides a systematic approach to training that starts with helping clients improve poor postural stability and **kinetic chain** mobility, and then incorporates programming and progressions to help people train for general fitness, strength, body building, and athletic performance. While many clients will not progress to training for athletic performance, using a training model that provides the exercise professional with the knowledge and tools to work with clients across a broad spectrum of movement skills and challenges is empowering. The ACE IFT Model Muscular Training component is divided into three phases, each with a title that defines its training focus (see Figure 6-2).

An overview of the primary objectives of Functional, Movement, and Load/Speed Training follows, while detailed information about muscular fitness assessments and programming associated with each training phase is presented in Chapters 7 and 8.

Functional Training

Functional Training focuses on the Muscular Training goals of establishing, or in many cases reestablishing, postural stability and kinetic chain mobility through the introduction of exercise programs that improve joint function through improved **muscular endurance,** flexibility, core function, static balance, and dynamic balance. This basic muscular function is typically gained as part of normal child development. Unfortunately, physical inactivity coupled with an increasingly technology-driven world has resulted in more adults having compromised posture, balance, and muscular function. Exercise selection for Functional

Training focuses on core and balance exercises that improve the strength and function of the muscles responsible for stabilizing the spine and **center of gravity (COG)** during static positions and dynamic movements. Exercises for Functional Training will initially use primarily body-weight resistance. As clients progress to Movement Training and Load/Speed Training, it is important to still include Functional Training exercises in their workouts. These can be included as part of either the warm-up or cool-down, or by incorporating progressions that increase the challenge of the Functional Training exercises by increasing the resistance or balance challenges.

Movement Training

The primary focus of Movement Training is on helping clients develop good movement patterns without compromising postural or joint stability. Movement Training focuses on the five primary movement patterns (Figure 6-3):

▸ *Bend-and-lift movements:* These movements are performed throughout the day as a person sits, stands, or squats down to lift an object off the floor.

▸ *Single-leg movements:* These movements involve single-leg balance and movement as performed during walking or going up and down stairs. In addition, lunging movements are performed when a person steps forward to reach down with one hand to pick up something small off the floor.

FIGURE 6-3
Five primary movement patterns

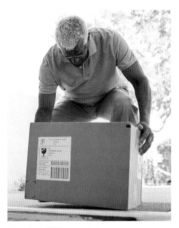
Bend-and-lift movement

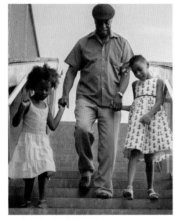
Single-leg movement

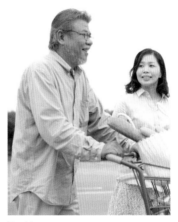
Pushing movement

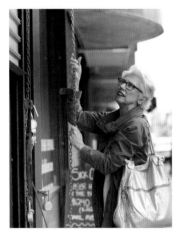
Pulling movement

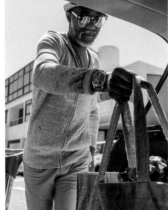
Rotational movement

▶ *Pushing movements:* These upper-body movements occur in four primary directions: forward (e.g., when pushing open a door), overhead (e.g., lifting something to a high shelf), **lateral** (e.g., lifting one's torso when getting up from a side-lying position), and downward (e.g., pushing oneself up and out of the side of a swimming pool).

▶ *Pulling movements:* These movements occur during exercises like a seated row or pull-up, or when pulling open a door.

▶ *Rotational movements:* These movements often occur in the torso as force transfers from the legs to the arms (e.g., throwing a ball) or during twisting movements like a dancer performing pirouettes or a golfer striking a ball.

Movement Training exercises should emphasize the proper sequencing of movements and control of the body's COG throughout the normal range of motion (ROM) being performed. Exercise professionals should integrate Functional Training exercises into Movement Training programs to help clients maintain and improve postural stability and kinetic chain mobility, as they are essential for performing the five primary movement patterns well. One option for including Functional Training exercises is to add them to the warm-up to prepare the body for the more rigorous movements that follow. Body-weight exercises are often used initially during Movement Training, with external resistance introduced typically to build muscular endurance with an emphasis on controlled motion. Professionals should make sure that clients can perform the five primary movement patterns well before adding external loads to the movement patterns to decrease the risk of injury that can result from loading poorly executed movements.

Load/Speed Training

The broad focus of Load/Speed Training is on applying external loads to movements that create a need for increased force production that results in muscular adaptations. Loads can be applied through resistance training, **high-intensity interval training (HIIT),** speed work, **plyometrics,** power lifting, and other sport-specific resistance (e.g., using swim training paddles or pedaling large gears while cycling uphill).

As with Movement Training, Load/Speed Training should integrate Functional Training exercises to help clients maintain and enhance postural stability and kinetic chain mobility to adequately support the increased workloads and force production. Load/Speed Training also integrates the five primary movements that are the focus of Movement Training, with the emphasis being on loading the movements through different planes of motion, angles, speeds, and combined movements.

Clients can have a variety of individual goals that are reached through Load/Speed Training. Fitness-related goals for this type of training include muscular strength, muscular endurance, muscle **hypertrophy,** decreased risk of **sarcopenia** and frailty, and positive changes in body composition. Exercise professionals can help clients reach their fitness-related Load/Speed Training goals by designing exercise programs for each client that incorporate appropriate muscular-training variables, including exercise selection and the frequency and intensity with which each exercise is performed.

Clients who have athletic performance goals can benefit from training that builds speed, **agility, quickness,** and power. Before advancing to training for athletic performance goals, clients should consistently exhibit good postural stability, kinetic chain mobility, and movement patterns. They should also have a good foundation of muscular strength to produce and control the force generated during athletic performance–focused exercises and drills. Exercise selection for clients with athletic performance goals can include power lifting, plyometrics, speed work, and drills for agility, coordination, and quickness.

Table 6-3 provides a summary of the three phases of Muscular Training.

TABLE 6-3
Muscular Training

Functional Training	<ul><li>Focus on establishing/reestablishing postural stability and kinetic chain mobility.</li><li>Exercise programs should improve muscular endurance, flexibility, core function, and static and dynamic balance.</li><li>Progress exercise volume and challenge as function improves.</li></ul>
Movement Training	<ul><li>Focus on developing good movement patterns without compromising postural or joint stability.</li><li>Programs should include exercises for all five primary movement patterns in varied planes of motion.</li><li>Integrate Functional Training exercises to help clients maintain and improve postural stability and kinetic chain mobility.</li></ul>
Load/Speed Training	<ul><li>Focus on application of external loads to movements to create increased force production to meet desired goals.</li><li>Integrate the five primary movement patterns through exercises that load them in different planes of motion and combinations.</li><li>Integrate Functional Training exercises to enhance postural stability and kinetic chain mobility to support increased workloads.</li><li>Programs should focus on adequate resistance-training loads to help clients reach muscular strength, endurance, and hypertrophy goals.</li><li>Clients with goals for athletic performance will integrate exercises and drills to build speed, agility, quickness, and power.</li></ul>

Applications for Older Adults

As individuals age, their motivations to begin, continue, or modify an exercise program may change. A competitive athlete may increase their interest in injury prevention, an occasional exerciser may choose to introduce more consistency to improve bone mineral density, and a previously physically inactive individual may elect to begin a program to improve declining health markers. Often, older adults have more time and sufficient financial stability to work with a health coach or exercise professional in creating a safe and effective exercise program, which makes serving this population a great business opportunity.

Although it is not yet possible to describe in detail exercise programs that will optimize physical functioning and health in all older adults, evidence suggests that the benefits of physical activity can minimize the physiological effects of aging that reduce exercise capacity and risk of physical disability that are often apparent with a sedentary lifestyle (Hamer, Lavoie, & Bacon, 2014).

The recommendations for exercise for older adults are consistent with the *Physical Activity Guidelines for Americans*, which state that regular physical activity is essential for healthy aging. Adults aged 65 years and older gain substantial health benefits from participation in regular physical activity, and it is never too late to start being more physically active. Moreover, promoting physical activity for older adults is especially important because this population is the least physically active of any age group (U.S. Department of Health & Human Services, 2018).

In general, exercise programming for older adults should include cardiorespiratory, muscle strengthening, balance, and flexibility exercises. Furthermore, individuals who are at risk for falling or mobility impairment should perform specific exercises to improve gait and coordination in addition to the other components of health-related physical fitness.

DEPENDENT/FRAIL OLDER ADULTS

The concept of frailty was briefly introduced in Chapter 3 as it relates to the physical-function continuum (see Figure 3-1, page 70). Although there are no clear definitions for the terms "frail" and "frailty" in the literature, the World Health Organization (WHO) defines frailty as a recognizable state in which the ability of older people to cope with acute or everyday stressors is compromised by increased vulnerability brought by age-associated declines in physical function and reserve across multiple organ systems (WHO, 2017). The components of frailty include physiological, psychological, social, and environmental factors (e.g., sarcopenia, functional impairment, cognitive impairment, and **depression**). From an exercise professional's perspective, the model first proposed by Fried et al. (2001) has practical application implications, as it encompasses five indicators of physical frailty: muscle weakness, subjective fatigue, reduced physical activity, slow gait speed, and weight loss (WHO, 2017). Using the criteria proposed by Fried and colleagues (2001), older adults presenting with no indicators for frailty are considered robust, up to two indicators are pre-frail, and three or more are considered frail.

Regardless of how it is defined, frailty can be treated to prevent the social and economic burden associated with this syndrome. Mounting evidence suggests that the adoption of a healthier lifestyle, including exercise interventions and good nutrition, can be used to restore and/or maintain functional ability and intrinsic capacity in older adults and may potentially prevent, delay, or reverse the frailty process (U.S. Department of Health & Human Services, 2018; WHO, 2017). In fact, the American College of Sports Medicine (ACSM) position stand on exercise and physical activity for older adults recommends that exercise programming for frail people is more beneficial than any other intervention (ACSM, 2009). Although specific program-design parameters are not provided, the ACSM guidelines also recommend that muscular and/or balance training should precede cardiorespiratory training for this population. The *Physical Activity Guidelines for Americans* suggest that multicomponent physical-activity programs performed on at least three days per week for 30 to 45 minutes for at least three to five months are most effective for increasing functional ability in frail older adults (U.S. Department of Health & Human Services, 2018).

A combination of cardiorespiratory- and muscular-training activities is more effective than either form of training alone in counteracting the detrimental effects of a sedentary lifestyle on the health and functioning of the cardiovascular and musculoskeletal systems in older adults (Hurst et al., 2019). Furthermore, higher-intensity exercise (rather than low-intensity activities) produces better treatment outcomes for several established diseases and geriatric syndromes (e.g., type 2 diabetes, clinical depression, **osteopenia,** sarcopenia, memory loss, and muscle weakness) (ACSM, 2009). However, it should be noted that lower-intensity programs provide enough exercise stimulus to reduce the risks of developing chronic cardiovascular and metabolic disease. Exercise professionals should consider these findings when developing exercise programs for older clients and approach program design with the intent to progress them along the function–health–fitness–performance continuum as far as they can safely and effectively do so. That is, once a client has made the appropriate physical gains to tolerate the minimum levels

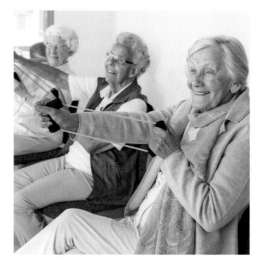

of recommended physical activity (e.g., 150 minutes per week), progressively increasing exercise intensity, whether through increased cardiorespiratory exertion or increased muscle-strengthening loads or volumes, is appropriate.

INDEPENDENT OLDER ADULTS

Individuals further along the function–health–fitness–performance continuum range from community-dwelling seniors who are able to independently perform ADL to those who are physically fit due to the continued performance of regular physical activity. Older adults in this population group fall within the health and fitness categories of the function–health–fitness–performance continuum. This group makes up the largest contingent of older adults, and also represents the largest variances in physical-fitness characteristics, which supports the notion that older adults are among the most heterogeneous population groups. As such, exercise professionals need to carefully interview and screen all older adults they service, as "one-size-fits-all" programming must be avoided. Furthermore, exercise professionals will most likely work with independent older adults (versus dependent/frail individuals), as they are more mobile and able to meet for exercise sessions at fitness facilities or other community locations. That said, clients of all levels of function may opt for virtual training sessions, where they exercise in their own homes while the health coach or exercise professional coaches or trains them via the internet. While leading exercise sessions remotely can provide some challenges, it can also be an empowering and effective way to reach clients who might not otherwise have the opportunity to work with an exercise professional.

FIT/ELITE OLDER ADULTS

Fit/elite older adults make up the smallest percentage of the senior population group. These highly fit seniors train on an almost daily basis to compete in sport tournaments, work in physically demanding jobs, or participate in recreational activities. They require exercise programming that helps them maintain their fitness levels and provides conditioning for improved performance in competition or in strenuous vocational or recreational activities. Programming should include general conditioning for muscular strength and endurance, flexibility, agility, and cardiovascular endurance. It also may include sport- or activity-specific training. Older adults at this level of fitness fall within the performance category of the function–health–fitness–performance continuum.

Supplying physically elite seniors with information concerning the adverse effects of **overtraining** and the need for appropriate recovery periods between workouts will help them prevent injury while training and competing. In addition, it is important to provide strategies for addressing injuries if they do occur.

⊶ EXPAND YOUR KNOWLEDGE ──────

Attracting Senior Clients to Fitness Programs: Marketing Strategies

Many older adults have the time to become loyal fitness participants while striving to maintain independence, health, and fitness. To keep this group engaged, programs need to offer useful information and education. The following list includes some best practices for successfully meeting the needs of older adult participants.

▸ **Programming should be enjoyable and address participant needs.** This strategy is important because fun programming that meets a specific need will keep participants interested and coming back for more. Consistency with physical activity is needed to truly see improvements in quality of life. When creating individual and group programs for older adults, it is important to consider how the programs can be delivered in a fun and safe manner and be mindful of the fact that they should also have a purpose that meets the needs of the clients. This includes offering options for both in-person and virtual or online programs.

▸ **Know and appreciate the uniqueness of the demographic.** When working with older adults, it is important to understand the unique perspectives, goals, and challenges of this population. In addition, it is important to enjoy working with older adults. Participants will appreciate the joy you bring into the individualized and group programming you create. It is also helpful to earn additional training or certifications focused on aging-specific topics.

▸ **Age is just a number, and it does not need a label.** While the older adult population is unique, seniors do not like to be reminded of their uniqueness all the time. It is important to avoid stereotypical names for programs, class names, events, and presentations. Being mindful with naming will enhance inclusiveness, increase comfort, and perhaps encourage other participants to join in the fun. Avoiding the use of stereotypical class descriptors is important and should be a top consideration for meeting the needs of this population and increasing one's ability to meet clients and class participants where they are in life's journey.

Special Considerations for Older Adults

Although there is no single exercise program appropriate for all seniors, multicomponent physical-activity programs that include balance training, muscular training, cardiorespiratory exercise, and flexibility exercise are more effective than doing any single type of activity for improving physical function and should be a focus in all older-adult programming.

BALANCE TRAINING

In Western civilization, falls in the older adult population place a heavy economic burden on society and are responsible for considerably reduced functional independence and quality of life (Jin, 2018). In 2014, 29% of adults 65 and older in the U.S. reported a fall. Falls are the leading cause of injury-related morbidity and mortality, with 37.5% of falls requiring medical treatment or restricted activity for at least one day. In 2015, falls caused an estimated 33,000 deaths, of which 25% occurred within six months if a hip was fractured

(U.S. Preventive Services Task Force, 2018). Falls are the second leading cause of accidental injury death worldwide (WHO, 2018). Annual costs attributed to falls are estimated at $50 billion for nonfatal fall injuries and $754 million on fatal falls, which accounts for 6% of Medicare expenditures, 8% of Medicaid expenditures, and 5% coming from other sources of payment [Centers for Disease Control and Prevention (CDC), 2020; Florence et al., 2018]. Additionally, falls have a critical influence on an individual's health status, especially in the elderly, with over 95% of hip fractures caused by falls (Alshammari et al., 2018). Furthermore, the risk of falling increases with age, a problem that is further exacerbated by the increasing proportion of elderly.

Exercise professionals who competently assess static and dynamic balance in older clients (see Chapter 7) can play a crucial role in identifying gait problems that could lead to falling. Gait instability is a major fall risk factor and walking is one of the most frequent dynamic ADL. Intrinsic factors (particularly impaired balance, loss of mobility, and muscle weakness) have consistently been identified as major risk factors for falling (CDC, 2017). If significant balance and gait deficits are present, the exercise professional should work closely with the client's healthcare provider to develop an exercise intervention strategy to address these problems. Chapter 8 provides in-depth programming guidelines as recommended in the ACE IFT Model for incorporating balance training into an older adult's multicomponent exercise routine.

EXPAND YOUR KNOWLEDGE

Fear of Falling

Unlike physical characteristics that contribute to an individual's balance, the fear of falling is a mindset that can increase an older adult's risk for suffering a fall and decrease quality of life. Many older adults lack confidence in their mobility and, as a result, are constantly afraid of falling, which leads to a restriction or avoidance of daily activities. In their review of the literature, Scheffer et al. (2008) reported that a fear of falling was prevalent in up to 85% of community-dwelling elders older than age 65. Other researchers have reported that the prevalence varies and is highest among those who have had a previous fall, are frail, are at an increased risk for hip fracture, have suffered a previous fall-related fracture, have chronic musculoskeletal pain, or require ambulation aides (Schoene et al., 2019).

The fear of falling manifests itself physically in older adults when they habitually stiffen their joints, causing unnecessary contraction of muscles and a flexed-forward posture. Many elderly people have an exaggerated fear of falling backward and hitting their heads or breaking their backs and hips. Consequently, the flexed-forward posture puts them at a more advantageous position to fall forward if a disruption in balance occurs, thereby resulting in potential fractures to the wrists and arms but protecting their backs and hips. A flexed posture does place the body in a more stable position, but because it requires more muscular force to maintain, there is an increased reliance on muscular strength and endurance.

Impaired mobility contributes to a fear of falling, which in turn can contribute to further decrements in mobility. If an individual is haunted by a fear of falling, they are likely to avoid walking and being physically active, which minimizes the use of the musculoskeletal system, thereby weakening the muscles that play an important role in maintaining balance. This reluctance to be active leads to more immobility and heightens an elderly person's lack of self-confidence in ambulation. Ironically, family and friends of older adults who fall often compound the problem by discouraging walking after a fall. Ultimately, a perceived sense of insecurity related to balance may actually increase the likelihood of a traumatic fall.

Importantly, exercise professionals can play an integral role in helping older adults who have a fear of falling alleviate some of their concerns. Multicomponent physical-activity programs that include balance, gait, coordination, muscle-strengthening, and moderate-intensity cardiorespiratory exercise are most successful at reducing falls and injuries (U.S. Department of Health & Human Services, 2018). A systematic review conducted by Sherrington et al. (2019) of 81 randomized controlled trials showed a 23% reduction in fall rate in those that performed exercise in general and that different types of exercise had different impacts on falls. Balance and functional exercises showed the greatest reduction, while the addition of muscular training probably also reduces fall rate. Furthermore, increased levels of physical activity contribute to improved self-efficacy and decreased fear of falling (Cho et al., 2015). Thus, with each successfully completed workout, exercise professionals can help their older clients who have concerns about falling move one step closer to increased self-confidence and an improved quality of life.

MUSCULAR TRAINING

Sarcopenia and muscular weakness significantly influence the pathogenesis of frailty and functional impairment that occurs with aging and contribute to numerous disease processes. This deterioration, which is typically attributed to reduced levels of activity or disuse due to disease, appears to increase in severity after the age of 65. Moreover, increased longevity has led to a higher frequency of sarcopenia and complications associated with declines in functional health and loss of independence (Shafiee et al., 2017; dos Santos et al., 2016).

However, because strength and muscle mass do not decrease concurrently, strength may be a superior indicator of muscular dysfunction. Indeed, a review of the literature suggests that the contribution of age-related decreased muscle mass to functional decline is mediated primarily by losses in muscle strength. In fact, losses of muscular strength are two to five times greater than decreases in muscle mass with age (Fragala et al., 2019). As such, resistance exercise may serve to directly improve **functional capacity** and could help older adults maintain independence, health, quality of life, and overall well-being (Fragala et al., 2019). For example, in their review of the literature, Fragala et al. (2019) found that participating in muscular training three times a week, with three sets of eight to 12 repetitions at a beginning intensity of 20 to 30% of **one-repetition maximum (1-RM)** and progressing to 80% 1-RM, can result in improved habitual gait velocity, levels of physical activity, and stair-climbing abilities, as well as gains in muscular strength and power and an overall improvement of physical function. In addition, 12 weeks of multicomponent exercise programs that include explosive muscular training can promote greater improvements in functional task performance by improving muscular power output, muscular strength, muscle fat infiltration, and muscle cross sectional area.

Maintaining physical function is directly related to muscular strength and power. In addition, research suggests that physical activity and exercise are associated with independent functioning, preserved quality of life, and delayed disability, with 30 minutes or more of exercise being the most effective for increasing ADL (Fragala et al., 2019). Unfortunately, it has been estimated that only 23% of the U.S. adult population meets physical-activity recommendations for both cardiorespiratory and muscular-strengthening activities (CDC, 2019), with participation rates dramatically lower for individuals aged 65 to 74 (16%), and likely as low as 10% for adults over 75 years old (CDC, 2019). Thus, increased public health efforts to facilitate the provision of muscular training among seniors are certainly warranted.

Exercise professionals can play an important role in promoting the benefits of improving strength through the programming of resistance exercise for their older clients. Programming guidelines following the ACE IFT Model for incorporating muscular training into an older adult's comprehensive exercise program are detailed in Chapter 8.

THINK IT THROUGH

The Importance of Muscular Training

How will you encourage your older clientele to engage in muscular training? Develop a brief explanation of the importance of muscular training for the maintenance of health and function in older adults. Plan on using this explanation in conversations with older clients if they have questions about adopting muscular training as a regular part of their programs.

APPLY WHAT YOU KNOW

Senior-friendly Resistance Exercise Equipment

Although selectorized weight machines are good options to use for older adults who need to increase muscular strength, exercise professionals might not always have access to this type of equipment, especially those who work with seniors in their homes or in retirement communities. In the absence of weight machines, elastic resistance bands and hand-held weights are useful for promoting strength. In addition, they are valuable for providing entry-level resistance work for those unable or unwilling to use machines.

Elastic resistance bands and tubes come in a variety of strengths, from light to heavy resistance. They can be ordered from most fitness supply companies and can be used to help develop both upper- and lower-body strength. Light ankle/wrist weights also are very useful for chair-based senior exercise classes. Ankle/wrist weights are more versatile than hand-held weights because they can be strapped on the ankle or around the wrist or held in the hand. Variable weights can be used individually or added together for increased resistance and work well for most seniors involved in chair exercise.

In the absence of resistance equipment, exercise professionals can use small plastic bottles filled with sand, or other household items such as soup cans, for resistance. Avoid partially filled containers that allow the contents to fall or slosh back and forth during use, and strongly emphasize the importance of proper joint alignment. Holding onto these objects may be awkward and movement of the contents can place undue stress on joints. Another household item—a wooden or plastic dowel—can be used in place of heavier weights or objects to promote proper movement and enhance flexibility in exercises such as the deadlift and shoulder press.

The underlying point to keep in mind is that a variety of objects can be used as part of a muscular-training program. As long as the weight of the object is appropriate for the ability of the exerciser, strength gains will be achieved.

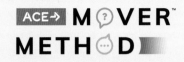

Working with a Client Who Is Hesitant to Progress

You have been working with Carl, a 62-year-old retired grandfather of three, once per week for the past five months. Initially, the focus was on establishing an aerobic base by increasing the frequency and duration of exercise until he was able to complete 20 continuous minutes of cardiorespiratory training, which he is now performing four days each week. During a recent session, the idea of increasing the intensity of cardiorespiratory training came up and Carl made it clear that he does not want to push himself too hard.

ACE→ ABC APPROACH

The following is an example of how the ACE Mover Method™ philosophy and ACE ABC Approach™ can be used to explore a client's hesitation for making changes to an existing exercise program.

Ask: Asking powerful open-ended questions can help the exercise professional find out more about a client's hesitation and current perspective in a nonjudgmental way.

Exercise Professional: You do not want to increase the intensity of your current cardiorespiratory exercise program. What is it about this progression that makes you uncomfortable?

Client: What I am doing currently when we meet for our weekly sessions and doing three times per week on my own feels very safe and appropriate and I am enjoying the addition of physical activity to my life. I am not getting any younger and don't want to push myself like the younger people I see in the gym. Walking or jogging faster does not seem like it would have a benefit for me since I am not at all concerned with competition. Making exercise harder does not seem wise to me.

Exercise Professional: Feeling comfortable and safe while exercising is important to you and the idea of increasing your intensity does not appear to have value. From where we started five months ago, you have already increased how often and for how long you can exercise and you are doing a great job! The program we have been working on mirrors movements you do in your daily life and enhances the function of your cardiorespiratory system to allow you to be more active for longer. Considering a typical week, how and when do you perform activities that require different levels of intensity?

Client: I do see how the movements we have been working on are similar to movements I do throughout my day and I have noticed that some of them are happening with less fatigue and I feel more confident. Moving feels less risky. When it comes to doing an activity at different intensities in a typical week, an example I can think of is yardwork, which includes everything from manually mowing the lawn to using heavy equipment to remove tree branches. However, I think the best reflection of this is when I am with my grandchildren. One minute, we are sitting down and the next minute they want to run around or race me in the swimming pool or in the yard. My grandkids are highly active and like me to go with them on walks, hikes, and bike rides. They are definitely my motivation for improving my health

Break down barriers: Ask additional open-ended questions to find out more about why the client does not want to act.

Exercise Professional: You can think of plenty of real-life examples involving changes in intensity and you are not sure that increasing the intensity of your current cardiorespiratory exercise will benefit you. The good news is that you can see improvement and the results of what we have been doing. What do you know about how the body adapts to the different demands that take place during exercise?

Client: I am not sure I know that much about how my body is changing due to exercise. One thing I can tell you though is that five months ago I was having a hard time completing a 10-minute bike ride or walk without having to take a break or sit for a few minutes. At this point, I can walk for at least 20 minutes without stopping and I am not completely exhausted afterward. In fact, I can now cover more distance in a 20-minute period than I could even a month ago. I think that means I am getting faster. Are there other changes that you think I should know about?

Exercise Professional: What you have described are some of the common changes you can expect to take place with exercise. If you recall, some of your initial goals were to increase the frequency and duration of exercise, which you have done! The body adapts to exercise in different ways and you have made some keen observations about these changes. You have noticed that you can exercise more often and for longer without stopping, have less exhaustion after exercise, and can cover more distance in a given amount of time. These changes mean that your body is adapting to the demands you are placing on it with exercise and you are moving more consistently and improving your endurance. Covering more distance in the same amount of time also lets us know that you are moving more quickly or walking at a greater intensity. You have naturally started to increase your intensity and your body is adapting positively! We will continue the work you are doing and gradually add different levels of intensity to your program that are personalized to your goals, abilities, and needs. Does all of this make sense to you?

Client: That is extremely helpful! I guess I did not consider the fact that moving faster means I am already working at a greater intensity. I did not realize that even at this age my body would respond so well to exercise. When you say increasing the exercise intensity will be personalized to me, what does that mean?

Exercise Professional: Great question! This means that we will always work within your ability level and plan our program according to your goals and needs. For example, a next step for us will be to assess a personalized marker of intensity based on your ability to talk while exercising. We will use that marker to gradually introduce some safe and appropriate intervals into your existing program that will bring your heart rate above that marker for a period and then back down to recover. You will always be in control of how hard you push yourself and can slow down or stop at any time. We will make sure this is something you can work on during our sessions together and that you have all the information to safely do this on your own, as well. Some of this training will mirror activities you described with your grandchildren in that it is stop-and-go exercise, where you are moving at one intensity and the next thing you know you are being challenged to a foot race. Remember, this is your program and you are the expert on yourself. It is my job to ensure that we are pairing evidence-based information with your goals to make sure we are on the right track and following the path that you ultimately choose.

Collaborate: Working together, find out what the client would like to do next now that he has more information and his concerns have been addressed.

Exercise Professional: Now that we have discussed how you are already increasing the intensity of your walks and how this relates to the activities you do with yardwork and with your grandchildren, how would you like to move forward with progressing your exercise program?

Client: This conversation was enlightening, and I appreciate you walking through my hesitation with me. I think I have a better understanding of what you mean by increasing my intensity through a personalized approach. At this point, I would like to assess the intensity marker you were telling me about and see what adding intervals to my existing program feels like. I am excited about this new progression! Is there still time during today's session to try it?

Exercise Professional: I appreciate your enthusiasm and I think we are on the same page! Today we can continue with our planned session and I can share with you more information about the assessment we will be doing that will allow us to program effective intervals. If it sounds good to you, I will show you what an interval looks like and we can do the assessment at our next session. Please let me know if you have any questions or concerns along the way. Let's get started!

In this example, the exercise professional observed a hesitation about programming from the client and used the ACE Mover Method philosophy and ACE ABC Approach to get on the same page with the client. The professional in this scenario respected the client's autonomy and explored the client's concerns without judgement and while using reflections and providing information when needed. Ultimately, the client remained in control of how the program moved forward and the professional was there to guide and support.

CARDIORESPIRATORY TRAINING

Cardiorespiratory fitness is a modifiable risk factor for long-term mortality. Increased cardiorespiratory fitness is associated with increased survival regardless of age and greater amounts of cardiorespiratory fitness is most notably beneficial and associated with long-term mortality in older adults (Mandsager et al., 2018). Cardiorespiratory fitness is considered a clinical vital sign by the American Heart Association (AHA) because of the link to cardiovascular disease risk and is an important predictor of health outcomes because it represents the ability of the body to transport oxygen from the atmosphere to the **mitochondria** to support physical work and is linked to pulmonary function, ventricular function, ventricular-arterial coupling (cardiovascular efficiency), efficient transport of blood from the heart to match demands for oxygen, and the ability of muscles to receive and use oxygen (Ross et al., 2016). In individuals 70 years or older, a higher capacity to perform a maximal treadmill exercise test is associated with reduction in all-cause mortality and may lead to reductions in overall frailty and continued physical independence (Mandsager et al., 2018). These findings support the aerobic hypothesis of Koch and Britton (2008)—a theory stating that the diminished capacity for energy transfer of oxygen at all levels of biological organization underlies complex disease, accelerated aging, and diminished longevity.

Physiological factors that are most frequently associated with longevity and successful aging include low blood pressure, low body mass index and central adiposity, preserved glucose tolerance, and a healthy blood lipid profile consisting of low triglyceride, low **low-density lipoprotein (LDL)** cholesterol, and high **high-density lipoprotein (HDL)** cholesterol concentrations (Waaijer et al., 2017; Deelen et al., 2016; Morrisette-Thomas et al., 2014). As such, ample evidence suggests that regular physical activity can slow physiologic changes of aging, optimize changes in body composition, promote psychological and cognitive well-being, decrease the risk of physical disability, better manage chronic disease, and increase longevity and quality of life (ACSM, 2018; Langhammer, Bergland, & Rydwik, 2018). In addition, cardiorespiratory exercise in older adults decreases resting and submaximal exercise heart rates, systolic blood pressure (SBP) and diastolic blood pressure, and increases **stroke volume.** Program participation of six months or more is recommended for improvements in cardiorespiratory fitness (Langhammer, Bergland, & Rydwik, 2018).

It is important to note that the acute effects of a single session of cardiorespiratory exercise are relatively short-lived, and the chronic adaptations to repeated sessions of exercise are quickly lost upon cessation of training, even in regularly active older adults (ACSM, 2009). Thus, exercise professionals should encourage their senior clients to participate in some form of cardiorespiratory-based activity on most, if not all, days of the week.

⁘ EXPAND YOUR KNOWLEDGE

Water Exercise

Exercise in the water provides a great alternative for both cardiorespiratory and muscular training for many older adults. Because water's buoyancy negates the impact of exercise, many older adults who cannot safely jog or jump on land can successfully perform those activities in the pool. Accessories made for in-pool use, such as water bells, paddles, webbed gloves, and ankle cuffs, can be incorporated to increase intensity and challenge strength or to provide more buoyancy to help an individual float during certain activities. A water temperature of 83 to 88° F (28 to 31° C) is suitable for most older adults, especially those who suffer from arthritis (ACSM, 2018).

Improved physiological and biomechanical factors affecting gait and performance of ADL have been shown in older adults who participate in a regular water-based functional training program. In a study featuring older adult women, researchers found that a 12-week water-based exercise program that featured three sessions per week resulted in significant increases in lower-body strength, power, flexibility, agility, and balance, and that a training effect was observed through a reduction in body weight and fat mass (Vale et al., 2020; Kim & O'sullivan, 2013). Another 12-week study showed that performing aquatic exercise two times per week at 50 minutes per session contributed to improvements in upper-body explosive strength, fat mass, and SBP (Neiva et al., 2018). Sufferers of chronic knee or hip pain related to **osteoarthritis** who participate in a water-exercise program experience reduced pain, stiffness, and difficulty performing physical functions, as well as improved self-efficacy (Fertelli, Mollaoglu, & Sahin, 2018). Thus, when clients are unable to exercise on land, or find land-based exercise intolerable, aquatic programs can provide an enabling alternative strategy.

For older clients diagnosed with osteoporosis, land-based training is preferable to water exercise for stimulating increases in bone mineral density. However, joint pain and disability may prohibit many clients with osteoporosis from performing functional activities on land. In these individuals, water-based exercise will help maintain or enhance joint ROM. Furthermore, with the use of the pool-based equipment, older adults can improve muscle strength, thereby improving functional abilities and reducing the risk of falls on land.

FLEXIBILITY EXERCISE

Overall flexibility decreases with age and can result in mobility limitations due to decreased ROM at the joints. Regularly performing flexibility exercise may help to alleviate some of the age-related changes in joint ROM, especially for the purposes of correcting or rehabilitating musculoskeletal problems. For example, the aging process tends to modify normal postural alignment, and flexed posture commonly increases with age. Age-related **hyperkyphosis** occurs in 20 to 40% of adults above age 60 and has been attributed to underlying osteoporosis and vertebral fractures (~30%); decreases in muscle mass, quality, and strength; decreased bone mineral density; and connective tissue fragility (Kado et al., 2004). Age-related changes to posture, such as hyperkyphosis, are important to understand because they may impact pulmonary function and physical function and lead to impaired balance and an increased risk for falling (Roghani et al., 2017). However, a focused program featuring both standing and side-lying end-range thoracic **extension** and rotation to mobilize the spine and strengthen supporting musculature in conjunction with stretches for the chest, spine, glutes, quadriceps, and thoracic and cervical spine when performed for eight weeks may improve hyperkyphosis posture and forward-head position (Bahrekazemi, Letafatkar, & Hadadnezhad, 2017).

Apart from corrective or rehabilitative stretching protocols, there is surprisingly little research on the potential benefits of flexibility-specific training for older adults who want to enhance functional abilities and/or experience general health benefits. Despite the lack of research, there is still a tendency in the literature to mention flexibility training as a beneficial adjunct to other forms of exercise. In their systematic review of the functional outcomes of flexibility-specific training in older adults, Stathokostas et al. (2012) found that flexibility-training interventions are often effective at increasing ROM in various joints and improving various functional outcomes in the older population. Research also suggests that the use of dynamic stretching with no load in the older adult population may improve hip **flexion** and hip extension ROM, both immediately post-stretch and for up to 60 minutes after the stretch force has been removed (Zhou et al., 2019). However, due to the incongruency of the protocols reviewed, conclusive recommendations regarding flexibility training specifically for older clientele, such as how long to hold a stretch, how many repetitions of each stretch to perform, and the type of stretches to do, are not available at this point. As such, exercise professionals should approach designing flexibility programs for their older clients based on individual client needs and goals. General stretching methods and protocols for older adults are discussed in Chapter 8.

SUMMARY

The vast heterogeneous characteristics of older adults makes designing an appropriate exercise program for this clientele very complex. Exercise professionals who integrate specific strategies for determining current levels of function, identify and prioritize specific needs at each functional level, and then provide exercise programming that effectively meets those needs without exposing older clients to unnecessary risks will be successful when working with the senior population. Additionally, utilizing the concepts of the ACE IFT Model and the ACE Mover Method philosophy will make the process of program design for an older client even more efficient and straightforward.

REFERENCES

Alshammari, S.A. et al. (2018). Falls among elderly and its relation with their health problems and surrounding environmental factors in Riyadh. *Journal of Family & Community Medicine*, 25, 1, 29–34.

American College of Sports Medicine (2018). *ACSM's Guidelines for Exercise Testing and Prescription* (10th ed.). Philadelphia: Wolters Kluwer.

American College of Sports Medicine (2009). Position stand: Exercise and physical activity for older adults. *Medicine & Science in Sports & Exercise*, 41, 7, 1510–1530.

Bahrekazemi, B., Letafatkar, A., & Hadadnezhad, M. (2017). The effect of eight weeks of global postural corrective exercises on kyphosis and forward head angle in elderly women with age-related hyperkyphosis. *International Journal of Medical Research & Health Sciences*, 6, 9, 40–44.

Centers for Disease Control and Prevention (2020). *Cost of Older Adult Falls.* https://www.cdc.gov/homeandrecreationalsafety/falls/data/fallcost.html

Centers for Disease Control and Prevention (2019). *Early Release of Selected Estimates Based on Data from the 2018 National Health Interview Survey.* https://www.cdc.gov/nchs/nhis/releases/released201905.htm#7A

Centers for Disease Control and Prevention (2017). *Risk Factors for Falls.* https://www.cdc.gov/steadi/pdf/Risk_Factors_for_Falls-print.pdf

Cho, J. et al. (2015). Effects of an evidence-based falls risk-reduction program on physical activity and falls efficacy among oldest-old adults. *Frontiers in Public Health*, 2, 182.

Deelen, J. et al. (2016). Employing biomarkers of healthy ageing for leveraging genetic studies into human longevity. *Experimental Gerontology*, 82, 166–174.

dos Santos, L. et al. (2017). Sarcopenia and physical independence in older adults: The independent and synergic role of muscle mass and muscle function. *Journal of Cachexia, Sarcopenia and Muscle*, 8, 2, 245–250.

Fertelli, T.K., Mollaoglu, M., & Sahin, O. (2018). Aquatic exercise program for individuals with osteoarthritis: Pain, stiffness, physical function, self-efficacy. *Rehabilitation Nursing: The Official Journal of the Association of Rehabilitation Nurses*, 44, DOI: 10.1097/rnj.0000000000000142.

Florence, C.S. et al. (2018). Medical costs of fatal and nonfatal falls in older adults. *Journal of the American Geriatrics Society*, 66, 693–698.

Fragala, M.S. et al. (2019). Resistance training for older adults: Position statement from the National Strength and Conditioning Association. *The Journal of Strength and Conditioning Research*, 33, 8, 2019–2052.

Fried, L.P. et al. (2001). Frailty in older adults: Evidence for a phenotype. *Journals of Gerontology A*, 56, 3, M146–M156.

Hamer, M., Lavoie, K.L., & Bacon, S.L. (2014). Taking up physical activity in later life and healthy ageing: The English longitudinal study of ageing. *British Journal of Sports Medicine*, 48, 239–243.

Hurst, C. et al. (2019). The effects of same-session combined exercise training on cardiorespiratory and functional fitness in older adults: A systematic review and meta-analysis. *Aging Clinical and Experimental Research*, 31, 1701–1717.

Jin, J. (2018). Prevention of falls in older adults. *Journal of the American Medical Association*, 319, 16, 1734.

Kado, D.M. et al. (2004). Hyperkyphotic posture predicts mortality in older community-dwelling men and women: A prospective study. *Journal of the American Geriatric Society*, 52, 1662–1667.

Kim, S.B. & O'sullivan, D.M. (2013). Effects of aqua aerobic therapy exercise for older adults on muscular strength, agility and balance to prevent falling during gait. *Journal of Physical Therapy Science*, 25, 8, 923–927.

Koch, L.G. & Britton, S.L. (2008). Aerobic metabolism underlies complexity and capacity. *Journal of Physiology*, 586, 83–95.

Langhammer, B., Bergland, A., & Rydwik, E. (2018). The importance of physical activity exercise among older people. *BioMed Research International*, Article ID: 7856823.

Mandsager, K. et al. (2018). Association cardiorespiratory fitness with long-term mortality among adults undergoing exercise treadmill testing. *JAMA Network Open*, 1, 6, e183605.

Morrisette-Thomas, V. et al. (2014). Inflamm-aging does not simply reflect increases in pro-inflammatory markers. *Mechanisms of Ageing and Development*, 139, 49–57.

Neiva, H.P. et al. (2018). The effect of 12 weeks of water-aerobics on health status and physical fitness: An ecological approach. *PLoS ONE*, 13, 5, e0198319.

Roghani, T. et al. (2017). Age-related hyperkyphosis: Update of its potential causes and clinical impacts—

Narrative review. *Aging Clinical and Experimental Research*, 29, 4, 567–577.

Ross, R. et al. (2016). Importance of assessing cardiorespiratory fitness in clinical practice: A case for fitness as a clinical vital sign: A scientific statement from the American Heart Association. *Circulation*, 134, 24, e653–e699.

Scheffer, A.C. et al. (2008). Fear of falling: Measurement strategy, prevalence, risk factors and consequences among older persons. *Age & Ageing*, 37, 1, 19–24.

Schoene, D. et al. (2019). A systematic review on the influence of fear of falling on quality of life in older people: Is there a role for falls? *Clinical Interventions in Aging*, 14, 701–719.

Shafiee, G. et al. (2017). Prevalence of sarcopenia in the world: A systematic review and meta-analysis of general population studies. *Journal of Diabetes and Metabolic Disorders*, 16, 21.

Sherrington, C. et al. (2019). Exercise for preventing falls in older people living in the community. *Cochrane Database of Systematic Reviews*, 1, Art. No. CD012424.

Stathokostas, L. et al. (2012). Flexibility training and functional ability in older adults: A systematic review. *Journal of Aging Research*, DOI: 10.1155/2012/306818.

U.S. Department of Health & Human Services (2018). *Physical Activity Guidelines for Americans* (2nd ed.). www.health.gov/paguidelines/

U.S. Preventive Services Task Force (2018). *Falls Prevention in Community-Dwelling Older Adults: Interventions.* https://www. uspreventiveservicestaskforce.org/uspstf/document/ RecommendationStatementFinal/falls-prevention-in-older-adults-interventions

Vale, F.A. et al. (2020). Balance as an additional effect of strength and flexibility aquatic training in sedentary lifestyle elderly women. *Current Gerontology and Geriatrics Research*, Article ID: 1805473.

Waaijer, M.E. et al. (2017). Assessment of health status by molecular measures in adults ranging from middle-aged to old: Ready for clinical use? *Experimental Gerontology*, 87, 175–181.

World Health Organization (2018). *Falls.* https://www. who.int/news-room/fact-sheets/detail/falls

World Health Organization (2017). *WHO Clinical Consortium on Healthy Ageing: Report of Consortium Meeting 1–2 December 2016 in Geneva Switzerland.* Geneva: World Health Organization.

Zhou, W-S. et al. (2019). Effects of dynamic stretching with different loads on hip joint range of motion in the elderly. *Journal of Sports Science and Medicine*, 18, 52–57.

SUGGESTED READINGS

American Council on Exercise (2020). *The Exercise Professional's Guide to Personal Training.* San Diego: American Council on Exercise.

American Council on Exercise (2019). *The Professional's Guide to Health and Wellness Coaching.* San Diego: American Council on Exercise.

American Council on Exercise (2015). *ACE Medical Exercise Specialist Manual.* San Diego: American Council on Exercise.

Centers for Disease Control and Prevention (2015). *A CDC Compendium of Effective Fall Interventions: What Works for Community-Dwelling Older Adults* (3rd ed.). Atlanta, Ga.: Centers for Disease Control and Prevention.

IN THIS CHAPTER

CHAPTER 7
Conducting Assessments

LEARNING OBJECTIVES

After reading this chapter, you will be able to:

▸ Select appropriate health-related resting measurements based on older clients' health history and goals

▸ Administer health-related resting assessments to older clients

▸ Select appropriate fitness assessments for older clients based on their functional abilities

▸ Administer fitness assessments for older clients based on functional abilities and client goals

▸ Implement effective strategies for delivering assessment results to older clients and determining the need for follow-up assessments

As increasing numbers of older adults see the value in becoming more physically active, health coaches and exercise professionals are likely to experience an increase in the number of senior clients. Virtually all healthcare professionals advocate some form of physical activity for the older population. But what does a recommendation to be more physically active mean in terms of practical application? How does an exercise program begin and what determines if it is adequate and appropriate? It all starts with the development of an exercise program, which is the successful integration of exercise science and behavioral support that leads to long-term program compliance and attainment of the individual's goals. The FITT principle (frequency, intensity, time, and type) identifies the components of an exercise program. But how are the questions "How often?" (frequency), "How hard?" (intensity), "How long?" (time/duration), and "Which exercise?" (type) answered? Will an exercise program for an active 80-year-old client with **cardiovascular disease** be the same as that for a 60-year-old client with **diabetes** who has little experience with physical activity?

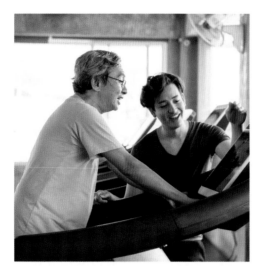

The answers to these questions become clearer during the preparticipation health screen, initial interview (see Chapter 5), and fitness assessment. Though the exercise program is a vital link to improving the quality of older adults' lives, it may not have a chance to succeed without some form of measurement to determine the individual's current fitness and/or functional status. For this reason, selecting and administering appropriate assessments at an appropriate time based on client goals, needs, and abilities allows the exercise professional to develop meaningful, safe, and effective exercise programming. This chapter provides a comprehensive rationale for administering a variety of assessment protocols and details a wide range of measurement and monitoring methods and tools.

The interpretation of assessment results in combination with client goals provides the guiding force for meaningful and effective exercise program design. By using the ACE Integrated Fitness Training® (ACE IFT®) Model, exercise professionals can determine which assessments are most appropriate based on initial placement within the Cardiorespiratory and Muscular Training components of the ACE IFT Model. If, for example, through the pre-exercise interview and screening, it is determined that an older adult is not consistently performing cardiorespiratory exercise for at least 20 continuous minutes on at least three days per week, they would begin in the Base Training phase. In this example, no cardiorespiratory assessments are necessary and the program focus would be on building duration and frequency of exercise bouts while emphasizing enjoyment and keeping the client excited about returning for the next session. Similarly, if an older client reports balance or mobility problems during the pre-exercise interview and health screen, they would be placed in the Functional Training phase and may be encouraged to perform functional assessments (as deemed appropriate) as part of a formal assessment process. Alternatively, the client with balance or mobility problems could be observed while performing exercises included in their initial programming that include opportunities for assessing postural stability and joint mobility, balance, and core function without going through a formal assessment process. Regardless of how assessments are introduced, it should be understood that many clients will begin exercise programs with very low self-efficacy for exercise ability and program success, so achieving the right balance between assessments and creating positive exercise experiences is important. Be mindful of the fact that not all clients need to undergo every assessment described in this chapter. It is up to the exercise professional and the client to determine which, if any, assessments are necessary for the initiation or progression of an exercise program. Deciding which assessments to use and when (or if) to use them is important for the ongoing development of the client–exercise professional relationship. Performing assessments should not become a barrier to regular exercise participation.

📖 APPLY WHAT YOU KNOW

A Client-centered Approach to Integrating Assessments into the Initial Exercise Session

The performance of assessments for health-related resting measures and Muscular and Cardiorespiratory Training offers valuable information on the physiological function of the heart, posture and joint alignment, muscle balance and function, static and dynamic balance and mobility, muscular endurance and muscular strength, and **ventilatory thresholds.** In turn, assessment results can be used by exercise professionals to design and progress Muscular and Cardiorespiratory Training programs according to the ACE IFT Model. However, it is common for many clients to commence an exercise program with very low self-efficacy for exercise ability and program success. It is imperative that exercise professionals strike the right balance between integration of assessments within the initial exercise session in order to acquire valuable health- and fitness-related information while simultaneously ensuring clients have a positive exercise experience and are looking forward to subsequent training sessions. The following considerations can assist exercise professionals with achieving this critical objective:

▶ In a client-centered approach, the client's goals and attributes should dictate all aspects of programming. Accordingly, exercise professionals should strategically determine which assessments (if any) are warranted that will best assist with getting clients moving.

▶ It is unnecessary for the first session to consist exclusively of assessments. An alternative is to intersperse select assessments with exercise training. Across subsequent sessions, additional assessments can gradually be performed as clients gain confidence in their exercise abilities.

▶ It is possible and recommended for exercise professionals to perform assessments that are concurrently part of the workout. For instance, the step up, onto, and over a 6-inch bench assessment (see page 217) can be completed as a balance and lower-body strength-training exercise for an older adult client. In fact, this strategy can be implemented for the completion of numerous Muscular Training assessments.

▶ When dealing with a client who opts out of being assessed, an exercise professional may simply move forward with exercise programming, carefully selecting exercises and intensities based on the client's health history and preferences. In this situation, the professional may have to be creative and collaborate with the client on benchmarks that show improvement due to training (e.g., improved back and shoulder function both at work and during exercise and feeling less daily muscular fatigue).

▶ Lastly, the exercise professional should be able to observe a client's movement proficiency improving over time. When a professional uses effective communication and coaching skills during training sessions to help the client enhance muscular conditioning, it will inevitably allow the client to experience improved function. Further, sharing with the client any noticeable improvements in exercise technique, along with advances in volume of exercise, may provide welcomed encouragement.

ACE→ MOVER METHOD

These strategies align perfectly with the ACE Mover Method™ philosophy wherein:

▸ Each professional interaction is client-centered, with a recognition that clients are the foremost experts on themselves. This is especially true for assessments, as exercise professionals must select the appropriate assessments to administer (if any) based on the client's willingness to perform them.

▸ Powerful open-ended questions and active listening are utilized in every session with clients. To select the appropriate assessments, an exercise professional must be skilled at communicating so that rapport is built and clients trust that their needs and preferences are heard and ultimately reflected in their personalized exercise programs.

▸ Clients are genuinely viewed as resourceful and capable of change. Appropriate assessment selection based on clients' preferences and goals is often the first opportunity for exercise professionals to give clients a task about which they can feel successful. Continued encouragement and positively reporting the results of assessments will allow clients to participate in the exercise program feeling confident that what they are doing is a positive step in self-care. When both the client and exercise professional view the client as successful, it empowers the client to succeed in behavior change and promotes client self-efficacy.

The purposes of conducting physical assessments are to collect baseline data, educate clients about current health and fitness status, use collected data to create personalized exercise programs, compare follow-up data to baseline data to monitor progress, and to serve as a source of motivation for setting appropriate goals [American College of Sports Medicine (ACSM), 2018]. Before performing any assessments, clients should be reminded to:

▸ Dress in comfortable clothing, including walking or running shoes

▸ Use walking aids if needed, such as a cane or walker

▸ Avoid consuming food, tobacco products, and caffeine three hours prior to testing

▸ Avoid vigorous exercise within two hours prior to testing

▸ Maintain adequate hydration

Health-related Resting Assessments

Prior to having clients perform any physical exertion, a preparticipation health screening and evaluation should be completed and exercise professionals should consider conducting several resting measures with their older clients. Assessments such as **anthropometry,** heart rate (HR), blood pressure (BP), and static posture can be administered during or before the first exercise session and can provide valuable insight to the client's state of physiological readiness to work out. Health-related resting assessments play an important role in exercise program design. Initial values and observations can be used to ensure clients are physiologically responding appropriately during exertion and as a means of comparison during reassessment. Some resting assessments, such as static posture, are directly related to placement within a particular phase of the ACE IFT Model, while other resting assessments, such as HR, may be used for determining appropriate exercise intensities within all phases of the Cardiorespiratory Training component of the ACE IFT Model. For ease of discussion, descriptions of how to measure exercise HR and BP are also included in this section.

ANTHROPOMETRIC MEASUREMENTS

Anthropometry is the study of human body measurements, especially on a comparative basis. Anthropometric measurements are a set of noninvasive, quantitative techniques for determining an individual's body dimensions by analyzing specific features of the body, such as body composition, skinfold thickness, height, body weight, and site-specific circumferences that together provide information about **overweight** and **obesity** classification and body size and shape and their associations with obesity-related diseases, morbidity, and mortality.

Body Composition

Body composition refers to the overall make-up of the body's total mass. Body-composition assessment determines the relative percentages of **lean body mass** and **fat mass.** Although increases in body weight tend to level off at about age 50 and even begin to decline in the seventh decade, body fat continues to increase and lean body mass decreases (Heo et al., 2012). The loss of muscle mass results in an accumulation of body fat (i.e., **sarcopenic obesity**).

Obesity has important functional implications in the older population because it can exacerbate the age-related decline in physical function. Hirani et al. (2017) found that **functional capacity,** particularly mobility, is markedly diminished in older adults with overweight and obesity as compared with adults of normal weight. Akune et al. (2014) found an increased incidence of nursing home admissions with an increase in sarcopenic obesity.

Exercise professionals who specialize in working with older adults should be aware of obesity-related functional declines and work toward improving body composition (i.e., reducing body fat and increasing lean mass) in clients with overweight or obesity.

It is worth noting that even in older individuals with a higher body mass index (BMI), regular physical activity can protect against health impairment. Villareal et al. (2011) determined a combination of weight loss and regular exercise improved physical function and decreased the incidence of frailty in older adults with obesity. In another study, it was determined that weight loss plus the combination of cardiorespiratory and muscular training was more effective than cardiorespiratory or muscular training alone for improving functional status in older adults with obesity (≥65 years of age) (Villareal et al., 2017).

Although excess body fat should be targeted for reduction, becoming physically active can help to maintain functional ability, as well as aid in weight-loss efforts, for older adults with obesity. There are a variety of methods used to measure body composition. **Hydrostatic weighing,** which is also called underwater weighing, and skinfold measurement are commonly used with younger populations, but there are notable disadvantages to using these methods with older adults. Hydrostatic weighing may make a person uneasy, as they must be completely submerged underwater while the reading is taken. More importantly, during the test, the individual must exhale all the air from the lungs and then wait for a signal before surfacing. In addition, there is a likelihood of gross inaccuracy due to the difficulty of remaining motionless and performing forced maximal expiration while submerged. Thus, only a small portion of the older adult population (e.g., competitive seniors) would fare well with this protocol.

The use of skinfold measurements to estimate body composition also is not optimal for older adults. As with hydrostatic weighing, the normative data used to determine the actual percentage of body fat are grouped together in a category listed as 60+ years. This general grouping cannot be considered reliable for a population that is so varied, since, realistically, the senior population potentially spans age 50 and above. Also, the pinching required by this method can create uneasiness and possible pain and may lead to a negative perception of exercise and cause program dropout. Nonetheless, for older clients who are interested in having their body composition measured, detailed information on the use of the assessment techniques described in this section can be found in *The Exercise Professional's Guide to Personal Training* (ACE, 2020).

An exercise professional can gain appreciable information about a client's health risks without using these techniques. Two methods that work well together and are easily performed are BMI and **waist circumference.**

BODY MASS INDEX

While not a means of assessing body composition, BMI compares weight in relation to stature and is calculated by dividing weight (kg) by height squared (m^2). A BMI conversion chart is found in Table 7-1.

The World Health Organization (WHO) defines overweight and obesity as BMIs ≥25 kg/m^2 and ≥30 kg/m^2, respectively (WHO, 2020). Guidelines recommend that all adults maintain a BMI between 18.5 and 24.9 kg/m^2, as there are increased health risks associated with having either a high or low BMI. A high BMI is associated with an increased risk for conditions such as diabetes, heart disease, and **hypertension.** However, research has found that a slightly higher BMI of 27 to 28 kg/m^2 has been associated with the lowest all-cause mortality rate for older adults (Winter et al., 2014). The researchers also found that the risk of all-cause death increased if the older adult had underweight compared to overweight.

Although BMI is widely adopted as an estimate of general adiposity, the failure to identify differences in body composition and body-fat distribution limits its usefulness. Specifically, in older individuals, an effect of age on percentage of body fat that is independent of BMI has been reported, such that there is a lack of classification accuracy for BMI in elderly people for whom there is a loss of lean tissue, particularly skeletal muscle, and increased fat mass (Batsis et al., 2016). In recognition that **visceral** fat accumulation increases the risk for **metabolic disease,** waist circumference has been promoted as an alternative surrogate measure of obesity. Because body-composition assessment in older adults is imperfect at best, it is useful to employ more than one technique for determining health risk associated with fat mass in this population.

WAIST CIRCUMFERENCE

The National Heart, Lung, and Blood Institute (NHLBI, 2020) and Centers for Disease Control and Prevention (CDC, 2020) recommend using waist circumference cut points of 40 inches (102 cm) in men and 35 inches (88 cm) in women to define central, or abdominal,

TABLE 7-1
Body Mass Index

	19	20	21	22	23	24	25	26	27	28	29	30	35	40
Height (inches)	**Weight (pounds)**													
58	91	95	100	105	110	115	119	124	129	134	138	143	167	191
59	94	99	104	109	114	119	124	128	133	138	143	148	173	198
60	97	102	107	112	118	123	128	133	138	143	148	153	179	204
61	100	106	111	116	121	127	132	137	143	148	153	158	185	211
62	104	109	115	120	125	131	136	142	147	153	158	164	191	218
63	107	113	118	124	130	135	141	146	152	158	163	169	197	225
64	110	116	122	128	134	140	145	151	157	163	169	174	203	233
65	114	120	126	132	138	144	150	156	162	168	174	180	210	240
66	117	124	130	136	142	148	155	161	167	173	179	185	216	247
67	121	127	134	140	147	153	159	166	172	178	185	191	223	255
68	125	131	138	144	151	158	164	171	177	184	190	197	230	263
69	128	135	142	149	155	162	169	176	182	189	196	203	237	270
70	132	139	146	153	160	167	174	181	188	195	202	209	243	278
71	136	143	150	157	165	172	179	186	193	200	207	215	250	286
72	140	147	155	162	169	177	184	191	199	206	213	221	258	294
73	144	151	159	166	174	182	189	197	204	212	219	227	265	303
74	148	155	163	171	179	187	194	202	210	218	225	233	272	311
75	152	160	168	176	184	192	200	208	216	224	232	240	279	319
76	156	164	172	180	189	197	205	213	221	230	238	246	287	328

Note: Find your client's height in the far left column and move across the row to the weight that is closest to the client's weight. The client's body mass index will be at the top of that column.

FIGURE 7-1
Waist circumference

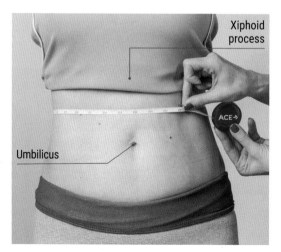

obesity. Increasingly, evidence suggests that central obesity is a better predictor of chronic disease (e.g., **type 2 diabetes,** hypertension, and **dyslipidemia**) and **metabolic syndrome** than BMI, even in individuals without obesity (Lukács et al., 2019; Tran et al., 2018). Thus, waist circumference may be more practical than BMI due to its higher predictive value for future health risks, ease of measurement, and understanding by the general public.

Waist circumference should be measured with the client standing upright, arms at the sides, feet together, and abdomen relaxed. A horizontal measure is taken at the narrowest part of the torso, above the umbilicus and below the xiphoid process (Figure 7-1).

A non-elastic yet flexible tape measure must be used. The tape should be periodically calibrated against a meter stick to ensure that it has not been stretched. When assessing clients with significant overweight, be sure to use a long enough tape so as to avoid embarrassing the client. Pull the tape tight enough to keep it in position without causing an indentation of the skin. There are tapes available that have a gauge that indicates the correct tension.

Many clients with overweight and obesity find the process of having their waist circumference measurement taken to be an unpleasant and demotivating experience. To help alleviate their uneasiness, exercise professionals should consider using an alternative technique that eliminates the numerical values that many clients find so upsetting. For example, the exercise professional can use a ribbon to measure the circumference, cutting the ribbon at the appropriate length. Then, when the measurement is repeated later in the program (and the ribbon is noticeably shorter), the exercise professional and the client have a very clear visual representation of the progress made.

HEART RATE

HR values are an effective assessment tool. Given their relatively linear relationship to $\dot{V}O_2max,$ HR measures are a beneficial guide for exercise intensity (ACSM, 2018). A great deal of information can be discerned when HR measures are used in conjunction with the rating of perceived exertion (RPE) scale.

The pulse rate (which in most people is identical to the HR) can be measured at any point on the body where an artery's pulsation is close to the surface. The following are some commonly palpated sites:

▸ *Radial artery:* The radial artery is located on the ventral aspect of the wrist on the side of the thumb (Figure 7-2). **Palpation** of the pulse at the radial artery can be performed by both clients and exercise professionals. In fact, intermittent palpation of the radial pulse, first by the client, followed by the professional, can help ensure accurate assessment of HR.

▸ *Carotid artery:* Located in the neck and lateral to the trachea, the carotid artery is more easily palpated when the neck is slightly extended (Figure 7-3). Clients often have an easier time finding their pulse at the carotid artery, which makes it an ideal anatomical location for self-assessment of HR during exercise. Note: Exercise professionals and clients should not push too hard on the carotid artery, as this may evoke a **vasovagal response** that actually slows down the HR.

FIGURE 7-2
Taking the pulse at the radial artery

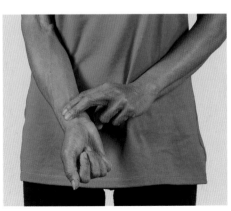

FIGURE 7-3
Taking the pulse at the carotid artery

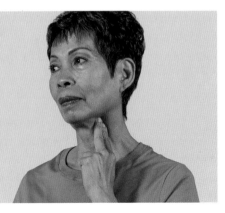

Measurement of HR is a valid indicator of work intensity or stress on the body, both at rest and during exercise. Lower resting and submaximal HRs may indicate higher fitness levels, since cardiovascular adaptations to exercise increase **stroke volume (SV),** thereby reducing HR. Conversely, higher resting and submaximal HRs are often indicative of poor physical fitness. **Resting heart rate (RHR)** is influenced by fitness status, fatigue, body composition, drugs and medication, alcohol, caffeine, and stress, among other things. A traditional classification system exists to categorize RHRs:

▸ Sinus bradycardia (slow HR): RHR <60 beats per minute (bpm)

▸ Normal sinus rhythm: RHR 60 to 100 bpm

▸ **Sinus tachycardia** (fast HR): RHR >100 bpm

While RHRs vary widely among individuals, it is important to note that females typically have slightly higher values for the following reasons:

▸ Smaller heart chamber size

▸ Lower blood volume circulating less oxygen throughout the body

▸ Lower hemoglobin levels in women

The following are some important notes about HR:

▸ Knowing a client's HR provides insight into the **overtraining syndrome,** as any elevation in RHR >5 bpm over the client's normal RHR that remains over a period of days is good reason to reduce or taper training intensities.

▸ Certain drugs, medications, and supplements can directly affect RHR. Individuals should abstain from consuming nonprescription stimulants or depressants for a minimum of 12 hours prior to measuring RHR.

▸ Body position affects RHR. Standing or sitting positions elevate HR more so than supine or prone positions due to the involvement of postural muscles and the effects of gravity.

▸ Digestion increases RHR, as the processes of absorption and digestion require energy, necessitating the delivery of nutrients and oxygen to the gastrointestinal tract.

▸ Environmental factors can affect RHR, as it is believed that noise, temperature, and sharing of personal information can place additional stress on the body, increasing HR as the body adjusts to the stressors.

During exercise, HR reflects exercise intensity. Because the heart plays a pivotal role in supplying oxygen and nutrients and removing waste products, HR is a valid indicator of the metabolic demands placed upon the body. Several methods are used to measure HR, both at rest and during exercise:

▸ 12-lead **electrocardiogram (ECG or EKG)**

▸ **Telemetry** (often two-lead, including commercial HR monitors)

▸ Palpation

▸ **Auscultation** with stethoscope

Palpation and auscultation are each accurate within 95% of an HR monitor.

Many cardiorespiratory fitness–testing protocols measure HR only at the end of an exercise bout. However, a 1-mile walking test may take an older adult anywhere from 15 to 40 minutes to complete, and a great deal of information can be gathered during this time. An HR measurement taken only at the end of the work squanders a valuable opportunity to collect revealing data. Additionally, because the normative data for evaluating older adults during tests such as this are unavailable beyond the seventh decade of life, the information extrapolated from it is of little use. HR and RPE measurements taken throughout the session could be the only reliable data available. If HR is considered an important measurement, then it must be monitored accurately throughout the testing and/or exercise session. Encouraging older clients to wear HR monitors during their workouts can provide this important information quickly and at-a-glance.

Procedure for Measuring Resting Heart Rate

True RHR is measured just before the client gets out of bed in the morning. Therefore, in most fitness environments, the exercise professional's assessment of RHR will not be reflective of true RHR. The pulsation heard through auscultation is generated by the expansion of the arteries as blood is pushed through after contraction of the left ventricle. This beat can be quite prominent in leaner individuals.

- The client should be resting comfortably for several minutes prior to obtaining RHR.
- The RHR may be measured indirectly by placing the fingertips on a pulse site (palpation), or directly by listening through a stethoscope (auscultation).
- Place the tips of the index and middle fingers (not the thumb, which has a pulse of its own) over the artery (typically, the radial artery is used) and lightly apply pressure.
- To determine the RHR, count the number of beats for 30 or 60 seconds and then convert that value to bpm, if necessary.
- When measuring by auscultation, place the bell of the stethoscope to the left of the client's sternum just above or below the nipple line. (It is important to be respectful of the client's personal space.)
- The client may also measure their own resting HR before rising from bed in the morning and report back.

Procedure for Measuring Exercise Heart Rate

- Measuring for 30 to 60 seconds is generally difficult during exercise. Therefore, exercise HRs are normally measured for shorter periods that are then converted to equal 60 seconds.
- Generally, a 10- to 15-second count is recommended over a six-second count, given the larger potential for error with the shorter count.
- Multiply the counted score by either six (for a 10-second count) or four (for a 15-second count).

Note: If the heart rhythm changes, exercise should immediately be terminated and the client should be referred to a physician.

RATING OF PERCEIVED EXERTION

RPE is used to subjectively quantify a client's overall feelings and sensations during the stress of physical activity. Subjective measures of exertion are useful since they can be compared with previous sessions and have been validated against the physiological measure of HR. RPE is preferable for determining exercise intensity for an older adult, as the prediction of maximal heart rate (MHR) is not always an accurate measure of exertion among the older adult population due to differences in the rate of structural and functional changes within the cardiorespiratory system, disease, and medication usage. RPE can be determined using the 0 to 10 category ratio scale (Figure 7-4).

0 Nothing at all	
0.5 Very, very weak	
1 Very weak	
2 Weak	
3 Moderate	
4 Somewhat strong	
5 Strong	VT1
6	VT2
7 Very strong	
8	
9	
10 Very, very strong	

FIGURE 7-4
Rating of perceived exertion: Category ratio scale

Note: VT1 = First ventilatory threshold; VT2 = Second ventilatory threshold

Common trends:

▸ Men tend to underestimate exertion, while women tend to overestimate exertion.

▸ The use of RPE has a significant learning curve that demonstrates deviation toward the mean as the client becomes more familiar with the scale.

▸ Initially, physically inactive individuals may find it difficult to use RPE charts, as they often find any level of exercise fairly hard.

▸ Conditioned individuals may under-rate their exercise intensity if they focus on the muscular tension requirement of the exercise rather than cardiorespiratory effort.

The solicitation of information about any discomfort in various parts of the body at discrete points during the assessment is prudent because it helps prevent possible injury if the problem was ignored. For example, a person who is closely monitored because they are expected to discontinue a walking assessment due to low functional capacity might have to quit because of lower-leg, hip, or back pain. Conversely, an unmonitored person who experiences discomfort in a quadriceps tendon halfway through the test, for example, but completes the exercise, may have begun to establish **tendinitis.** Even if the pain never becomes significant, it still may induce a negative mindset about exercise and lead to dropout.

When working with older clients, it may be prudent to discuss the concept of perception, specifically as it applies to discomfort or pain. It may be directly or indirectly related to the physical assessment and can manifest itself in a variety of ways.

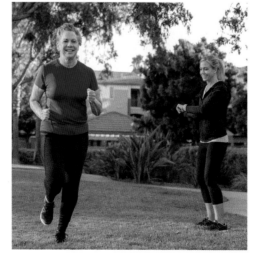

BLOOD PRESSURE

ACSM (2018) considers BP measurement an integral component of the pretest evaluation. BP is defined as the force of blood distending the arteries and is measured in millimeters of mercury (mmHg). It is determined by **cardiac output** and **total peripheral resistance (TPR)** and, therefore, can be elevated by an increase in either or both (ACSM, 2018).

BP readings are divided into a top (systolic) and bottom (diastolic) number. The systolic blood pressure (SBP) represents the maximal pressure created by the heart during ventricular contraction. The diastolic blood pressure (DBP) value is the minimum pressure that remains in the arteries during the filling phase of the cardiac cycle, which occurs when the heart relaxes.

BP assessment can be influenced by client anxiety over unfamiliar surroundings and other stressors, so it may be helpful to let the individual relax quietly for several minutes prior to taking the measurement. With the client seated, place the cuff of the sphygmomanometer around the upper portion of the bare arm, about 1 inch above the crease of the elbow joint. The middle of the bladder should be over the brachial artery on the inner part of the upper arm. Have the client rest their arm comfortably on a table or arm of a chair at heart level. Place the bell of the stethoscope firmly on the brachial artery, which can be located by feeling for a pulse at the inner portion of the elbow joint. Interfering noise, called artifact, can occur if the stethoscope comes in contact with anything during the reading.

While listening to the pulse through the stethoscope, pump the cuff until the pulse disappears. Release the pressure from the cuff at a rate that will cause the pressure to fall about 2 to 3 mmHg per second. If the pressure is released too fast, it will be difficult to obtain an accurate reading. If released too slowly, pressure builds within the arm and causes discomfort and an inaccurate reading. The BP assessment must be performed within 60 seconds of inflating the bladder to avoid the likelihood of falsely elevated readings. Table 7-2 lists other potential sources of error in BP assessment.

TABLE 7-2
Potential Sources of Error in Blood Pressure Assessment

▸ Inaccurate sphygmomanometer	▸ Experience of technician
▸ Improper cuff size	▸ Reaction time of technician
▸ Auditory acuity of technician	▸ Improper stethoscope placement or pressure
▸ Rate of inflation or deflation of cuff pressures	▸ Background noise
▸ Certain physiological abnormalities (e.g., damaged brachial artery, subclavian steal syndrome, and arteriovenous fistula)	▸ Allowing the client to hold exercise equipment handrails

As the pressure falls, the **Korotkoff sounds** can be heard. The first sound represents the SBP reading. As the mercury continues to fall, the sound becomes louder and changes to a sharp tapping.

The point at which the sound disappears is the DBP reading. During exercise, there may be an audible muffling of sound instead of complete disappearance; this is the diastolic reading. Table 7-3 lists the BP classification for adults age 18 and older.

TABLE 7-3

Categories of Blood Pressure in Adults*

Category	SBP		DBP
Normal	<120 mmHg	and	<80 mmHg
Elevated	120–129 mmHg	and	<80 mmHg
Hypertension			
Stage 1	130–139 mmHg	or	80–89 mmHg
Stage 2	≥140 mmHg	or	≥90 mmHg

Note: SBP = Systolic blood pressure; DBP = Diastolic blood pressure

*Individuals with SBP and DBP in two different categories should be designated to the higher BP category. BP is based on an average of two or more careful readings obtained on two or more occasions.

Reprinted with permission from Whelton, P.K. et al. (2017). 2017 ACC/AHA/AAPA/ABC/ACPM/AGS/APhA/ASH/ASPC/NMA/PCNA guideline for the prevention, detection, evaluation, and management of high blood pressure in adults: A report of the American College of Cardiology/American Heart Association Task Force on Clinical Practice Guidelines. *Journal of the American College of Cardiology,* Nov 7. pii: S0735-1097 (17) 41519-1.

Procedure for Measuring Blood Pressure

Equipment:

▶ Sphygmomanometer (BP cuff)

▶ Stethoscope

▶ Chair

Procedure:

▶ Have the client sit with both feet flat on the floor for five minutes. Note: If the client is seated on an exam table as opposed to a chair, DBP may be increased by 6 mmHg. Crossing the legs or other changes in body position may affect SBP readings.

Cuff placement:

▶ While the right arm is considered standard, many individuals favor placing the cuff on the left arm due to the increased proximity to the heart, which amplifies the heart sounds.

  ▪ Smoothly and firmly wrap the BP cuff around the arm with its lower margin about 1 inch (2.5 cm) above the antecubital space (i.e., the inside of the elbow). The tubes should cross the antecubital space.

  ▪ Since BP cuffs come in a variety of sizes, it is important to ensure the correct size is used, as clients with large muscle mass or who have obesity may have falsely elevated BP readings, while clients with thin, small frames may have falsely low BP readings, with a standard-sized cuff. The bladder in the cuff should encircle at least 80% of the upper arm.

▶ The client's arm should be supported either on an armchair or by the exercise professional at an angle of 0 to 45 degrees. Note: Positioning the arm above or below heart level can sway the reading by 2 mmHg. If the arm is elevated, BP readings may be reduced; if the arm is too low, BP readings may be increased.

Measuring BP at rest:

▸ Turn the bulb knob to close the cuff valve (turning it all the way to the right, no more than finger tight) and rapidly inflate the cuff to 160 mmHg, or 20 to 30 mmHg above the point where the pulse can no longer be felt at the wrist.

▸ Place the stethoscope over the brachial artery using minimal pressure (do not distort the artery).

  ▪ The stethoscope should lie flat against the skin and should not touch the cuff or the tubing.

  ▪ The client's arm should be relaxed and straight at the elbow.

▸ Release the pressure at a rate of about 2 mmHg per second by slowly turning the knob to the left, listening for the Korotkoff sounds. Note: Deflation rates >2 mm per second can lead to a significant underestimation of SBP and overestimation of DBP.

  ▪ SBP is determined by reading the dial at the first perception of sound (a faint tapping sound).

  ▪ DBP is determined by reading the dial when the sounds cease to be heard or when they become muffled.

▸ If a BP reading needs to be repeated on the same arm, allow approximately five minutes between trials so that normal circulation can return to the area.

▸ Share measurements with the client, as well as the classification of values (see Table 7-3).

Note: If abnormal readings result, repeat the measurement on the opposite arm. In fact, many within the medical community are recommending that BP measurements be taken in both arms. If there is a significant discrepancy (>10 mmHg) between readings from arm to arm, it could represent a circulatory problem, and the client should be referred to their physician for medical evaluation (McManus & Mant, 2012).

Measuring BP during exercise:

▸ BP is very difficult to measure during exercise due to the excessive amount of movement and noise, unless the person is riding a stationary bicycle.

▸ Traditionally, when exercise BP measurements are justified, they are usually measured before and following exercise (to monitor against excessive **hypotension**).

▸ A sphygmomanometer with a stand and a hand-held gauge is a better choice for measuring BP during exercise.

▸ If SBP drops during exercise, it should immediately be remeasured prior to terminating the session, just to ensure accuracy in measurement. If the client was anxious prior to the cardiorespiratory assessment, it is likely that the initial exercise SBP reading will drop.

Exercise Response

SBP increases at the onset of exercise at a rate of approximately 10 mmHg per 1 **metabolic equivalent (MET)** (ACSM, 2018). As exercise intensity increases, SBP increases linearly (Wielemborek-Musial et al., 2016). An excessive rise in BP (SBP >250 mmHg) is considered a hypertensive response to exercise. A drop in SBP (>10 mmHg) or below resting levels occurring with increased exercise intensity is considered a hypotensive response and should be viewed as abnormal. Contrary to the normal rise in SBP that occurs during dynamic exercise, DBP should remain constant or decrease slightly. If DBP increases by >10 mmHg during exercise or above pretest values, this is an abnormal response (ACSM, 2018). The ACSM (2018) considers ongoing unstable **angina** to be an absolute contraindication for maximal exercise testing and resting hypertension, with a SBP reading above 200 mmHg or a DBP reading above 110 mmHg being considered a relative contraindication.

EXPAND YOUR KNOWLEDGE

Blood Pressure and Cardiovascular Disease

The relationship between elevated BP and cardiovascular events (e.g., **myocardial infarction** or **cerebrovascular accident**) is unmistakable. For individuals 40 to 70 years old, each 20-mmHg increase in resting SBP or each 10-mmHg increase in resting DBP above normal doubles the risk of cardiovascular disease (ACSM, 2018). A difference of 15 mmHg or more between arms increases the risk of **peripheral vascular disease** and **cerebrovascular disease** and is associated with a 70% risk of dying from heart disease (McManus & Mant, 2012). If the exercise professional discovers an abnormal BP reading, either at rest or during exercise, it is prudent to recommend that the client visit their personal physician.

BP can be reduced with certain behavioral modifications (i.e., exercise, weight loss, sodium restriction, smoking cessation, and stress management) or medication. For those with elevated blood pressure, BP can realistically be reduced with lifestyle interventions; for those with clinical hypertension (see Table 7-3), it is likely that their personal physicians will want to treat the hypertension with medication and lifestyle interventions. The exercise professional can provide guidance and motivation on appropriate lifestyle-modification practices.

STATIC POSTURAL ASSESSMENT

New clients often enter a supervised exercise program with a desire to lose weight, increase energy levels, tone their muscles, or even reduce certain health risks, such as hypertension or cancer. Exercise is an integral component in achieving any of these goals. Nonetheless, both cardiorespiratory and muscular training activities place extra stress upon the body. For this reason, it is important to assess potential areas of dysfunction so as not to exacerbate any underlying conditions.

The initial physical assessments may begin with a basic assessment of standing posture and movement efficiency to allow exercise professionals to observe the alignment of the body's segments and identify suspected muscle imbalances and the client's ability to control mobility without compromising postural and joint stability while performing the five primary movement patterns. When clients have adequate movement efficiency, which is positively influenced by proper posture and good muscular balance and control, the performance of activities of daily living (ADL) as well as sports and fitness activities requires less energy and poses a reduced risk for musculoskeletal injury. Muscular imbalances, such as those that can be detected through basic postural assessments, should be addressed prior to initiating any physical activities. The following list presents three examples of how imbalances can lead to musculoskeletal problems.

▸ If a client has excessive ankle **pronation,** continuous treadmill walking may reinforce this dysfunctional movement pattern and place undue stress on the knee joint.

▸ If a client comes into the program with weak core muscles, many movement patterns may be altered under physical stress. For example, a weak core can cause the lower back to arch excessively when performing an overhead press, placing undue stress on the lumbar spine.

▸ Posture can be compromised when the body's frame is carrying excessive amounts of body weight. Excessive abdominal fat can contribute to **lordosis** of the lower back that may lead to back pain and dysfunction over time.

Information gained from a thorough postural and movement assessment can be used to address musculoskeletal dysfunction and areas of instability, thus improving movement efficiency and overall postural stability and kinetic chain mobility.

Good posture occurs when body parts are symmetrically balanced in all planes. Ideal postural alignment allows the body's muscles, joints, and nerves to function efficiently and effectively. Even digestion and breathing are enhanced by good posture. The structural integrity of the body relies mostly on the deeper, stabilizing muscles of the core that are capable of **isometric** muscle activation for extended periods of time. Improper training techniques, poor body mechanics, or prolonged periods of inactivity (such as sitting at a desk) can create muscle imbalances throughout the body. Muscular imbalance often contributes to a decreased range of motion (ROM) at the joints, dysfunctional movement patterns, joint instability, and eventually pain.

Muscle imbalances and postural deviations are often correctable, especially if these are due to certain lifestyle factors and behaviors. Correctable factors include the following:

▸ Muscular overload, often from repetitive movements (e.g., long-distance running)

▸ Awkward positions or movements (e.g., slouching)

▸ Side dominance (as in tennis players or golfers)

▸ Lack of joint stability

▸ Lack of joint mobility

▸ Imbalanced strength-training programs

▸ Non-correctable factors include congenital conditions like **scoliosis,** trauma, skeletal deviations, and certain diseases or dysfunctions, like **rheumatoid arthritis**

Determinants of Postural Alignment

With chronic poor posture, the supporting musculature eventually adapts by either shortening or lengthening. Prolonged misalignment adversely affects the structure and function of nerve tissue as well.

Occupational and sports-related activities often contribute to postural deviations. Prolonged sitting or standing may cause muscle imbalance. Repetitive motions and heavy manual labor may also be harmful, especially if proper body mechanics are not employed. Wearing high heels and restrictive clothing, as well as sleeping on nonsupportive mattresses, can also lead to postural problems.

In older adults, postural changes can occur from a general weakening of the musculoskeletal system that is associated with a decline in physical activity. Age-related limitations caused by poor posture include difficulty with the following actions:

▸ Walking or standing for prolonged periods

▸ Stooping, crouching, or kneeling

▸ Getting in and out of a car

▸ Reaching or extending the arms overhead

Osteoporosis is also a concern in the aging population and can certainly lead to postural changes such as **kyphosis** and related compensations [including a shift in center of gravity (COG), shortening of stride length in gait, and decreased physical activity].

Observing posture is an important and ongoing process for recognizing postural changes. Exercise professionals need to develop interventions to minimize both postural deviations and limitations. If not addressed, joint misalignments and muscular dysfunction can become more pronounced.

Procedure for Assessing Static Posture

A basic postural assessment provides a good starting point to determine muscular imbalances. Figure 7-5 illustrates proper alignment and anatomical positioning in all three **planes of motion**:

▸ **Sagittal plane:** A longitudinal line that divides the body or any of its parts into right and left sections

▸ **Frontal plane:** A longitudinal line dividing the body or any of its parts into **anterior** and posterior sections

▸ **Transverse plane:** A horizontal line that divides the body or any of its parts into superior and inferior sections

Since all movement is based on a person's posture, an exercise professional should be able to recognize the important characteristics associated with proper spinal alignment and good overall posture. The following represent what an exercise professional should look for when assessing a client's standing posture.

Frontal Views (Anterior and Posterior)

▸ For the anterior view, good posture presents as a line of gravity that bisects the right and left sides of the body equally, falling between the feet and ankles, and intersecting the pubis, umbilicus, sternum, mandible (chin), maxilla (face), and frontal bone (forehead) (Figure 7-6a).

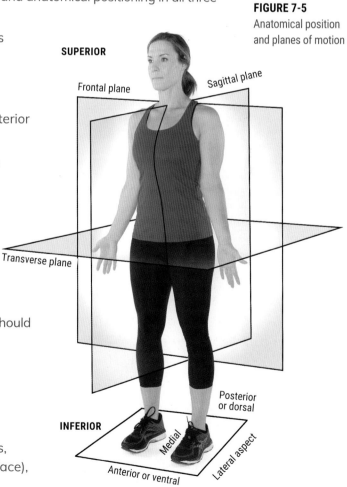

FIGURE 7-5
Anatomical position and planes of motion

SUPERIOR

Frontal plane

Sagittal plane

Transverse plane

INFERIOR

Posterior or dorsal

Medial

Anterior or ventral

Lateral aspect

▸ For the posterior view, good posture is indicated if the line of gravity bisects the sacrum and overlaps the spinous processes of the vertebrae, leaving the right and left sides of the body equally balanced (Figure 7-6b).

Sagittal View

▸ Observing the client from the side, good posture presents as a line of gravity that passes through the anterior third of the knee, the greater trochanter of the femur, and the acromioclavicular (AC) joint, and slightly anterior to the mastoid process of the temporal bone of the skull (in line with, or just behind, the ear lobe) (Figure 7-6c).

Transverse View

▸ All transverse plane observations of the limbs and torso are performed from the frontal- and sagittal-view positions and include observing rotation, pronation, and **supination.**

▸ For the anterior view, good posture presents as the palms facing the lateral aspect of the thighs with the thumbs visible, the patellae pointing straight ahead, and the feet pointing straight ahead or turned slightly outward.

▸ For the posterior view, good posture is indicated when the calcaneus is oriented perpendicular to the floor and the palms of the hands are not visible (as they are facing the lateral aspect of the thighs with the pinky side of the hand visible).

▸ For the sagittal view, good posture presents as the feet pointing forward, the knees facing neither outward nor inward, and the backs of the hands visible, as the palms are facing the lateral aspect of the thighs.

FIGURE 7-6

Assessing a client's posture

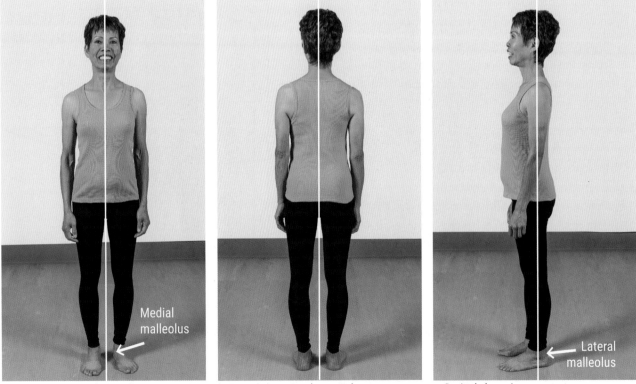

a. Frontal plane view (anterior)   b. Frontal plane view (posterior)   c. Sagittal plane view

     American Council on Exercise

The exercise professional should keep in mind that the body is rarely symmetrical. Therefore, it is important to focus on areas of obvious muscle imbalance and gross deviations that differ from ideal alignment by more than 1/4 inch (0.6 cm). Client health history will provide valuable information on past injuries and/or musculoskeletal problems. The visual and manual observations from the postural assessment will enable a targeted focus on any problematic areas.

It is important to maintain professional courtesy and respect personal boundaries and scope of practice. An exercise professional is not qualified to diagnose any condition and should be vigilant in referring to a healthcare professional when necessary. If a client reports persistent musculoskeletal pain (i.e., lasting longer than two weeks), or if a structural or congenital condition (e.g., scoliosis) is suspected, the client should be referred to their primary healthcare professional and receive medical clearance prior to engaging in a new exercise program.

Application of Static Postural Assessment Results

It is important for the exercise professional to initially assess and identify any postural deviations and/or accompanying pain. The next step is to discuss the specific observations made and educate the client on the long-term ramifications. Using the guidelines presented in Chapter 8, along with recommendations from the client's allied health and medical team, exercise professionals should develop and implement a personalized exercise program to strengthen and lengthen appropriate muscle groups. Keen observation and feedback will facilitate client awareness on key postural issues. Exercise professionals should monitor body mechanics throughout each training session. The goal is to foster healthier habits that will not only improve the body's structure and function, but also reduce the likelihood of pain, injury, and dysfunction. Additional assessments of joint ROM may be conducted. For further information on techniques and acceptable parameters, refer to *The Exercise Professional's Guide to Personal Training* (ACE, 2020).

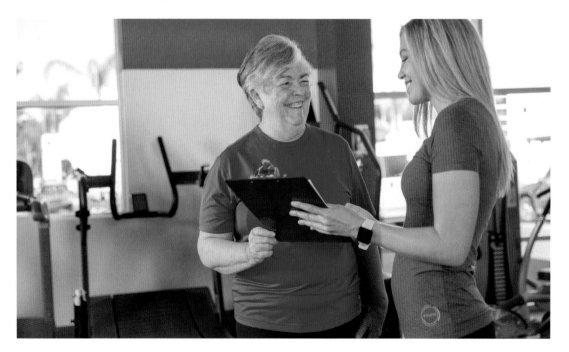

📖 APPLY WHAT YOU KNOW

Kinetic Chain: Subtalar Position and Tibial and Femoral Rotation

Because the body is one continuous kinetic chain, the position of the subtalar joint will impact the position of the tibia and femur. Barring structural differences in the skeletal system (e.g., tibial **torsion** or **femoral anteversion**), a pronated subtalar joint position typically forces internal rotation of the tibia and slightly less internal rotation of the femur (Figure 7-7 and Table 7-4). To demonstrate this point, stand with shoes off and place the hands firmly on the fronts of the thighs. Notice what happens to the orientation of the knees and thighs when moving between pronation and supination. Additionally, notice how the calcaneus everts as the subtalar joint is pronated.

FIGURE 7-7
Foot pronation and supination and the effects up the kinetic chain

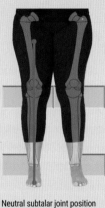 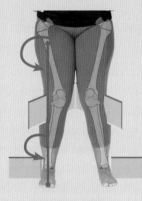 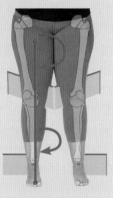

Neutral subtalar joint position with neutral knee alignment

Pronation with internal rotation of the knee

Supination with external rotation of the knee

TABLE 7-4

Subtalar Joint Pronation/Supination and the Effect on the Feet, Tibia, and Femur

Subtalar Joint Movement	Foot Movement	Tibial (Knee) Movement	Femoral Movement	Frontal Plane
Pronation	Eversion	Internal rotation	Internal rotation	Anterior view
Supination	Inversion	External rotation	External rotation	Anterior view

Subtalar joint pronation forces internal rotation at the tibia, flexion at the knee, and hip flexion and internal rotation when weight bearing. Additional stresses on some knee ligaments and the integrity of the joint itself may lead to injury during ambulation if the joint remains in pronation (Houglum, 2016). Additionally, closed-chain pronation tends to move the calcaneus into **eversion,** which may actually lift the outside of the heel slightly off the ground (moving the ankle into **plantar flexion**). In turn, this may tighten the calf muscles and potentially limit ankle **dorsiflexion,** but exercise professionals should keep in mind that the opposite is also true: A tight gastrocnemius and soleus complex (triceps surae) may force **calcaneal eversion** in an otherwise neutral subtalar joint position (Gray & Tiberio, 2007).

To illustrate this point, stand barefoot facing a wall with the feet 36 inches (0.9 m) away. Extend both arms in front of the body, placing the hands on the wall for support. Slowly lean forward, flexing the elbows and dorsiflexing the ankles while keeping both heels firmly pressed into the floor. Observe for any movement in the feet (e.g., appearance of the arch collapsing with calcaneal eversion). As a tight gastrocnemius and soleus complex reach the limit of their extensibility, the body may need to evert the calcaneus to allow further movement. This scenario may occur repeatedly in gait immediately prior to the push-off phase if the gastrocnemius and soleus complex are tight, forcing calcaneal eversion and subtalar joint pronation.

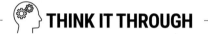 **THINK IT THROUGH**

A Client Who Is Reluctant to Undergo Assessment

Upon visiting with a client during the initial interview process, you observe that they have noticeable kyphosis while completing the health-history questionnaire. During the interview, they confide that they do not want to undergo any formal physical-fitness testing because it makes them uncomfortable to be scrutinized and compared to norms. What would you do in this situation? How would you handle the topic of postural assessment with this client? How would you approach the training program if the client refuses to participate in a baseline postural assessment?

Fitness Assessments

There is an art to the physical-fitness assessment of the older adult and it lies in understanding this unique population. The preparticipation interview is conducted through comfortable dialogue, yet in such detail as to determine what physical activity the individual has been engaged in on a *regular* basis, program expectations, and the client's personal goals. Once this has been established, the exercise professional can decide the best way to proceed with the physical-fitness assessment. The information gathered from this initial conversation can help an exercise professional to be aware of potential limitations and dysfunction and apply this knowledge when making decisions about conducting assessments, thus helping to prevent new injury and/or aggravate old ones. For example, if a client explains that he has a difficult time walking due to arthritis of the lower back and knees, administering a cardiorespiratory fitness test based on walking is inappropriate and could cause harm. In contrast, an older client who is physically active and routinely participates in endurance events, such as 5K runs or master's cycling competitions, would probably enjoy the challenge and competitive aspects of certain types of physical assessments. The exercise professional must decide on appropriate assessments (if any) for measuring the physical fitness of an older client. Fitness assessments may be used prior to the initial program design and/or as a means for establishing appropriate intensity markers as a program progresses. Fortunately, the ACE IFT Model provides guidance on when specific assessments may be administered based on the phase in which a client begins and when a client is progressing from one phase to the next. Ultimately, it is up to the exercise professional to interpret all

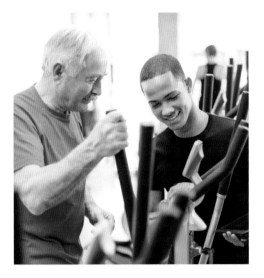

information gathered about a client, determine if and when assessments are needed, and decide on an appropriate starting point within the Cardiorespiratory and Muscular Training components of the ACE IFT Model.

The risk of heart attack and sudden cardiac death during exercise among individuals who participate in regular physical activity, though very low, still exists. The risk can be further reduced with appropriate pre-exercise screening and careful observation of clients during and following exercise. $\dot{V}O_2$max is an excellent measure of cardiorespiratory efficiency, or the body's ability to use oxygen for energy, and is closely related to the functional capacity of the heart and circulatory system. Measuring $\dot{V}O_2$max in a laboratory involves the collection and analysis of exhaled air during maximal exercise. Conducting a cardiorespiratory assessment at maximal effort is not always feasible and can actually place certain individuals at risk. Therefore, it is recommended that submaximal tests, which are the types of tests presented in this chapter, be used in the fitness setting.

If any negative signs or symptoms arise during exercise testing, the client's personal physician should be notified immediately. Emergency medical services (EMS) should be activated when severe signs or symptoms arise, including the following (ACSM, 2018):

▸ Onset of angina, chest pain, or angina-like symptoms

▸ Significant drop (≥10 mmHg) in SBP) despite an increase in exercise intensity or a decrease in SBP below the value obtained in the same position prior to assessment

▸ Excessive rise in BP: SBP reaches >250 mmHg and/or DBP reaches >115 mmHg

▸ Shortness of breath, or wheezing (does not include heavy breathing due to intense exercise)

▸ Signs of poor **perfusion**: lightheadedness, confusion, **ataxia,** pallor (pale skin), **cyanosis** (bluish coloration, especially around the mouth), nausea, or cold and clammy skin

▸ Failure of HR to increase with increased exercise intensity

▸ Noticeable change in heart rhythm by palpation or auscultation

▸ Subject requests to stop

▸ Physical or verbal manifestations of severe fatigue

THE SENIOR FITNESS TEST

Rikli and Jones (2013) created the Senior Fitness Test as an answer to the need for a simple, easy-to-use battery of test items that assess the functional fitness of older adults. It measures the key physical abilities needed to perform common, everyday activities. The test, which is considered safe and enjoyable for older adults, meets scientific standards for reliability and validity, and has accompanying performance norms based on actual tests of more than 700 men and women between the ages of 60 and 94. It is the first test of its kind to provide normative data for the older adult such that individuals can see how they compare to their age-appropriate population. Exercise professionals can refer to Rikli and Jones (2013) for tables of performance norms and standards. That said, the true value of these tests when working with clients is that they provide a series of baseline data against which the exercise professional can compare future performance. Any improvements in performance can be empowering to older clients, as they represent an increase in physical function.

30-Second Chair Stand

Purpose: To assess lower-body strength, which is needed for numerous tasks such as climbing stairs, walking, and getting out of a chair, tub, or car. Also reduces the chance of falling.

Description: Number of full stands that can be completed in 30 seconds with arms folded across chest

Arm Curl

Purpose: To assess upper-body strength, which is needed for performing household and other activities involving lifting and carrying things such as groceries, suitcases, and grandchildren

Description: Number of biceps curls that can be completed in 30 seconds holding a hand weight of 5 lb (2.27 kg) for women or 8 lb (3.63 kg) for men

6-Minute Walk

Purpose: To assess aerobic endurance, which is important for walking distances, stair climbing, shopping, sightseeing while on vacation, etc.

Description: Number of yards/meters that can be walked in 6 minutes around a 50-yard (45.7-meter) course

The following protocol was developed by Rikli and Jones (2013) as part of their Senior Fitness Test for community-dwelling older adults and should be appropriate for exercise professionals to administer to most of their clients. This assessment provides valuable information about the cardiorespiratory endurance of an older client.

Contraindications

This type of testing is not recommended for:

▸ Individuals with unstable angina and myocardial infarction during the previous month

▸ Individuals with an RHR >120 bpm

▸ Individuals with an SBP >180 mmHg and a DBP >100 mmHg

Note: Clients with any of these findings should be referred to their physicians for further evaluation.

Equipment:

▸ Four cones

▸ Stopwatch

Protocol:

▸ Place four cones on a flat surface so that they create a rectangle measuring 20 x 5 yards (18.3 x 4.6 m) (Figure 7-8).

▸ Place a mark with masking tape on the floor at every 5-yard (4.57-m) increment to make scoring easier.

▸ Demonstrate the correct path around the rectangle using proper heel-to-toe walking keeping one foot in contact with the floor at all times (to ensure no running).

▸ Ask the client to stand at the starting line.

▸ Start the stopwatch and simultaneously give the instruction to "Go."

▸ Have the client walk continuously around the 50-yard (45.7-m) rectangular course for 6 minutes, or until the client decides to stop walking, whichever comes first.

▸ The score is the number of laps walked multiplied by 50 yards (45.7 m), plus the number of extra yards or meters [indicated by the closest 5-yard (4.57-m) marker].

FIGURE 7-8
6-minute walk test cone placement

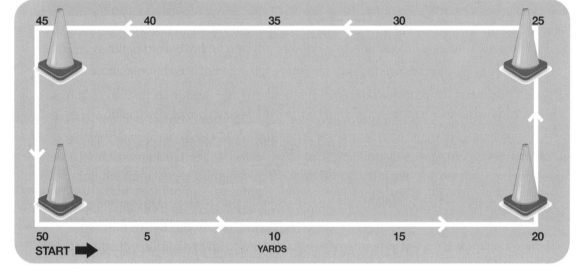

Note: When administering the Senior Fitness Test in its entirety, the 6-minute Walk Test should always be given last.

2-Minute Step

Purpose: This is an alternate aerobic-endurance test, for use when conducting the 6-minute walk test is not feasible.

Description: Number of full steps completed in 2 minutes, raising each knee to a point midway between the patella (kneecap) and iliac crest (top of hip bone). The score is the number of times the right knee reaches the required height.

Chair Sit-and-Reach

Purpose: To assess lower-body (primarily hamstrings) flexibility, which is important for good posture, normal gait patterns, and various mobility tasks such as getting in and out of a bathtub or car

Description: From a sitting position at the front of a chair, with one leg extended (the client's preferred leg, or the leg that will result in a better score) and hands reaching toward toes, the number of inches (or cm) (+ or –) between the extended fingers and the tips of the toes (i.e., if the fingertips do not reach the toes, this is recorded as a – score, and if the fingertips reach beyond the toes, this is recorded as a + score)

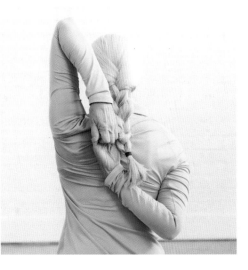

Back Scratch

Purpose: To assess upper-body (shoulder) flexibility, which is important in tasks such as combing one's hair, putting on overhead garments, and reaching for a seat belt

Description: With one hand reaching over the shoulder and one up the middle of the back (the client's preferred arm reaches up, or the arm that will result in a better score), the number of inches (or cm) (+ or –) between extended middle fingers (i.e., if the fingers touch but do not overlap, this is a score of 0; if they overlap, the distance between the middle fingertips is recorded as a + score; if they do not touch, the distance between the middle fingertips is recorded as a – score)

8-Foot Up-and-Go

Purpose: To assess agility/dynamic balance, which is important in tasks that require quick maneuvering such as getting off a bus in time, or getting up to attend to something in the kitchen, go to the bathroom, or answer the phone

Description: Number of seconds required to get up from a seated position, walk 8 feet (2.44 m), turn, and return to the seated position

Height and Weight

Purpose: To assess body weight relative to height, because of the importance of weight management for functional mobility

Description: Involves measuring height and weight, then using a conversion table to determine BMI (see Table 7-1)

BALANCE AND GAIT ASSESSMENTS

Multidirectional Reach Test

The purpose of the Multidirectional Reach Test (MDRT) is to measure the distance a person is able or willing to lean in a forward, backward, and lateral direction (Newton, 2001). The only equipment needed for this test is a yardstick and a wall. After reviewing the test administration that follows, refer to Table 7-5 for reference values and Figure 7-9 for a scoring form.

FORWARD REACH

▸ Position a yardstick on a wall at the height of the acromion process (top of the shoulder).

- Instruct the individual to stand in a comfortable position with feet shoulder-width apart.
- Instruct the individual to raise one arm in front to shoulder height (hand extended, palm turned to face medially) and not to touch the yardstick.
- Instruct the individual to reach forward as far as possible without raising the heels from the floor. Record the location of the middle fingertip.
- Now, instruct the individual to stop reaching and return to the starting position.
- Subtract the end number from the starting position number to obtain the length reached.
- Pause before the next trial.
- Provide one practice trial before the start of the three test trials.

BACKWARD REACH

Repeat all instructions for the forward reach but ask the individual to lean backward as far as possible without raising the toes from the floor. Record the location of the middle fingertip.

LATERAL REACH TO THE RIGHT

- Position a yardstick on a wall at the height of the acromion process (top of the shoulder).
- Instruct the individual to stand in a comfortable position with feet shoulder-width apart.
- Instruct the individual to raise one arm horizontally to shoulder height (hand extended, palm turned to face medially) and not to touch the yardstick.
- Instruct the individual to reach sideways to the right as far as possible. Record the location of the middle fingertip.
- Now, instruct the individual to stop reaching and return to the starting position.
- Subtract the end number from the starting position number to obtain the number of inches reached.
- Pause before the next trial.
- Provide one practice trial before the start of the three test trials.

LATERAL REACH TO THE LEFT

Repeat all instructions for the lateral reach to the right but ask the individual to reach sideways to the left as far as possible. Record the location of the middle fingertip.

TABLE 7-5

Multidirectional Reach Test (MDRT) Reference Values

	Above average	Below average
Forward direction (Mean: 8.9 in.) (SD: ± 3.4 in.)	>12.2 in.	<5.6 in.
Backward direction (Mean: 4.6 in.) (SD: ± 3.1 in.)	>7.6 in.	<1.6 in.
Right lateral direction (Mean: 6.9 in.) (SD: ± 3.0 in.)	>9.4 in.	<3.8 in.
Left lateral direction (Mean: 6.6 in.) (SD: ± 2.9 in.)	>9.4 in.	<3.8 in.

Source: Newton, R.A. (2001). Validity of the multidirectional reach test: A practical measure for limits of stability in older adults. *Journal of Gerontology: Medical Sciences,* 56A, 4, M248–M252.

Scoring Form for Multidirectional Reach Test (MDRT)

FORWARD REACH

Distance reached

Trial 1_____

Trial 2_____

Trial 3_____

Mean:_____

Movement strategy

hip_____ ankle_____trunk rotation_____

scapular protraction_____other_____

hip_____ ankle_____trunk rotation_____

scapular protraction_____other_____

hip_____ ankle_____trunk rotation_____

scapular protraction_____other_____

BACKWARD REACH

Distance reached

Trial 1_____

Trial 2_____

Trial 3_____

Mean:_____

Movement strategy

hip_____ ankle_____trunk rotation_____

scapular protraction_____other_____

hip_____ ankle_____trunk rotation_____

scapular protraction_____other_____

hip_____ ankle_____trunk rotation_____

scapular protraction_____other_____

LATERAL REACH TO THE RIGHT

Distance reached

Trial 1_____

Trial 2_____

Trial 3_____

Mean:_____

Movement strategy

hip_____ ankle_____trunk rotation_____

scapular protraction_____other_____

hip_____ ankle_____trunk rotation_____

scapular protraction_____other_____

hip_____ ankle_____trunk rotation_____

scapular protraction_____other_____

LATERAL REACH TO THE LEFT

Distance reached

Trial 1_____

Trial 2_____

Trial 3_____

Mean:_____

Movement strategy

hip_____ ankle_____trunk rotation_____

scapular protraction_____other_____

hip_____ ankle_____trunk rotation_____

scapular protraction_____other_____

hip_____ ankle_____trunk rotation_____

scapular protraction_____other_____

FIGURE 7-9

Score sheet for the Mulidirectional Reach Test

Fullerton Advanced Balance Scale

The Fullerton Advanced Balance (FAB) Scale is used to assess a variety of proprioceptive challenges, including the following (Rose, 2010):

▸ Ability to use ground cues to maintain upright balance while standing with a reduced **base of support**

▸ Ability to lean forward to retrieve an object without altering the base of support

▸ Ability to turn a full circle in both directions in the fewest number of steps without loss of balance

▸ Ability to dynamically control **center of mass** with an altered base of support

▸ Ability to maintain upright balance while standing on a compliant surface (e.g., foam pad) with eyes closed

After reviewing the tests, refer to Figure 7-13 on pages 220–221 for a score sheet for the Fullerton Advanced Balance Scale and Table 7-6 on pages 222–223 for an interpretation of the individual test items. The Fullerton Advanced Balance Scale is designed to measure changes in multiple dimensions of balance in independent, fit, or elite community-dwelling older adults.

1. STAND WITH FEET TOGETHER AND EYES CLOSED

Purpose: To assess the ability to use ground cues to maintain upright balance while standing with a reduced base of support

Equipment: Stopwatch

Testing procedures: Demonstrate the correct test position and then instruct the client to move the feet independently until they are together. If some clients are unable to achieve the correct position due to lower-extremity joint problems, encourage them to bring their heels together even though the fronts of the feet are not touching. Have clients adopt a position that will ensure their safety as the arms are folded across the chest and they prepare to close the eyes. Begin timing as soon as the client closes the eyes. (Instruct clients to open the eyes if they feel so unsteady that a loss of balance is imminent.)

Verbal instructions: "Bring your feet together, fold your arms across your chest, close your eyes when you are ready, and remain as steady as possible until I instruct you to open your eyes."

2. REACH FORWARD TO RETRIEVE AN OBJECT (PENCIL) HELD AT SHOULDER HEIGHT WITH AN OUTSTRETCHED ARM

Purpose: To assess the ability to lean forward to retrieve an object without altering the base of support; measure of stability limits in a forward direction

Equipment: Pencil and 12-inch ruler

Testing procedures: Instruct the client to raise the preferred arm to 90° and extend it with fingers outstretched. (Follow with a demonstration of the correct action.) Use the ruler to measure a distance of 10 inches from the end of the fingers of the outstretched arm. Hold the object (pencil) horizontally and level with the height of the client's shoulder. Instruct the client to reach forward, grasp the pencil, and return to the initial starting position without moving the feet, if possible (Figure 7-10). (It is acceptable to raise the heels, as long as the feet do not move while reaching for the pencil.) If the client is unable to reach the pencil within two or three seconds of initiating the forward lean, indicate to the client that it is okay to move the feet in order to reach the pencil. Record the number of steps taken by the client in order to retrieve the pencil.

Verbal instructions: "Try to lean forward to take the pencil from my hand and return to your starting position without moving your feet from their present position." After allowing two or three seconds of lean time: "You can move your feet in order to reach the pencil."

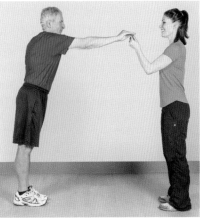

3. TURN 360° IN RIGHT AND LEFT DIRECTIONS

Purpose: To assess the ability to turn in a full circle in both directions in the fewest number of steps without loss of balance

Equipment: None

Testing procedures: Verbally explain and then demonstrate the task to be performed, making sure to complete each circle in four steps or less and pause briefly between turns. Instruct the client to turn in a complete circle in one direction, pause, and then turn in a complete circle in the opposite direction. Count the number of steps taken to complete each circle. Allow for a small correction in foot position before a turn in the opposite direction is initiated.

Verbal instructions: "Turn around in a full circle, pause, and then turn in a second full circle in the opposite direction."

4. STEP UP, ONTO, AND OVER A 6-INCH BENCH

Purpose: To assess the ability to control COG in dynamic task situations; also a measure of lower-body strength and control

Equipment: 6-inch-high bench (18- by 18-inch stepping surface)

Testing procedures: Verbally explain and demonstrate how to step up, onto, and over the bench in both directions before the client performs the test. Instruct the client to step onto the bench with the right foot, lift the left leg directly up and over the bench, and step off the other side, then repeat the movement in the opposite direction with the left leg leading the action.

During the performance of the test, watch to see that the client's trailing leg (a) does not make contact with the bench or (b) swing around, as opposed to directly over, the bench.

Verbal instructions: "Step up onto the bench with your right leg, lift your left leg directly up and over the bench, and step off the other side. Repeat the movement in the opposite direction with your left leg as the leading leg."

5. TANDEM WALK

Purpose: To assess the ability to dynamically control the center of mass with an altered base of support

Equipment: Masking tape

Testing procedures: Verbally explain and demonstrate how to perform the test correctly before the client attempts to perform it. Instruct the client to walk on the line in a tandem position (heel-to-toe) until they are told to stop. Allow the client to repeat the test one time if unable to achieve a tandem stance position within the first two steps. The client may elect to step forward with the opposite foot on the second trial. Score as interruptions any instances where the client (a) takes a lateral step away from the line when performing the tandem walk or (b) is unable to achieve correct heel-to-toe position during any step taken along the course. Do not ask the client to stop until 10 steps have been completed.

Verbal instructions: "Walk forward along the line, placing one foot directly in front of the other such that the heel and toe are in contact on each step forward. I will tell you when to stop."

6. STAND ON ONE LEG

Purpose: To assess the ability to maintain upright balance with a reduced base of support

FIGURE 7-11
Stand on one leg

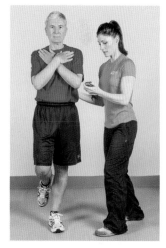

Equipment: Stopwatch

Testing procedures: Instruct the client to fold the arms across the chest, lift the preferred leg off the floor, and maintain balance until instructed to return the foot to the floor (Figure 7-11). Begin timing as soon as the client lifts the foot from the floor. Stop timing if the legs touch, the preferred leg contacts the floor, or the client removes the arms from the chest before 20 seconds have elapsed. Allow the client to perform the test a second time with the other leg if they are unsure as to which is the preferred limb.

Verbal instructions: "Fold your arms across your chest, lift your preferred leg off the floor (without touching the other leg), and stand with your eyes open as long as you can."

7. STAND ON FOAM WITH EYES CLOSED

Purpose: To assess the ability to maintain upright balance while standing on a compliant surface (e.g., foam pads) with eyes closed

Equipment: Stopwatch; two foam pads, with a length of nonslip material placed between the two pads and an additional length of nonslip material between the floor and first pad if the test is being performed on an uncarpeted surface

Testing procedures: Instruct the client to step onto the foam pads without assistance, fold the arms across the chest, and close the eyes when ready. (Demonstrate the correct standing position on the foam pads). Make sure the position adopted ensures the safety of the client. Position the foam pads close to a wall in all cases and in a corner of the room if the client appears unsteady. Begin timing as soon as the eyes close. Stop the trial if the client (a) opens the eyes before the timing period has elapsed, (b) lifts the arms off the chest, or (c) loses balance and requires manual assistance to prevent falling. (Instruct clients to open their eyes if they feel so unsteady that a loss of balance is imminent.)

Verbal instructions: "Step up onto the foam pads and stand with your feet shoulder-width apart. Fold your arms over your chest and close your eyes when you are ready. I will tell you when to open your eyes."

8. TWO-FOOTED JUMP FOR DISTANCE

Purpose: To assess upper- and lower-body coordination and lower-body power

Equipment: 36-inch ruler

Testing procedures: Instruct the client to jump as far but as safely as possible while maintaining a two-footed stance. Demonstrate the correct movement prior to the client performing the jump. (The exercise professional should not jump much more than twice the length of their own feet when demonstrating.) Observe whether the client leaves the floor with both feet and lands with both feet. Use the ruler to measure the length of the foot and then multiply by two to determine the ideal distance to be jumped.

Verbal instructions: "Try to jump as far but as safely as you can."

9. WALK WITH HEAD TURNS

Purpose: To assess the ability to maintain dynamic balance while walking and turning the head

Equipment: Metronome set at 100 bpm

Testing procedures: After first demonstrating the test, allow the client to practice turning the head in time with the metronome while standing in place. Encourage the client to turn the head at least 30° in each direction (e.g., "Turn your head to look into each corner of the room.") (Figure 7-12). Observe how far the client is able to turn the head during the standing head turns. A 30° head turn is required during the walking trial. Instruct the client to walk forward while turning the head from side to side and in time with the auditory tone. Begin counting steps as soon as the client attempts to turn the head with the beat of the metronome. The ultimate goal is for the client to achieve 10 steps. Observe whether the client deviates from a straight path while walking or is unable to turn the head the required distance to the timing of the metronome.

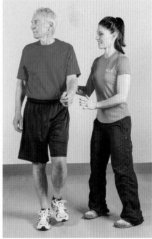

FIGURE 7-12
Walk with head turns

Verbal instructions: "Walk forward while turning your head from left to right with each beat of the metronome. I will tell you when to stop."

10. REACTIVE POSTURAL CONTROL

Purpose: To assess the ability to efficiently restore balance following an unexpected perturbation

Equipment: None

Testing procedures: Instruct the client to stand with their back to you. Extend your arm with the elbow locked and place the palm of your hand against the client's back between the scapulae. Instruct the client to lean back slowly against your hand until you tell them to stop. Quickly flex your elbow until your hand is no longer in contact with the client's back at the moment you estimate that a sufficient amount of force has been applied to require a movement of the feet to restore balance.

You may actually begin releasing your hand while you are still giving the instructions. This release should be unexpected, so do not prepare the client for the moment of release. Always stand in close proximity as a precaution to prevent falling.

Verbal instructions: "Slowly lean back into my hand until I ask you to stop."

SCORE SHEET FOR
FULLERTON ADVANCED BALANCE (FAB) SCALE

Name:_____ Date of Test:_____

1. Stand with feet together and eyes closed
- ☐ 0 Unable to obtain the correct standing position independently
- ☐ 1 Able to obtain the correct standing position independently but unable to maintain the position or keep the eyes closed for more than 10 seconds
- ☐ 2 Able to maintain the correct standing position with eyes closed for more than 10 seconds but less than 30 seconds
- ☐ 3 Able to maintain the correct standing position with eyes closed for 30 seconds but requires close supervision
- ☐ 4 Able to maintain the correct standing position safely with eyes closed for 30 seconds

2. Reach forward to retrieve an object (pencil) held at shoulder height with outstretched arm
- ☐ 0 Unable to reach the pencil without taking more than two steps
- ☐ 1 Able to reach the pencil but needs to take two steps
- ☐ 2 Able to reach the pencil but needs to take one step
- ☐ 3 Can reach the pencil without moving the feet but requires supervision
- ☐ 4 Can reach the pencil safely and independently without moving the feet

3. Turn 360° in right and left directions
- ☐ 0 Needs manual assistance while turning
- ☐ 1 Needs close supervision or verbal cueing while turning
- ☐ 2 Able to turn 360° but takes more than four steps in both directions
- ☐ 3 Able to turn 360° but unable to complete in four steps or fewer in one direction
- ☐ 4 Able to turn 360° safely taking four steps or fewer in both directions

4. Step up, onto, and over a 6-inch bench
- ☐ 0 Unable to step up onto the bench without loss of balance or manual assistance
- ☐ 1 Able to step up onto the bench with leading leg, but trailing leg contacts the bench or leg swings around the bench during the swing-through phase in both directions
- ☐ 2 Able to step up onto the bench with leading leg, but trailing leg contacts the bench or swings around the bench during the swing-through phase in one direction
- ☐ 3 Able to correctly complete the step up and over in both directions but requires close supervision in one or both directions
- ☐ 4 Able to correctly complete the step up and over in both directions safely and independently

5. Tandem walk
- ☐ 0 Unable to complete the 10 steps independently
- ☐ 1 Able to complete the 10 steps with more than five interruptions
- ☐ 2 Able to complete the 10 steps with five or fewer interruptions
- ☐ 3 Able to complete the 10 steps with two or fewer interruptions
- ☐ 4 Able to complete the 10 steps independently and with no interruptions

FIGURE 7-13
Score sheet for the Fullerton Advanced Balance Scale

6. Stand on one leg

☐ 0 Unable to try or needs assistance to prevent falling

☐ 1 Able to lift leg independently but unable to maintain position for more than 5 seconds

☐ 2 Able to lift leg independently and maintain position for more than 5 but less than 12 seconds

☐ 3 Able to lift leg independently and maintain position for more than 12 but less than 20 seconds

☐ 4 Able to lift leg independently and maintain position for the full 20 seconds

7. Stand on foam with eyes closed

☐ 0 Unable to step onto foam or maintain standing position independently with eyes open

☐ 1 Able to step onto foam independently and maintain standing position but unable or unwilling to close eyes

☐ 2 Able to step onto foam independently and maintain standing position with eyes closed for at least 10 seconds

☐ 3 Able to step onto foam independently and maintain standing position with eyes closed for more than 10 seconds but less than 20 seconds

☐ 4 Able to step onto foam independently and maintain standing position with eyes closed for 20 seconds

8. Two-footed jump for distance

☐ 0 Unable to attempt or attempts to initiate two-footed jump, but one or both feet do not leave the floor

☐ 1 Able to initiate two-footed jump, but one foot either leaves the floor or lands before the other

☐ 2 Able to perform two-footed jump, but unable to jump farther than the length of their own feet

☐ 3 Able to perform two-footed jump and achieve a distance greater than the length of their own feet

☐ 4 Able to perform two-footed jump and achieve a distance greater than twice the length of their own feet

9. Walk with head turns

☐ 0 Unable to walk 10 steps independently while maintaining 30° head turns at an established pace

☐ 1 Able to walk 10 steps independently but unable to complete required number of 30° head turns at an established pace

☐ 2 Able to walk 10 steps but veers from a straight line while performing 30° head turns at an established pace

☐ 3 Able to walk 10 steps in a straight line while performing head turns at an established pace but head turns less than 30° in one or both directions

☐ 4 Able to walk 10 steps in a straight line while performing required number of 30° head turns at established pace

10. Reactive postural control

☐ 0 Unable to maintain upright balance; no observable attempt to step; requires manual assistance to restore balance

☐ 1 Unable to maintain upright balance; takes fewer than two steps and requires manual assistance to restore balance

☐ 2 Unable to maintain upright balance; takes fewer than two steps, but is able to restore balance independently

☐ 3 Unable to maintain upright balance; takes one to two steps, but is able to restore balance independently

☐ 4 Unable to maintain upright balance but able to restore balance independently with only one step

FIGURE 7-13 (continued)

TABLE 7-6

Interpretation of the Individual Test Items on the Fullerton Advanced Balance (FAB) Scale for Possible Underlying Impairments

Item	Possible Impairments	Recommended Exercises
1. Stand with feet together and eyes closed	Weak hip abductors/adductors	Lateral weight shifts against resistance; side leg raises against gravity/resistance
	Poor COG control	Seated/standing balance activities emphasizing weight shifts in multiple directions
	Poor use of somatosensory cues	Standing balance activities with eyes closed (controlled sway in A-P and lateral directions)
2. Reach forward to object	Reduced limits of stability	Seated/standing COG control activities
	Reduced ankle ROM	Ankle circles, heel lifts, and drops from height
	Fear of falling	Confidence-building activities—high success
	Lower-body muscle weakness	Wall sits; lower-body exercises with resistance
3. Turn in a full circle	Poor dynamic COG control	Standing weight-transfer activities; gait pattern enhancement (turns, directional changes)
	Possible vestibular impairment (e.g., dizziness)	Head and eye movement coordination exercises
	Lower-body weakness	Lower-body exercises with resistance; emphasize hip and knee flexion; hip abduction/adduction
4. Step up and over	Poor dynamic COG control	Seated/standing balance activities emphasizing backward weight shifts
	Lower-body weakness	Lower-body exercises with resistance (own body/resistance band; emphasize sustained unilateral stance positions)
	Reduced ROM at ankle, knee, hip	Flexibility exercises emphasizing hip/knee/ankle flexion; seated and standing
5. Tandem walk	Poor dynamic COG control	Standing/moving COG control activities; emphasize A-P control during weight shifts
	Poor use of vision	Activities emphasizing gaze-stabilization techniques
	Weak hip abductors/adductors	Side leg raise against gravity/resistance; lateral weight shift and lunge activities
6. Stand on one leg	Poor COG control	Standing A-P weight shifts and transfers; reduced BOS activities
	Lower-body muscle weakness	Lower-body exercises with resistance (body/resistance band); emphasize hip abductors/adductors
	Poor use of vision	Activities emphasizing gaze stabilization
7. Stand on foam with eyes closed	Poor use of vestibular inputs for balance	Seated/standing activities performed with reduced/absent vision on altered surfaces
	Lower-body muscle weakness	Lower-body exercises with resistance (body/resistance band); emphasize quadriceps, gastrocnemius/soleus muscles
	Heightened fear of falling when vision absent	Confidence-building activities with progressive reduction in availability of vision

TABLE 7-6 *(continued)*

Item	Possible Impairments	Recommended Exercises
8. Two-footed jump	Poor dynamic COG control	Standing/moving COG activities emphasizing leaning away from and back to midline
	Poor upper- and lower-body coordination	Selected exercises to improve upper- and lower-body coordination; multiple task activities
	Lower-body muscle weakness	Lower-body exercises with resistance (body/resistance band) performed at progressively faster speeds
9. Walk with head turns	Possible vestibular impairment	Head and eye movement coordination exercises; gait pattern enhancement (turns, directional changes)
	Poor use of vision	Activities emphasizing gaze stabilization
	Poor dynamic COG control	Standing/moving activities with head turns; progressively increase speed and frequency of head turns
10. Reactive postural test	Absent postural strategy (i.e., step)	Activities emphasizing step strategy (i.e., resistance band release activity)
	Poor COG control	Standing COG control activities; volitional stepping activities in multiple directions
	Lower-body muscle weakness	Lower-body exercises with resistance; emphasize hip and knee flexion; hip abduction/adduction.

Note: COG = Center of gravity; A-P = Anterior-posterior direction; ROM = Range of motion

Stork-stand Balance Test

Source: Johnson & Nelson, 1986

Objective: To assess static balance by standing on one foot in a modified stork-stand position

Equipment:

▸ Firm, non-slip surface

▸ Stopwatch

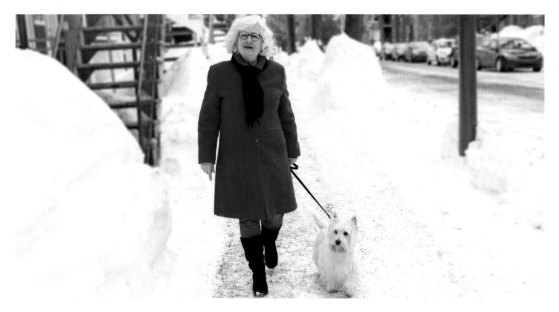

Test protocol and administration:

▶ Explain the purpose of the test.

▶ Ask the client to remove their shoes and stand with feet together and hands on the hips.

▶ Instruct the client to raise one foot off the ground and bring that foot to lightly touch the inside of the stance leg, just below the knee (Figure 7-14).

   ▪ The client must raise the heel of the stance foot off the floor and balance on the ball of the foot (Figure 7-15).

   ▪ Stand behind the client for support if needed.

   ▪ Allow 1 minute of practice trials.

   ▪ After the practice trials, perform the test, starting the stopwatch as the heel lifts off the floor.

▶ Repeat with the opposite leg.

▶ Allow up to three trials per leg and record the best performance on each side.

Observations:

▶ Timing stops when any of the following occurs:

   ▪ The hand(s) come off the hips.

   ▪ The stance or supporting foot inverts, everts, or moves in any direction.

   ▪ Any part of the elevated foot loses contact with the stance leg.

   ▪ The heel of the stance leg touches the floor.

   ▪ The client loses balance.

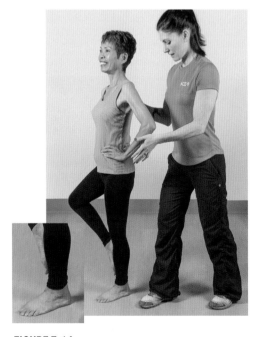

FIGURE 7-14
Stork-stand balance test: Starting position

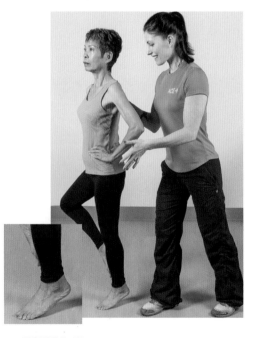

FIGURE 7-15
Stork-stand balance test: Test position

General interpretation:

▸ Currently, this test does not have standardized norms for older adults. However, an exercise professional can use the findings of this test for independent, fit, or elite older adults as a comparative baseline measurement during reassessment efforts as the fitness program progresses.

▸ As a point of reference, maintaining balance with good postural control (without excessive swaying) and not exhibiting any of the test-termination criteria for 25 to 30 seconds is an "average" score for younger individuals.

Sharpened Romberg Test

Sources: Black et al., 1982; Newton, 1989

Objective: To assess static balance and postural control while standing on a reduced base of support while removing visual sensory perception

Equipment:

▸ Firm, flat, non-slip surface

▸ Stopwatch

Test protocol and administration:

▸ Explain the purpose of the test.

▸ Instruct the client to remove their shoes and stand with one foot directly in front of the other (tandem or heel-to-toe position), with the eyes open.

▸ Ask the client to fold their arms across the chest, touching each hand to the opposite shoulder (Figure 7-16).

▸ Allow sufficient practice trials. Once the client feels stable, instruct the client to close their eyes. Start the stopwatch to begin the test.

▸ Always stand in close proximity as a precaution to prevent falling.

▸ Continue the test for 60 seconds or until the client exhibits any test-termination cue, as listed in the "Observations" section below.

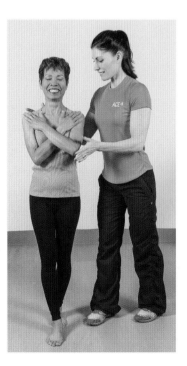

FIGURE 7-16
Sharpened Romberg test

▸ Allow up to two trials per lead leg position and record the best performance on each side.

Observations:

▸ Continue to time the client's performance until one of the following occurs:

  ▪ The client loses postural control and balance.

  ▪ The client's feet move on the floor.

  ▪ The client's eyes open.

  ▪ The client's arms move from the folded position.

  ▪ The client exceeds 60 seconds with good postural control.

General interpretations:

▸ The client needs to maintain their balance with good postural control (without excessive swaying) and not exhibit any of the test-termination criteria for 30 or more seconds.

▸ The inability to reach 30 seconds is indicative of inadequate static balance and postural control.

Tinetti Gait Evaluation

Tinetti (1986) devised a simple, scored screening scale to detect and quantify problems with gait (Table 7-7). It is beneficial for looking specifically at the biomechanical patterning of walking.

TABLE 7-7
Tinetti Gait Evaluation*

Initiation of gait after told to "go"	Any hesitancy or multiple attempts to start	=0
	No hesitancy	=1
Step length and height	a) Right swing foot	
	Does not pass left stance foot	=0
	Passes left stance foot with step	=1
	Right foot does not clear floor completely with step	=0
	Right foot completely clears floor	=1
	b) Left swing foot	
	Does not pass right stance foot	=0
	Passes right stance foot with step	=1
	Left foot does not clear floor completely with step	=0
	Left foot completely clears floor	=1
Step symmetry	Right and left step length not equal (estimate)	=0
	Right and left step appear equal	=1
Step continuity	Stopping or discontinuity between steps	=0
	Steps appear continuous	=1
Path†	Marked deviation	=0
	Mild/moderate deviation or uses walking aid	=1
	Straight without walking aid	=2
Trunk	Marked sway or uses walking aid	=0
	No sway but flexion of knees or back or spreads arms while walking	=1
	No sway, no flexion, no use of arms, and no use of walking aid	=2
Walk stance	Heels apart	=0
	Heels almost touching while walking	=1

*The subject stands with the examiner. The subject then walks down a hallway or across the room, first at their usual pace, then back at a rapid, but safe pace (using usual walking aid such as a cane or walker). The maximal gait score is 12.

†Estimate path in relation to floor tiles. Observe excursion of one foot over about 10 feet of the course.

Modified with permission from from M. Tinetti (1986). Performance-oriented assessment of mobility problems in elderly patients. *Journal of the American Geriatrics Society,* 34, 2, 119–126.

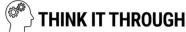

THINK IT THROUGH

Practicing Assessments

The physical-fitness assessments presented in this chapter represent a comprehensive approach to testing the various body systems to gather information about how the senior client will respond to the initiation of an exercise program. Before conducting these assessments with your clients, determine how you will first practice the protocols with others. It is always a good idea to have at least some practical experience administering a physical-fitness assessment on someone other than a paying client (e.g., family member or friend) before you incorporate it into your practice. Furthermore, participating in the assessment yourself, as if you were the client, is a tremendously valuable practice experience to understand firsthand what the test requires of the subject. Take the time to practice each of the assessments presented in this section before you conduct them with your clients. What did you learn from the experience?

CARDIORESPIRATORY ASSESSMENTS

Ventilatory threshold assessment is based on the physiological principle of ventilation. During submaximal exercise, ventilation increases linearly with oxygen (O_2) uptake and carbon dioxide (CO_2) production. This occurs primarily through an increase in **tidal volume.** At higher or near-maximal intensities, the frequency of breathing becomes more pronounced and **minute ventilation ($\dot{V}_E$)** rises disproportionately to the increase in O_2 uptake (Figure 7-17).

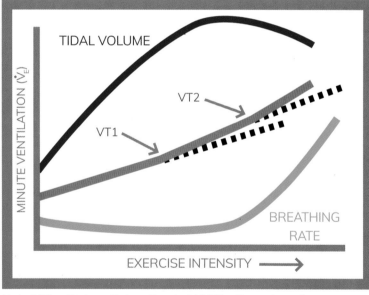

FIGURE 7-17
Ventilatory effects during aerobic exercise

Note: VT1 = First ventilatory threshold; VT2 = Second ventilatory threshold

This disproportionate rise in breathing rate represents a state of ventilation that is no longer directly linked with O_2 demand at the cellular level and is generally termed the ventilatory threshold. The overcompensation in breathing frequency results from an increase in CO_2 production related to the **anaerobic glycolysis** that predominates during near-maximal-intensity exercise. During strenuous exercise, breathing frequency may increase from 12 to 15 breaths per minute at rest to 35 to 45 breaths per minute, while tidal volume increases from resting values of 0.4 to 1.0 L up to 3 L or greater (McArdle, Katch, & Katch, 2019).

As exercise intensity increases, ventilation increases in a somewhat linear manner, demonstrating deflection points at certain intensities associated with metabolic changes within the body. One point, called the "crossover" point, or VT1, represents a level of intensity at which blood lactate accumulates faster and must be offset by blood buffers, which are compounds that neutralize acidosis in the blood and muscle fibers. This metabolic change causes the person to alter breathing in an effort to blow off the extra CO_2 produced by the buffering of acid metabolites. The cardiorespiratory challenge to the body at this point lies primarily with inspiration and not with the expiration of additional amounts of CO_2 (associated with buffering lactate in the blood). The need for O_2 is met primarily through an increase in tidal volume and not respiratory rate. As exercise intensity continues to increase past the crossover point, ventilation rates begin to increase exponentially as O_2 demands outpace the O_2-delivery system and lactate begins to accumulate in the blood. Consequently, respiratory rates increase.

The second disproportionate increase in ventilation—VT2, sometimes called the **respiratory compensation threshold**—occurs at the point where lactate is rapidly increasing with intensity and results in hyperventilation even relative to the extra CO_2 that is being produced. This second threshold represents the point at which blowing off the CO_2 is no longer adequate to buffer the increase in acidity that is occurring with progressively intense exercise.

In well-trained individuals, VT1 is approximately the highest intensity that can be sustained for one to two hours of exercise. In elite marathon runners, VT1 is very close to their competitive pace. The VT2 is the highest intensity that can be sustained for 30 to 60 minutes in well-trained individuals.

An important note for assessment purposes is that the exercise intensity associated with the ability to talk comfortably is highly related to VT1. As long as the exerciser can speak comfortably, they are almost always below VT1. The first point where it becomes more difficult to speak approximates the intensity of VT1, and the point at which speaking is definitely not comfortable approximates the intensity of VT2.

The majority of exercise professionals will not have access to metabolic analyzers for identifying VT1 and VT2 and will need valid field assessments to identify these markers. As such, the most useful and practical approaches for assessing cardiorespiratory fitness are presented here. This section reviews field assessments for measuring HR at VT1 and VT2.

Contraindications

This type of assessment is not recommended for:

▸ Individuals with certain breathing problems [asthma or **chronic obstructive pulmonary disease (COPD)**]

▸ Individuals prone to panic/anxiety attacks, as the labored breathing may create discomfort or precipitate an attack

▸ Those recovering from a recent respiratory infection

▸ Individuals who are not fit enough to perform or benefit from the assessment

Talk Test

Following up on suggestions from a generation ago, several groups have explored the value of the **talk test** as a method of monitoring (and controlling) exercise training intensity (Cannon et al., 2004; Persinger et al., 2004; Recalde et al., 2002; Voelker et al., 2002; Porcari et al., 2001; Dehart et al., 2000). The usual experience with the talk test is that if two people are exercising and having a conversation, one of them will eventually turn to the other and say something like, "If we are going to keep talking, you are going to have to slow down." The talk test works on the premise that at about the intensity of VT1, the increase in ventilation is accomplished by an increase in breathing frequency. One of the requirements of comfortable speech is to be able to control breathing frequency. Thus, at the intensity of VT1, it is no longer possible to speak comfortably.

The simple talk test has been shown to work fairly well as an index of the exercise intensity at VT1. Options include asking clients to recite something familiar, such as reciting the alphabet or "A is for apple, B is for boy, etc.," then answer the question, "Can you speak comfortably?" If the answer is yes, the intensity is below the VT1. At the first response that is less than an unequivocal "yes," the intensity is probably right at that of the VT1, and if the answer is "no," the intensity is probably above VT1. When the client can no longer say more than a word or two between breaths, they are at or above VT2.

The talk test has several advantages as a method of programming and monitoring exercise compared to a given $\%\dot{V}O_2max$ or $\%MHR$, since it is based off an individual's unique metabolic or ventilatory responses to exercise. Thus, for most people, training at intensities at which the answer to the question, "Can you speak comfortably?" becomes less than an unequivocal "yes" may represent the ideal training intensity marker. Therefore, the talk test is an appropriate marker to use for many individuals, especially for those seeking to lose weight or develop their cardiorespiratory efficiency. Training at or near this intensity (unique to the individual's own metabolism) increases the likelihood of a better exercise experience. Higher-intensity training for those individuals with performance goals can be regulated in terms of VT2.

Submaximal Talk Test for VT1

This test is best performed using HR telemetry (HR strap and watch) for continuous monitoring. To avoid missing VT1, the exercise increments need to be small, increasing steady-state HR by approximately 5 bpm per stage. Consequently, this test will require some preparation to determine the appropriate increments that elicit a 5-bpm increase. Once the increments are determined, the time needed to reach steady-state HR during a stage must also be determined (60 to 120 seconds per stage is usually adequate).

The end point of the test is not a predetermined HR but is instead based on monitoring changes in breathing rate (technically metabolic changes) that are determined by the client's ability to recite a predetermined combination of phrases. Note: Reading, as opposed to reciting from memory, is not advised, as it compromises balance if testing is being performed on a treadmill.

The objectives of the test are to measure the HR response at VT1 by progressively increasing exercise intensity and achieving steady state at each stage, as well as to identify the HR where the ability to talk continuously becomes compromised. This point represents the intensity where the individual can continue to talk while breathing with minimal discomfort and reflects an associated increase in tidal volume that should not compromise breathing rate or the ability to talk. Progressing beyond this point where breathing rate increases significantly, making continuous talking difficult, is not necessary and will render the test inaccurate.

Equipment:

▶ Treadmill, cycle ergometer, elliptical trainer, or arm ergometer

▶ Stopwatch

▶ HR monitor (optional)

▶ Predetermined text that the individual will recite (e.g., alphabet)

Pre-test procedure:

▶ As this test involves small, incremental increases in intensity specific to each individual, the testing stages need to be predetermined. The goal is to incrementally increase workload in small quantities to determine VT1. Large incremental increases may result in the individual passing through VT1, thereby invalidating the test:

  ▪ Recommended workload increases are approximately 0.5 mph, 1% grade, or 10 to 20 watts.

  ▪ The objective is to increase steady-state HR at each stage by approximately 5 bpm.

  ▪ Plan to complete this test within eight to 16 minutes to ensure that localized muscle fatigue from longer durations of exercise is not an influencing factor.

▶ Measure pre-exercise HR and BP (if necessary), both sitting and standing, and then record the values on the testing form.

▶ Describe the purpose of this graded exercise test, review the predetermined protocol and the passage to be recited, and allow the client the opportunity to address any questions or concerns. Each stage of the test lasts one to two minutes to achieve a steady-state HR at each workload.

▶ Allow the client to walk on the treadmill or use the ergometer to warm up and get used to the apparatus. If using a treadmill, they should avoid holding the handrails. If the client is too unstable without holding onto the rails, consider using another testing modality, as this will invalidate the test results.

▶ Take the client through a light warm-up (RPE of 0.5 to 2 on the 0 to 10 scale) for three to five minutes, maintaining an intensity comfortably below a moderate level.

Test protocol and administration:

▶ Once the client has warmed up, adjust the workload intensity so the client is working at a moderate intensity level (RPE of 3 to 4 on the 0 to 10 scale).

▶ Toward the latter part of each stage (i.e., last 20 to 30 seconds), measure/record the HR and then ask the client to recite the predetermined passage. Upon completion of the recital, ask the client to identify whether they felt this task was easy or uncomfortable-to-challenging. Note: Conversations with questions and answers are not suggested, as the test needs to evaluate the challenge of talking continuously, not in brief bursts as in conversation. Also, reading, as opposed to reciting from memory, is not advised, as it may compromise balance if testing is being performed on a treadmill.

- The test concludes when the client reports that they can speak, but not entirely comfortably.

▸ If VT1 is not achieved, progress through the successive stages, repeating the protocol at each stage until VT1 is reached.

▸ Once the HR at VT1 is identified, progress to the cool-down phase (matching the warm-up intensity) for three to five minutes.

▸ This test should ideally be conducted on two separate occasions with the same exercise modality to determine an average VT1 HR.

- HR varies between treadmills, bikes, etc., so it is important to conduct the tests with the exercise modality that the client uses most frequently.

- The VT1 HR will also be noticeably higher if the test is conducted after weight training due to fatigue and increased metabolism. Therefore, clients should be tested before performing muscular-training exercises.

VT2 Threshold Assessment

VT2 is equivalent to another important metabolic marker called the **onset of blood lactate accumulation (OBLA),** the point at which blood lactate accumulates at rates faster than the body can buffer and remove it (blood lactate >4 mmol/L). This marker represents an exponential increase in the concentration of blood lactate, indicating an exercise intensity that can no longer be sustained for long periods, and represents the highest sustainable level of exercise intensity, a strong marker of exercise performance. Continually measuring blood lactate is an accurate method to determine OBLA and the corresponding VT2. However, the cost of lactate analyzers and handling of biohazardous materials make it impractical for most exercise professionals. Consequently, field tests have been created to challenge an individual's ability to sustain high intensities of exercise for a predetermined duration to *estimate* VT2. This method of testing requires an individual to sustain the highest intensity possible during a single bout of steady-state exercise. This obviously mandates high levels of conditioning and experience in pacing. Consequently, VT2 testing is *only* recommended for well-conditioned individuals with fitness and performance goals.

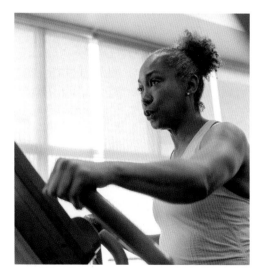

Well-trained individuals can probably estimate their own HR response at VT2 during their training by identifying the highest intensity they can maintain for an extended duration. In cycling, coaches often select a 10-mile time trial or 60 minutes of sustained intensity, whereas in running, a 30-minute run is often used. Given that testing for 30 to 60 minutes is impractical in most fitness facilities, exercise professionals can opt to use shorter single-stage tests of highest sustainable intensity to estimate the HR response at VT2.

In general, the intensity that can be sustained for 15 to 20 minutes is higher than what could be sustained for 30 to 60 minutes in conditioned individuals. To predict the HR response at VT2 using a 15- to 20-minute test, professionals can estimate that the corrected HR response would be equivalent to approximately 95% of the 15- to 20-minute HR average. For example, if an individual's average sustainable HR for a 20-minute bike test is 168 bpm, their HR at VT2 would be 160 bpm (168 bpm x 0.95).

This assessment is best performed using an HR-monitoring device for continuous measurements. Individuals participating in this test need experience with the selected modality to effectively pace themselves at their maximal sustainable intensity for the duration of the bout. In addition, this test should only be performed by clients who are cleared for exercise and ready for Performance Training.

Pre-assessment procedure:

▸ Briefly explain the purpose of the assessment, review the predetermined protocol, and allow the client the opportunity to address any questions or concerns.

▸ Take the client through a light warm-up (2- to 3-out-of-10 effort) for three to five minutes, maintaining an HR below 120 bpm.

Assessment protocol and administration:

▸ Begin the assessment by increasing the intensity to the predetermined level.

  ▪ Allow the individual to make changes to the exercise intensity as needed during the first few minutes of the bout. Remember, they need to be able to maintain the selected intensity for 20 minutes.

▸ During the last five minutes of exercise, record the HR at each minute interval.

▸ Use the average HR collected over the last five minutes to account for any **cardiovascular drift** associated with fatigue, thermoregulation, and changing blood volume.

▸ Multiply the average HR attained during the 15- to 20-minute high-intensity exercise bout by 0.95 to determine the VT2 estimate.

Application of Information from Cardiorespiratory Fitness Testing

Once a client's cardiorespiratory fitness level has been established, and any cardiovascular health risks have been ruled out, it is important to understand how to safely and effectively improve upon the client's current level of fitness. Exercise professionals should keep in mind that cardiorespiratory assessments are not used to determine in which phase of the ACE IFT Model a client begins, but rather are used to establish appropriate intensity levels within each phase of the Model. For example, if a client is insufficiently active (i.e., not performing at least 20 minutes of moderate-intensity cardiorespiratory exercise on at least three days per week), cardiorespiratory assessments are not needed because the client will begin in the Base Training phase and the talk test or RPE will be used to ensure that the client is training at an appropriate intensity. It is not until clients are ready to progress to the Fitness Training phase that the submaximal talk test for VT1 is administered, while the VT2 threshold test is used to establish an exercise intensity if and when clients progress to the Performance

Training phase. As with younger adults, physical fitness exists on a continuum for older adults, ranging from sedentary or deconditioned to highly fit or peak sports performance. The time and energy commitments required to improve sport performance are obviously much more involved than the requirements for improving overall health.

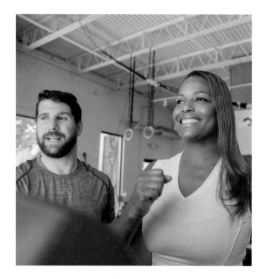

The *Physical Activity Guidelines for Americans* suggest that all adults should participate in structured cardiorespiratory-related physical activity at a moderate intensity for at least 150 minutes per week or a vigorous intensity for at least 75 minutes per week to meet recommended physical-activity guidelines. In addition, it is recommended that most adults incorporate muscle-strengthening activities at least two days a week (U.S. Department of Health and Human Services, 2018).

For clients who are not capable of achieving these recommendations at the outset, reaching this level of activity should be the primary goal during the initial conditioning stage, or the Base Training phase of the ACE IFT Model. It is prudent for the exercise professional to support and encourage regular participation in cardiorespiratory activities. Chapter 8 provides guidelines for developing safe and effective cardiorespiratory exercise plans. For beginning exercisers, or those who are returning after a significant break, intensity should be kept low to promote positive experiences and exercise adherence.

If the cardiorespiratory testing was unremarkable, or if the client does not have cardiovascular health risks requiring medical clearance, an appropriate fitness program can be initiated. For novice exercisers and those who are deconditioned, improving cardiorespiratory fitness should be addressed in a twofold manner. The first goal is to establish an aerobic base by gradually increasing exercise duration and frequency through positive exercise experiences that encourage clients to exercise regularly. This allows the body to adapt to the new demands of exercise and respond accordingly (e.g., increase in capillary density, increase in mitochondrial size/number, and enhanced ability to remove lactic acid). Initially, training volume can be increased by 5 to 10% per week until the desired training volume is achieved.

For those who do not have contraindications for higher-intensity exercise, already have a solid cardiorespiratory training base, and are completing at least 20 minutes of moderate-intensity cardiorespiratory exercise on at least three days per week, the Fitness Training phase is appropriate. In this phase, increasing aerobic efficiency through the integration of vigorous-intensity intervals and increased frequency and duration based on client goals are the focus. From there, clients may progress to the Performance Training phase if they are motivated and seeking to achieve endurance-performance objectives. This phase incorporates higher-intensity steady-state training as well as interval training and is typically reserved for those with competitive endurance goals requiring specialized training.

CORE FUNCTION ASSESSMENTS

McGill's Torso Muscular Endurance Test Battery

Optimally functioning core muscles help clients perform ADL like lifting a heavy laundry basket or recreational activities like swinging a golf club. Further, back dysfunction may be reversed by having a conditioned core. To evaluate balanced core endurance and stability, it is important to assess all sides of the torso. Each of the following assessments is performed individually, then evaluated collectively. Poor endurance capacity of the torso muscles or an imbalance among these muscle groups is believed to contribute to low-back dysfunction and core instability.

TRUNK FLEXOR ENDURANCE TEST

The trunk flexor endurance test is the first in the battery of three tests and assesses muscular endurance of the trunk flexors (i.e., rectus abdominis, external and internal obliques, and transverse abdominis). It is a timed test involving isometric activation of the anterior muscles, stabilizing the spine until the individual exhibits fatigue and can no longer hold the assumed position. This test may not be suitable for individuals who suffer from low-back pain, have had recent back surgery, and/or are in the midst of an acute low-back flare-up.

Equipment:

▸ Stopwatch

▸ Board (or step)

▸ Strap (optional)

Pre-assessment procedure:

▸ After explaining the purpose of the flexor endurance test, describe the proper body position.

  ▪ The starting position requires the client to be seated, with the hips and knees bent to 90 degrees, aligning the hips, knees, and second toe.

  ▪ Instruct the client to fold their arms across the chest, touching each hand to the opposite shoulder, lean against a board positioned at a 50- to 60-degree incline, and keep the head in a neutral position (Figure 7-18).

  ▪ It is important to ask the client to press the shoulders into the board and maintain this "open" position throughout the test after the board is removed.

FIGURE 7-18
Trunk flexor endurance test

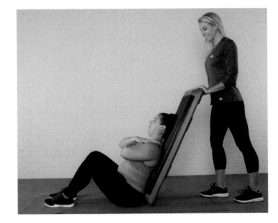 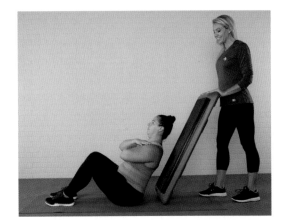

- Instruct the client to engage the abdominals to maintain a flat-to-neutral spine. The back should never be allowed to arch during the test.

- The exercise professional can anchor the toes under a strap or manually stabilize the feet if necessary.

▸ The goal of the test is to hold this 50- to 60-degree position for as long as possible without the benefit of the back support.

▸ Encourage the client to practice this position prior to attempting the test.

Assessment protocol and administration:

The exercise professional starts the stopwatch as they move the board about 4 inches (10 cm) back, while the client maintains the 50- to 60-degree, suspended position.

▸ Terminate the test when there is a noticeable change in the trunk position:

- Watch for a deviation from the neutral spine (i.e., the shoulders rounding forward) or an increase in the low-back arch.

- No part of the back should touch the back rest.

▸ Record the client's time on the testing form.

TRUNK LATERAL ENDURANCE TEST

The trunk lateral endurance test, also called the side-bridge test, assesses muscular endurance of the lateral core muscles (i.e., transverse abdominis, obliques, quadratus lumborum, and erector spinae). This timed test involves isometric muscle activation of the lateral muscles on each side of the trunk that stabilize the spine. This test may not be suitable for individuals with shoulder pain or weakness and who suffer from low-back pain, have had recent back surgery, and/or are in the midst of an acute low-back flare-up.

Equipment:

▸ Stopwatch

▸ Mat (optional)

Pre-assessment procedure:

▸ After explaining the purpose of this test, describe the proper body position.

- The starting position requires the client to be on their side with extended legs, aligning the feet on top of each other.

- Have the client place the lower arm under the body and the upper arm on the side of the body.

- When the client is ready, instruct them to assume a full side-bridge position, keeping both legs extended and the sides of the feet on the floor. The elbow of the lower arm should be positioned directly under the shoulder with the forearm facing out (the forearm can be placed palm down for balance and support) and the upper arm should be resting along the side of the body or across the chest to the opposite shoulder.

- The hips should be elevated off the mat and the body should be in straight alignment (i.e., head, neck, torso, hips, and legs). The torso should only be supported by the client's foot/feet and the elbow/forearm of the lower arm (Figure 7-19).

> *Modification:* If a client is unable to support their full body weight while balancing on the feet, an alternative is for the client to rest on the side of the lower leg with both knees bent in the hook-lying position (Figure 7-20), thereby shortening the lever of the legs and increasing the surface area on which to balance. If this modification is used, be sure to perform subsequent assessments in the modified position so that the results are comparable. Because McGill's original test battery was not performed using this modification, the scoring and reliability of results will vary.

▸ The goal of the test is to hold this position for as long as possible. Once the client breaks the position, the test is terminated.

▸ Encourage the client to practice this position prior to attempting the test.

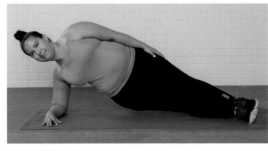

FIGURE 7-19
Trunk lateral endurance test

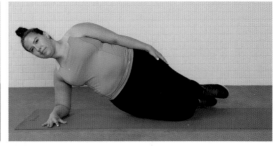

FIGURE 7-20
Trunk lateral endurance test: Modified hook-lying position

Assessment protocol and administration:

▸ The exercise professional starts the stopwatch as the client moves into the side-bridge position.

▸ Terminate the test when there is a noticeable change in the trunk position
- A deviation from the neutral spine (i.e., the hips dropping downward)
- The hips shifting forward or backward in an effort to maintain balance and stability

▸ Record the client's time on the testing form.

▸ Repeat the test on the opposite side and record this value on the testing form.

TRUNK EXTENSOR ENDURANCE TEST

The trunk extensor endurance test is generally used to assess muscular endurance of the torso extensor muscles (i.e., erector spinae and multifidi). This is a timed test involving a static, isometric contraction of the trunk extensor muscles that stabilize the spine. This test may not be suitable for a client with major strength deficiencies, where the individual cannot even lift the torso from a forward flexed position to a neutral position, a client with a high body mass, in which case it would be difficult for the exercise professional to support the client's suspended upper-body weight, and a client who suffers from low-back pain, has had recent back surgery, and/or is in the midst of an acute low-back flare-up.

Equipment:

▸ Elevated, sturdy exam table

▸ Nylon strap

▸ Stopwatch

Pre-assessment procedure:

▸ After explaining the purpose of the test, review the proper body position.

  ▪ The starting position requires the client to be prone, positioning the iliac crests at the table edge while supporting the upper extremity on the arms, which are placed on the floor or on a riser.

  ▪ While the client is supporting the weight of the upper body, anchor the client's lower legs to the table using a strap. If a strap is not used, the exercise professional will have to use their own body weight to stabilize the client's legs (Figure 7-21a).

▸ The goal of the test is to hold a horizontal, prone position for as long as possible. Once the client falls below horizontal, the test is terminated.

▸ Encourage the client to practice this position prior to attempting the test.

Assessment protocol and administration:

▸ When ready, the client lifts/extends the torso until it is parallel to the floor with the arms crossed over the chest (Figure 7-21b).

  ▪ *Modification:* If a client is unable to support their body weight while hanging off the edge of a table, an alternative is for the client to lie prone on the floor and come into spinal extension (Figure 7-22), thereby eliminating the need for a table and strap (or for the exercise professional to hold the client's legs). The client should be instructed to keep the thighs in contact with the floor throughout the duration of the assessment. If this modification is used, be sure to perform subsequent assessments in the modified position so that the results are comparable. Because McGill's original test battery was not performed using this modification, the scoring and reliability of results will vary.

▸ Start timing as soon as the client assumes this position.

▸ Terminate the test when the client can no longer maintain the position.

▸ Record the client's time on the testing form.

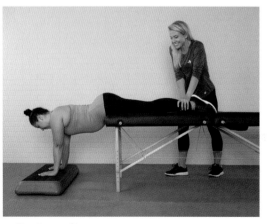

a. Starting position

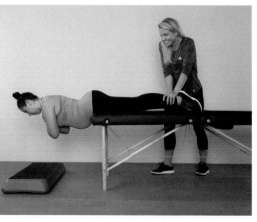

b. Test position

FIGURE 7-21
Trunk extensor endurance test

FIGURE 7-22
Trunk extensor
endurance test:
Modified position

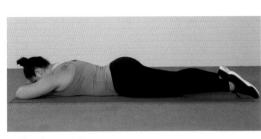

a. Starting position

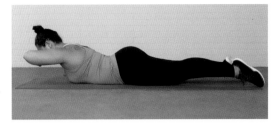

b. Test position

TOTAL TEST BATTERY INTERPRETATION

Each individual test in this testing battery is not a primary indicator of current or future back problems. McGill (2016) has shown that the relationships among the test results are more important indicators of muscle imbalances that can lead to back pain compared to looking at the individual results of each test because the torso extensors, flexors, and lateral musculature are involved in virtually all tasks. In fact, even in a person with little or no back pain, the ratios can still be off, suggesting that low-back pain may eventually occur without diligent attention to a solid core-conditioning program. McGill (2016) suggests the following ratios indicate balanced endurance among the muscle groups:

▸ Flexion:extension ratio should be less than 1.0

  ▪ For example, a flexion score of 120 seconds and extension score of 150 seconds generates a ratio score of 0.80

▸ Right-side bridge (RSB):left-side bridge (LSB) scores should be no greater than 0.05 from a balanced score of 1.0 (i.e., 0.95 to 1.05)

  ▪ For example, a RSB score of 88 seconds and an LSB score of 92 seconds generates a ratio score of 0.96, which is within the 0.05 range from 1.0

▸ Side bridge (either side):extension ratio should be less than 0.75

  ▪ For example, a RSB score of 88 seconds and an extension score of 150 seconds generates a ratio score of 0.59

Demonstrated deficiencies in these core functional assessments should be addressed during exercise programming as part of the foundational exercises for a client.

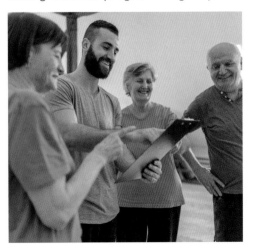

The goal is to create ratios consistent with McGill's recommendations. Muscular endurance, more so than muscular strength or even ROM, has been shown to be an accurate predictor of back health (McGill, 2016). When working with clients with low-back dysfunction, it is prudent to include daily stabilization exercises in their home exercise plans (see pages 270–271). After completing all elements of McGill's torso muscular endurance test battery, exercise professionals can use Figure 7-23 to record the client's data.

Trunk flexor endurance test

Time to completion: _____

Trunk lateral endurance test

Right side time to completion: _____ Left side time to completion: _____

Trunk extensor endurance test

Time to completion: _____

Ratio of Comparison	Criteria for Good Relationship between Muscles
Flexion:extension	Ratio less than 1.0
Right-side bridge:left-side bridge	Scores should be no greater than 0.05 from a balanced score of 1.0
Side bridge (each side):extension	Ratio less than 0.75

Flexion:extension ratio: _____ Rating: ☐ Good   ☐ Poor

Right-side bridge:left-side bridge ratio: _____ Rating: ☐ Good   ☐ Poor

Side-bridge (each side):extension ratio: _____ Rating: ☐ Good   ☐ Poor

FIGURE 7-23
McGill's torso muscular endurance test battery—record sheet

Front Plank

The front plank test assesses the core musculature's ability hold the spine in neutral alignment when the body is in a forearm plank position. To perform the assessment, the client adopts a prone plank position in which the forearms and toes are in contact with the floor. The elbows should be aligned directly underneath the shoulders and the body should maintain a straight line from shoulders to heels (i.e., the hips should not rise above or fall below shoulder level) (Figure 7-24a). Clients can also be given the option of supporting the lower body using the knees instead of the toes if they feel that attempting to hold the position on the toes will be too challenging (Figure 7-24b).

Equipment:

▸ Stopwatch

▸ Exercise mat

Pretest procedure:

▸ After explaining the purpose of the front plank test, explain and demonstrate the proper technique.

▸ Allow for adequate warm-up and stretching if needed.

Test protocol and administration:

▸ Instruct the client to adopt the forearm plank position. As soon as the client is in the position and exhibiting proper alignment, start the stopwatch and cue the client to hold the position for as long as possible up to 30 seconds.

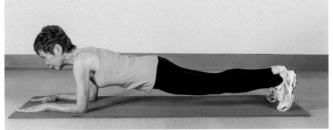

a. Good alignment

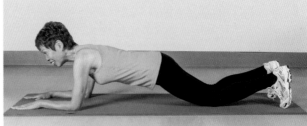

b. Modification

FIGURE 7-24
Front plank

▸ The goal of the test is to hold the forearm plank position with the body in proper alignment for as long as possible, up to 30 seconds. If the client breaks form and comes out of proper position, terminate the test and record the number of seconds attained.

Test evaluation:

▸ After the test is complete, ask the client where they felt the muscles working the most. That is, did the client feel the work mainly in the lower back or the abdomen?

- If the client felt it mainly in the lower back, it is an indication that they lack appropriate core stability.

- If the client reports feeling it mainly in the abdominal muscles, it is an indication that they are recruiting the appropriate musculature to support the spine in the forearm plank position.

▸ If the client is able to hold proper alignment throughout the duration of the test, it is an indication that their core muscles are able to effectively stabilize the spine. Evaluate the muscular fitness of the core using the following criteria:

- Unable to hold proper alignment for 30 seconds (poor)

- Able to hold proper alignment for 30 seconds (good)

MOVEMENT ASSESSMENTS

Movement Training focuses on establishing efficient movement through healthy ROMs specific to each client, essentially teaching clients to perform the five primary movement patterns effectively in all three planes of motion without compromising postural or joint stability. Thus, the movement assessments introduced here are designed to help the exercise professional observe a client's ability to control mobility as they perform the five primary movements:

▸ *Bend-and-lift:* Hip hinging and squatting movements performed throughout the day (e.g., sitting on or standing up from a chair or squatting down to lift up an object off the floor)

▸ *Single-leg:* Movements done while balancing on one leg, including lunging [e.g., alternate foot stance during walking (gait cycle), stepping forward to reach down with one hand to pick up something off the floor, or walking down/up a flight of stairs)]

▸ *Pushing:* Movements performed in a forward direction (e.g., during a push-up exercise or when pushing open a door), in an overhead direction (e.g., during an overhead press or when putting an item on a high shelf), or in a lateral direction (e.g., pushing open double sliding doors or lifting one's torso when getting up from a side-lying position)

▸ *Pulling:* Movements performed during an exercise such as a bent-over row or pull-up or during a movement like pulling open a car door

▸ *Rotation:* Movements, such as the rotation of the thoracic spine during gait or reaching across the body to pick up an object on one's left side and placing it on the right side (e.g., when putting on a seatbelt in a car)

Bend-and-Lift Assessment: Squat Pattern

Objective: To assess symmetrical lower-extremity mobility and stability and trunk mobility and stability during a bend-and-lift movement

Equipment:

▸ None

Instructions:

▸ Briefly discuss the protocol so the client understands what is required.

▸ Ask the client to stand with the feet shoulder-width apart with the arms hanging freely to the sides.

▸ Ask the client to perform five to 10 bend-and-lift movements (i.e., squats), lowering as deep as is comfortable. It is important not to cue the client to use good technique, but instead observe their natural movement.

Observations (Table 7-8):

▸ Anterior view (Figure 7-25):

▪ *Feet:* Is there evidence of pronation, supination, eversion, or **inversion**?

▪ *Knees:* Do they move inward or outward?

▪ *Torso:* How is the overall symmetry of the entire body over the base of support? Is there evidence of a lateral shift or rotation?

▸ Side view (Figure 7-26):

▪ *Feet:* Do the heels remain in contact with the floor throughout the movement?

▪ *Hip and knee:*

> Does the client exhibit "glute" or "quadriceps dominance" (i.e., is the descent initiated by pushing the hips backward or by driving the knees forward)?

> Does the client achieve a parallel position between the top of the thighs and the floor?

> Does the client control the descent to avoid resting the hamstrings against the calves at the bottom of the squat?

▪ *Lumbar and thoracic spine:* Does the client exhibit an exaggerated curve in the lumbar (i.e., "lumbar dominance") or thoracic spine during the descent?

▪ *Head:* Are any changes in the position of the head observed during the movement?

Interpretation:

▸ Identify origin(s) of movement limitation or compensation.

▸ Evaluate the impact on the entire kinetic chain.

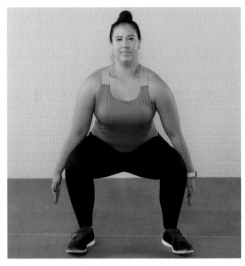

FIGURE 7-25

Bend-and-lift assessment (squat pattern): Anterior view

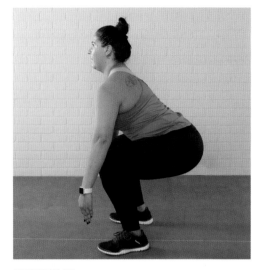

FIGURE 7-26

Bend-and-lift assessment (squat pattern): Side view

TABLE 7-8

Bend-and-Lift Assessment: Squat Pattern

View	Location	Compensation	Key Suspected Compensations: Overactive (Tight)	Key Suspected Compensations: Underactive (Lengthened)
☐ Anterior	Feet	Lack of foot stability: Ankles collapse inward/feet turn outward	Soleus, lateral gastrocnemius, peroneals	Medial gastrocnemius, gracilis, sartorius, tibialis group
☐ Anterior	Knees	Move inward	Hip adductors, tensor fascia latae	Gluteus medius and maximus
☐ Anterior	Torso	Lateral shift to a side	Side dominance and muscle imbalance due to potential lack of stability in the lower extremity during joint loading	
☐ Side	Feet	Unable to keep heels in contact with the floor	Plantar flexors	None
☐ Side	Hip and knee	Initiation of movement	Movement initiated at knees may indicate quadriceps and hip flexor dominance, as well as insufficient activation of the gluteus group	
☐ Side	Hip and knee	Unable to achieve tops of thighs parallel to the floor	Poor mechanics, lack of dorsiflexion due to tight plantar flexors (which normally allow the tibia to move forward)	
	Contact behind knee	Hamstrings contact back of calves	Muscle weakness and poor mechanics, resulting in an inability to stabilize and control the lowering phase	

TABLE 7-8 *(continued)*

View	Location	Compensation	Key Suspected Compensations: Overactive (Tight)	Key Suspected Compensations: Underactive (Lengthened)
☐	Side	Lumbar and thoracic spine	Back excessively arches (i.e., lumbar dominance)	Hip flexors, back extensors, latissimus dorsi	Core, rectus abdominis, gluteal group, hamstrings
			Back rounds forward	Latissimus dorsi, teres major, pectoralis major and minor	Upper back extensors
☐	Side	Head	Downward	Increased hip and trunk flexion	
			Upward	Compression and tightness in the cervical extensor region	

Sources: Kendall, F.P. et al. (2005). Muscles Testing and Function with Posture and Pain (5th ed.). Baltimore, Md.: Lippincott Williams & Wilkins; Cook, G. (2003). Athletic Body in Balance. Champaign, Ill.: Human Kinetics; Donnelly, D.V. et al. (2006). The effect of directional gaze on kinematics during the squat exercise. Journal of Strength and Conditioning Research, 20, 145–150; Fry, A.C., Smith J.C., & Schilling, B.K. (2003). Effect of knee position on hip and knees torques during the barbell squat. Journal of Strength and Conditioning Research, 17, 629–633; Abelbeck, K.G. (2002). Biomechanical model and evaluation of a linear motion squat type exercise. Journal of Strength and Conditioning Research, 16, 516–524; Sahrmann, S.A. (2002). Diagnosis and Treatment of Movement Impairment Syndromes. St. Louis, Mo.: Mosby.

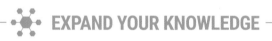 **EXPAND YOUR KNOWLEDGE**

Movement Patterns during a Squat

The gluteals and core musculature play an important role in the squat movement, during which individuals can exhibit "lumbar dominance," "quadriceps dominance," or "glute dominance."

▸ *Lumbar dominance:* This implies a lack of core and gluteal muscle strength to counteract the force of the hip flexors and erector spinae as they pull the pelvis forward during a squat movement. In this scenario, the individual experiences excessive loads within the lumbar spine as it moves into extension during the squat. The muscles of the abdominal wall and gluteal complex do not contribute enough in this situation to spare the back and foster proper execution of the squat (McGill, 2017). Chronically tight hip flexors, such as those experienced by individuals who sit for prolonged periods throughout the day, may also contribute to the problem.

▸ *Quadriceps dominance:* This implies reliance on loading the quadriceps group during a squat movement. The first 10 to 15 degrees of the downward phase are initiated by driving the tibia forward, creating shearing forces across the knee as the femur slides over the tibia. In this lowered position, the gluteus maximus does not eccentrically load and cannot generate much force during the upward phase. Quadriceps-dominant squatting transfers more pressure into the knees, placing greater loads on the **anterior cruciate ligament (ACL)** (Wilthrow et al., 2005).

▸ *Glute dominance:* This implies reliance on eccentrically loading the gluteus maximus during a squat movement. The first 10 to 15 degrees of the downward phase are initiated by pushing the hips backward, creating a hip hinge (Figure 7-27). In the lowered position, this maximizes the eccentric loading on the gluteus maximus to generate significant force during the upward, **concentric** phase.

The glute-dominant squat pattern is the preferred method of squatting, as it spares the lumbar spine and relieves undue stress on the knees. Glute dominance also helps activate the hamstrings, which pull on the posterior surface of the tibia and help unload the ACL to protect it from potential injury (Hauschildt, 2008).

FIGURE 7-27
Hip hinge

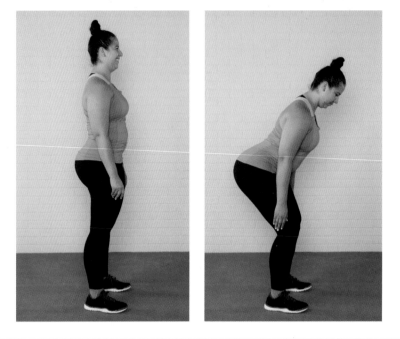

Single-leg Assessment: Step-up

Objective: To assess symmetrical lower-extremity mobility and stability and trunk mobility and stability during a single-leg (step-up) movement

Equipment:

▸ Bench; select a bench height that allows the client to start with the hip and knee at approximately a 90-degree angle.

Instructions:

▸ Briefly discuss the protocol so the client understands what is required.

▸ Ask the client to stand with the feet shoulder-width apart with the arms hanging freely to the sides.

▸ Instruct the client to place one leg up squarely on the bench while maintaining an upright posture.

▸ Instruct the client to push off with the heel of the foot on the bench while simultaneously bringing the opposite leg up to a 90-degree angle.

▸ Instruct the client to return slowly to the starting position in a one-two-three rhythm.

▸ Ask the client to perform five to 10 single-leg (step-up) movements.

▸ Switch the leg positioned on the bench and repeat the above steps.

▸ It is important not to cue the client to use good technique, but instead observe their natural movement.

Observations (Table 7-9):

▸ Anterior view (Figure 7-28):

  ▪ *First repetition:* Observe the stability of the foot (i.e., evidence of pronation, supination, eversion, or inversion).

  ▪ *Second repetition:* Observe the alignment of the stance-leg knee over the foot (i.e., evidence of knee movement in any plane).

  ▪ *Third repetition:* Watch for excessive hip adduction greater than 2 inches (5.1 cm) as measured by excessive stance-leg adduction or downward hip-tilting toward the opposite side.

  ▪ *Fourth repetition:* Observe the stability of the torso.

  ▪ *Fifth repetition:* Observe the alignment of the moving leg (i.e., lack of dorsiflexion at the ankle, deviation from the sagittal plane at the knee or ankle, or hiking of the moving hip).

▸ Side view (Figure 7-29):

  ▪ *First repetition:* Observe the stability of the torso and stance leg.

  ▪ *Second repetition:* Observe the mobility of the hip (i.e., allowing 70 degrees of hip flexion without compensation—anterior tilting) of the moving leg.

Interpretation:

▸ Identify origin(s) of movement limitation or compensation.

▸ Evaluate the impact on the entire kinetic chain.

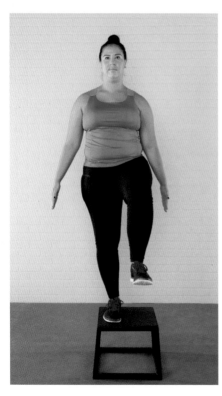

FIGURE 7-28
Step-up: Anterior view

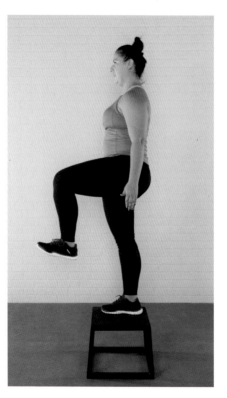

FIGURE 7-29
Step-up: Side view

TABLE 7-9

Single-leg Assessment: Step-up

View	Location	Compensation	Key Suspected Compensations: Overactive (Tight)	Key Suspected Compensations: Underactive (Lengthened)
☐ Anterior	Feet	Lack of foot stability: Ankles collapse inward/feet turn outward	Soleus, lateral gastrocnemius, peroneals	Medial gastrocnemius, gracilis, sartorius, tibialis group, gluteus medius and maximus—inability to control internal rotation
☐ Anterior	Knees	Move inward	Hip adductors, tensor fascia latae	Gluteus medius and maximus
☐ Anterior	Hips	Hip adduction* >2 inches (5.1 cm) Stance-leg hip rotation (inward)	Hip adductors, tensor fascia latae Stance-leg or raised-leg internal rotators	Gluteus medius and maximus Stance-leg or raised-leg external rotators
☐ Anterior	Torso	Lateral tilt, forward lean, rotation	Lack of core stability	
☐ Anterior	Raised-leg	Limb deviates from sagittal plane Hiking the raised hip	Ankle plantar flexors Raised-leg hip extensors Stance-leg hip flexors—limiting posterior hip rotation during raise	Ankle dorsiflexors Raised-leg hip flexors
☐ Side	Pelvis and low back	Lack of ankle dorsiflexion Anterior tilt with forward torso lean Posterior tilt with hunched-over torso	Stance-leg hip flexors Rectus abdominis and hip extensors	Rectus abdominis and hip extensors Stance-leg hip flexors

*Hip adduction involves weight transference over the stance leg while preserving hip, knee, and foot alignment. This weight transference requires a 1- to 2-inch (2.5- to 5-cm) lateral shift over the stance-leg, with a small hike in the stance-hip of 4 to 5 degrees or less.

Sources: Kendall, F.P. et al. (2005). *Muscles Testing and Function with Posture and Pain* (5th ed.). Baltimore, Md.: Lippincott Williams & Wilkins; Cook, G. (2003). *Athletic Body in Balance*. Champaign, Ill.: Human Kinetics; Sahrmann, S.A. (2002). *Diagnosis and Treatment of Movement Impairment Syndromes*. St. Louis, Mo.: Mosby.

Push Assessment: Shoulder Push Stabilization

Objective: To assess stabilization of the scapulothoracic joint and core control during closed-kinetic-chain pushing movements

Instructions:

▸ Briefly discuss the protocol so the client understands what is required.

  ▪ The client presses their body off the ground as the exercise professional evaluates the ability to stabilize the scapulae against the thorax (rib cage)

during pushing-type movements (Figure 7-30).

■ Instruct the client to lie prone on the floor with arms abducted in the push-up position or bent-knee push-up position.

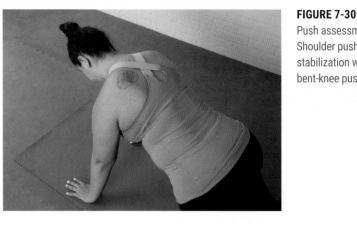

▸ Ask the client to perform several push-ups to full arm extension.

■ Subjects should perform full push-ups; modify to bent-knee push-ups if necessary.

■ It is important to remember not to cue the client to use good technique, but instead observe their natural movement.

■ Repetitions need to be performed slowly and with control.

Observations (Table 7-10):

▸ Observe any notable changes in the position of the scapulae relative to the rib cage at both end-ranges of motion (i.e., the appearance of scapular "winging").

▸ Observe for lumbar hyperextension in the press position.

General interpretations:

▸ Identify the origin(s) of movement limitation or compensation.

▸ Evaluate the impact on the entire kinetic chain.

TABLE 7-10

Push Assessment: Shoulder Push Stabilization

View		Joint Location	Compensation	Key Suspected Compensations
☐	Side	Scapulothoracic	Exhibits "winging" during the push-up movement	Inability of the parascapular muscles (i.e., serratus anterior, trapezius, levator scapula, rhomboids) to stabilize the scapulae against the rib cage. Can also be due to a flat thoracic spine.
☐	Side	Trunk	Hyperextension or "collapsing" of the low back	Lack of core, abdominal, and low-back strength, resulting in instability

Sources: Kendall, F.P. et al. (2005). Muscles Testing and Function with Posture and Pain (5th ed.). Baltimore, Md.: Lippincott Williams & Wilkins; Sahrmann, S.A. (2002). Diagnosis and Treatment of Movement Impairment Syndromes. St. Louis, Mo.: Mosby.

Pull Assessment: Standing Row

Objective: To assess movement efficiency and potential muscle imbalances during pulling movements

Equipment:

▸ Selectorized cable machine with handle attachments or resistance band with handles

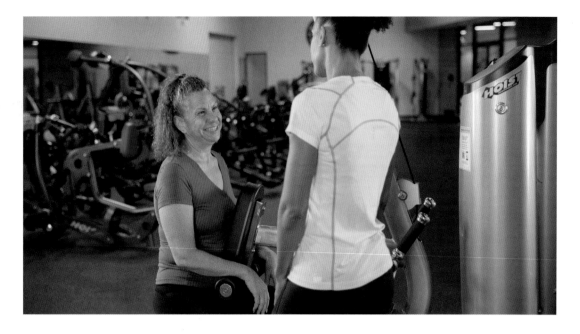

Instructions:

▸ Briefly discuss the protocol so the client understands what is required.

▸ A light resistance appropriate for the client should be selected.

▸ Ask the client to stand with feet shoulder-width apart and knees slightly bent.

▸ Position the anchor point at a height that aligns with the client's xiphoid process.

▸ Instruct the client to grab the handles.

▸ Instruct the client to pull the bar or handle toward their pectoral muscles/torso while keeping the chest forward and back straight (Figure 7-31). The client should briefly pause and then return to the starting position.

▸ Ask the client to perform several repetitions slowly and with control

▸ It is important to remember not to cue the client to use good technique, but instead observe their natural movement.

FIGURE 7-31
Pull assessment:
Standing row

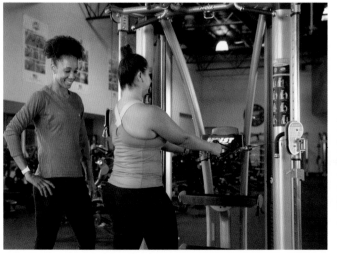
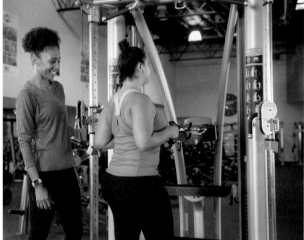

TABLE 7-11

Pull Assessment: Standing Row

View		Location	Compensation	Key Suspected Compensations: Overactive (Tight)	Key Suspected Compensations: Underactive (Lengthened)
☐	Side	Lumbar spine	Hyperextension	Hip flexors, back extensors	Core, rectus abdominis, gluteal group, hamstrings
☐	Posterior	Scapulothoracic	Elevation	Upper trapezius, levator scapulae, rhomboid major and minor	Mid and lower trapezius
☐	Side	Head	Migrates forward (protraction)	Cervical spine extensors, upper trapezius, levator scapulae	Cervical spine flexors
☐	Posterior	Scapulothoracic	Abduction (protraction)	Serratus anterior, anterior scapulohumeral muscles, upper trapezius	Rhomboid major and minor, middle trapezius

Observations (Table 7-11):

▸ Observe for shoulder elevation or the head migrating forward.

▸ Observe for lumbar hyperextension in the pull position.

General interpretations:

▸ Identify the origin(s) of movement limitation or compensation.

▸ Evaluate the impact on the entire kinetic chain.

Rotation Assessment: Thoracic Spine Mobility

Objective: To assess bilateral mobility of the thoracic spine. Lumbar spine rotation is considered insignificant, as it offers only approximately 15 degrees of rotation.

Equipment:

▸ Chair

▸ Squeezable ball or block

▸ 48-inch (1.2-m) dowel

Instructions:

▸ Briefly discuss the protocol so the client understands what is required.

▸ Instruct the client to sit upright toward the front edge of the seat with the feet together and firmly placed on the floor. The client's back should not touch the backrest.

▸ Place a squeezable ball or block between the knees and a dowel across the front of the shoulders, instructing the client to hold the bar in the hands (i.e., front barbell squat grip) (Figure 7-32a).

▸ While maintaining an upright and straight posture, the client squeezes the block to immobilize the hips and gently rotates left and right to an end-ROM without any bouncing (Figure 7-32b).

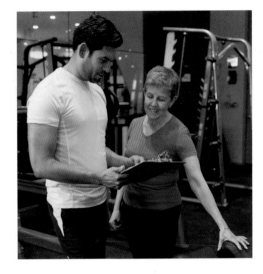

▸ It is important to remember not to cue the client to use good technique, but instead observe their natural movement.

▸ Ask the client to perform a few repetitions in each direction, slowly and with control.

Observation (Table 7-12):

▸ Observe any bilateral discrepancies between the rotations in each direction.

General interpretations:

▸ Identify the origin(s) of movement limitation or compensation. As an individual rotates, the facet joints of each vertebra experience shearing forces against each other. One way to reduce this force and promote greater movement is to laterally flex the trunk during the movement or at the end-range of movement. This assessment evaluates trunk rotation in the transverse plane. Therefore, any lateral flexion of the trunk (dowel tilting up or down) must be avoided.

▸ Evaluate the impact on the entire kinetic chain. Remember that the lumbar spine generally exhibits limited rotation of approximately 15 degrees (Sahrmann, 2002), with the balance of trunk rotation occurring through the thoracic spine. If thoracic spine mobility is limited, the body strives to gain movement in alternative planes within the lumbar spine (e.g., increase in lordosis to promote greater rotation).

FIGURE 7-32
Rotation assessment: Thoracic spine mobility

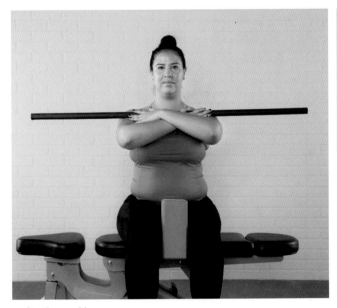

a. Starting position

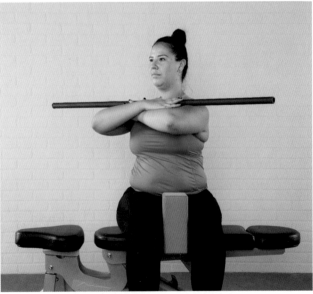

b. Assessment position

TABLE 7-12

Rotation Assessment: Thoracic Spine Mobility

View	Location	Compensation	Possible Biomechanical Problems
☐ Anterior or posterior	Trunk	None if trunk rotation achieves 45 degrees in each direction	
☐ Anterior or posterior	Trunk	Bilateral discrepancy (assuming no existing congenital issues in the spine)	Side-dominance Differences in paraspinal development Torso rotation, perhaps associated with some hip rotation Note: Lack of thoracic mobility will negatively impact glenohumeral mobility

Source: Sahrmann, S.A. (2002). *Diagnosis and Treatment of Movement Impairment Syndromes*. St. Louis, Mo.: Mosby.

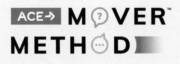

For the past three months, you have been working with Ben, who is an 82-year-old retiree who hired you because he was interested in improving lower-body strength and endurance after noticing that rising from a chair was becoming more of a challenge. Ben has consistently showed up for scheduled exercise sessions, has progressed through Functional Training, and has begun making progress in Movement Training. Until this point in the program, no formal assessments of muscular fitness have been performed because Ben did not want to start the program with assessments. Therefore, the program focus has been on promoting postural stability, joint mobility, and moving more efficiently. At his most recent exercise session, Ben showed interest in performing the 30-second chair stand test to assess lower-extremity muscular endurance, so you and he decided to give it a try.

Observations from this assessment include the following:

▸ Ben was able to perform nine complete repetitions (thighs reached parallel to the floor).

▸ Ben attempted a tenth repetition, at which time a full repetition was not achieved.

▸ Valgus tendencies appeared during the tenth repetition and the thighs did not reach parallel to the floor.

The following is an example of how the ACE Mover Method can be applied when discussing assessment results with clients.

ACE→ ABC APPROACH

Ask: Asking powerful open-ended questions to initiate the discussion around assessment results enables the client to play an active role in the assessment evaluation and interpretation process, which is important now and when it is time to reassess.

Exercise Professional: Great job with your exercise session today Ben! You worked hard and maintained postural stability when we focused on the five primary movement patterns. We also introduced the 30-second chair stand test to gather some initial information about the endurance of your leg muscles, which was a specific concern for you when we first started working together. What observations did you make about your chair stand test performance?

Client: I enjoyed our workout and felt like my energy level was high. I was excited to try the chair stand test today because I feel more comfortable and wanted to push myself to see what I could achieve. For the first three or four repetitions, my legs felt strong and my body felt the same as it does when we do this exercise during our workout sessions. By the fifth repetition, I felt like I was working much harder to maintain good posture and to take my squat low enough to reach the chair. I was able to get out a few more repetitions after this point but by the end, I could not get low enough and my posture felt off. My goal was to get to 10 repetitions and I almost made it. My leg muscles felt fatigued. I also noticed that about halfway through, I really started to feel the work being done in the top of my thighs. They were burning! I could not have done this type of test when I first started. I probably would have quit immediately! What did you think of my overall performance?

Exercise Professional: Thank you for all of the insight you provided. Your observations during the assessment match what I noticed, which lets me know that you are recognizing the difference between moving efficiently and moving with dysfunction like we have been talking about. After the ninth repetition, when your exercise form changed dramatically, a key observation was that the alignment of your knees changed and moved inward. This lets me know that we need to continue to strengthen your hip and knee muscles to better support efficient movement. You also mentioned that for the last few repetitions you began to feel more of a challenge in your upper thighs, which may indicate that movement was becoming more quadriceps dominant as fatigue set in. In other words, you began to lower yourself by moving your knees forward instead of your hips back. Overall, performing nine repetitions is going to be our baseline. Moving forward, we are going to work together to increase the number of completed repetitions in the 30-second time frame. What else would you like to know?

Client: That was very helpful, and I am glad to know what my baseline squat performance is, so I have something to compare against later. I am more self-assured now and I am curious to know how my performance compares to others.

Exercise Professional: While we are mainly focused on your individual performance and achieving your personal goals, we can also look at where the number of repetitions you completed places you compared to others in your age group. You performed nine repetitions with good posture, which is already an improvement from your starting point three months ago when you could not perform a single body-weight squat with postural stability and good form. According to the general normative values, your score categorizes you as below average compared to other 80- to 89-year-olds. We can use this information to update the exercise program and formulate goals, based on your input.

Break down barriers: Asking more open-ended questions provides an opportunity to discover what the client perceives to be an obstacle to better performance and play an active role in exercise program design.

Exercise Professional: Now that we have discussed all this information, what do you think would help improve your performance?

Client: I did not realize how much we could learn from performing this assessment and I am glad we took the time to incorporate this into our program. Even though my overall score places me in the below average category, I am more focused on the fact that I can now do nine repetitions with good form. I would like to increase this number and see if I can improve to a better category score as well. My main barriers to getting a higher score were fatigue and poor posture. I think I need to be stronger in my legs and work on adding more repetitions to our workouts, and maybe we should even use some weights. What are your thoughts?

Exercise Professional: Focusing on your individual performance is important to you and increasing your strength and adding more repetitions to your workouts seem like good ideas to you. These are great observations and align with the model for exercise program design that we are using. In fact, increasing the number of repetitions for the primary movement patterns and gradually loading those movements is the next step. In addition, there are some very effective exercises and stretches we can incorporate that will support better alignment of your knee joints to protect against unnecessary wear and tear, while leading us toward your goal of getting into and out of a chair with ease.

Collaborate: Now it is time to work together to decide on next steps while at the same time ensuring the client feels understood and respected.

Exercise Professional: Improving your lower-body endurance is important to you for moving with ease as you lower and raise yourself from a chair and you recognize that doing more repetitions and adding weight to specific exercises may help to reach this goal. What specific goals would you like to work on next to help you move more efficiently?

Client: That is correct. I am interested to see what new exercises we add to our exercise program and I am excited for the addition of weight to the foundational movements we are working on. You mentioned earlier about giving me some home exercises to do on my off days, but I was not ready at that time. Would some of the exercises and stretches for supporting better joint alignment be something I can do at home? I enjoy showing up to the gym for our workouts three times per week and believe I am ready to do more on the days I am not at the gym.

This scenario demonstrates that assessments do not always need to be done at the beginning of your relationship with a client but should instead be strategically timed so that the client is both physically and mentally ready to complete them. In addition, the scenario exhibits a cohesive partnership between the client and exercise professional, as they explored the 30-second chair stand test performance and results. The exercise professional used open-ended questions to make sure the client had opportunities to share his experience, which led to collaboration on the exercise program, next steps, and goals. This personalized program design, coupled with appropriate progressions, help to ensure self-efficacy on the part of the client and rapport building between the exercise professional and client.

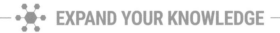 **EXPAND YOUR KNOWLEDGE**

When and Why Should Assessments Be Repeated?

Assessments are not exclusively relegated to the initial phase of training. The performance of follow-up assessments is valuable for numerous reasons. For example, repeated assessments may be warranted to account for favorable training adaptations that have occurred in order to make the necessary adjustments to various Muscular Training variables. Moreover, effective goal setting should include SMART goals, as this strategy can be effective for promoting positive behavior change, including initiation and maintenance of regular physical activity. Accordingly, measurable and time-bound goals that have been established can be evaluated with follow-up assessments that have been mutually agreed upon by the client and exercise professional.

◀ **SUMMARY** ▶

Physical-fitness assessments for older adults are just as important as (if not more important than) those for younger clients. It is well established that maximal effort performed with deconditioned muscle tissue is unwise and unnecessary in the field setting. Furthermore, when attempting to establish a total-body training program for an older adult, maximal results in a few exercises do not adequately represent the specifics of the entire body, nor will they transfer well into a precise exercise program of sets, repetitions, and loads.

Using the individual's perception of exertion to help determine a prudent level of exercise has long been accepted in the health and fitness community. It may appear too conservative by comparison to clinical standards, but the field setting is the "real world" where individual differences tend to dictate the success of an exercise program. While relying on perception may prevent the individual from achieving a true baseline intensity in the first few weeks of the exercise program, this is acceptable because, regardless of the intensity, the exercise performed is definitely more physiological "work" than the individual will have performed recently. Therefore, the experience is positive and adherence to the program and lifestyle change is more likely.

REFERENCES

Abelbeck, K.G. (2002). Biomechanical model and evaluation of a linear motion squat type exercise. *Journal of Strength and Conditioning Research*, 16, 516–524.

Akune, T. et al. (2014). Incidence of certified need of care in the long-term care insurance system and its risk factors in the elderly of Japanese population-based cohorts: The ROAD study. *Geriatrics & Gerontology International*, 14, 695–701.

American College of Sports Medicine (2018). *ACSM's Guidelines for Exercise Testing and Prescription* (10th ed.). Philadelphia: Wolters Kluwer.

American Council on Exercise (2020). *The Exercise Professional's Guide to Personal Training*. San Diego: American Council on Exercise.

Batsis, J.A. et al. (2016). Diagnostic accuracy of body mass index to identify obesity in older adults: NHANES 1999–2004. *International Journal of Obesity (London)*, 40, 5, 761–767.

Black, F.O. et al. (1982). Normal subject postural sway during the Romberg test. *American Journal of Otolaryngology*, 3, 309–318.

Cannon, C. et al. (2004). The talk test as a measure of exertional ischemia. *American Journal of Sports Medicine*, 6, 52–57.

Centers for Disease Control and Prevention (2020). *Assessing Your Weight*. https://www.cdc.gov/healthyweight/assessing/index.html

Cook, G. (2003). *Athletic Body in Balance*. Champaign, Ill.: Human Kinetics.

Dehart, M. et al. (2000). Relationship between the talk test and ventilatory threshold. *Clinical Exercise Physiology*, 2, 34–38.

Donnelly, D.V. et al. (2006). The effect of directional gaze on kinematics during the squat exercise. *Journal of Strength and Conditioning Research*, 20, 145–150.

Fry, A.C., Smith J.C., & Schilling, B.K. (2003). Effect of knee position on hip and knees torques during the barbell squat. *Journal of Strength and Conditioning Research*, 17, 629–633.

Gray, G. & Tiberio, D. (2007). *Chain Reaction Function*. Adrian, Mich.: Gray Institute.

Hauschildt, M. (2008). Landing mechanics: What, why and when? *NSCA's Performance Training Journal*, 7, 1, 13–16.

Heo, M. et al. (2012). Percentage of body fat cutoffs by sex, age, and race-ethnicity in the US adult population from NHANES 1999–2004. *American Journal of Clinical Nutrition*, 95, 594–602.

Hirani, V. et al. (2017). Longitudinal associations between body composition, sarcopenic obesity and outcomes of frailty, disability, institutionalisation and mortality in community-dwelling older men: The Concord Health and Ageing in Men Project. *Age Ageing*, 46, 413–420.

Houglum, P.A. (2016). *Therapeutic Exercise for Musculoskeletal Injuries* (4th ed.). Champaign, Ill.: Human Kinetics.

Johnson, B.L. & Nelson, J.K. (1986). *Practical Measurement for Evaluation in Physical Education* (4th ed.). Minneapolis, Minn.: Burgess.

Kendall, F.P. et al. (2005). *Muscles: Testing and Function with Posture and Pain* (5th ed.). Baltimore, Md.: Lippincott Williams & Wilkins.

Lukács, A. et al. (2019). Abdominal obesity increases metabolic risk factors in non-obese adults: A Hungarian cross-sectional study. *BMC Public Health*, 19, Article No. 1533.

McArdle, W., Katch, F., & Katch, V. (2019). *Exercise Physiology: Nutrition, Energy, and Human Performance* (8th ed.). Philadelphia: Lippincott, Williams & Wilkins.

McGill, S.M. (2017). *Ultimate Back Fitness and Performance* (6th ed.). Waterloo, Canada: www.Backfitpro.com

McGill, S.M. (2016). *Low Back Disorders: Evidence-Based Prevention and Rehabilitation* (3rd ed.). Champaign, Ill.: Human Kinetics.

McManus, R.J. & Mant, J. (2012). Do differences in blood pressure between arms matter? *The Lancet*, 379, 9819, 872–873.

National Heart, Lung, and Blood Institute (2020). *Classification of Overweight and Obesity by BMI, Waist Circumference, and Associated Disease Risks*. https://www.nhlbi.nih.gov/health/educational/lose_wt/BMI/bmi_dis

Newton, R.A. (2001). Validity of the multidirectional reach test: A practical measure for limits of stability in older adults. *Journal of Gerontology: Medical Sciences*, 56A, 4, M248–M252.

Newton, R. (1989). Review of tests of standing balance abilities. *Brain Injury*, 3, 4, 335–343.

Persinger, R. et al. (2004). Consistency of the talk test for exercise prescription. *Medicine & Science in Sports & Exercise*, 36, 1632–1636.

Porcari, J.P. et al. (2001). Prescribing exercise using the talk test. *Fitness Management*, 17, 9, 46–49.

Recalde, P.T. et al. (2002). The talk test as a simple marker of ventilatory threshold. *South African Journal of Sports Medicine*, 9, 5–8.

Rikli, R.E. & Jones, J.C. (2013). *Senior Fitness Test Manual* (2nd ed.). Champaign, Ill.: Human Kinetics.

Rose, D.J. (2010). *Fallproof!* (2nd ed.). Champaign, Ill.: Human Kinetics.

Sahrmann, S.A. (2002). *Diagnosis and Treatment of Movement Impairment Syndromes*. St. Louis, Mo.: Mosby.

Tinetti, M.E. (1986). Performance-oriented assessment of mobility problems in elderly patients. *Journal of the American Geriatric Society*, 34, 119–226.

Tran, N.T.T. et al. (2018). The importance of waist circumference and body mass index in cross-sectional relationships with risk of cardiovascular disease in Vietnam. *PLoS ONE*, 13, 5, e0198202.

U.S. Department of Health & Human Services (2018). *Physical Activity Guidelines for Americans* (2nd ed.). www.health.gov/paguidelines

Villareal, D.T. et al. (2017). Aerobic or resistance exercise, or both in dieting obese older adults *New England Journal of Medicine*, 376, 1943–1955.

Villareal, D.T. et al. (2011). Weight loss, exercise, or both and physical function in obese older adults. *New England Journal of Medicine*, 364, 1218–1229.

Voelker, S.A. et al. (2002). Relationship between the talk test and ventilatory threshold in cardiac patients. *Clinical Exercise Physiology*, 4, 120–123.

Whelton, P.K. et al. (2017). 2017 ACC/AHA/AAPA/ABC/ACPM/AGS/APhA/ASH/ASPC/NMA/PCNA guideline for the prevention, detection, evaluation, and management of high blood pressure in adults: A report of the American College of Cardiology/American Heart Association Task Force on Clinical Practice Guidelines. *Journal of the American College of Cardiology*, Nov 7. pii: S0735-1097 (17) 41519-1.

Wielemborek-Musial, K. et al. (2016). Blood pressure response to submaximal exercise test in adults. *BioMed Research International*, 5607507.

Wilthrow, T.J. et al. (2005). The relationship between quadriceps muscle force, knee flexion and anterior cruciate ligament strain in an in vitro simulated jump landing. *American Journal of Sports Medicine*, 34, 2, 269–274.

Winter, J.E. et al. (2014). BMI and all-cause mortality in older adults: A meta-analysis. *The American Journal of Clinical Nutrition*, 99, 4, 875–890.

World Health Organization (2020). *Obesity and Overweight*. https://www.who.int/news-room/fact-sheets/detail/obesity-and-overweight

SUGGESTED READINGS

American Council on Exercise (2020). *The Exercise Professional's Guide to Personal Training*. San Diego: American Council on Exercise.

American Council on Exercise (2019). *The Professional's Guide to Health and Wellness Coaching*. San Diego: American Council on Exercise.

Rikli, R.E. & Jones, J.C. (2013). *Senior Fitness Test Manual* (2nd ed.). Champaign, Ill.: Human Kinetics.

Rose, D.J. (2010). *Fallproof!* (2nd ed.). Champaign, Ill.: Human Kinetics.

CHAPTER 8

Exercise Programming

LEARNING OBJECTIVES

After reading this chapter, you will be able to:

▶ Implement warm-up and cool-down techniques appropriate for older adults

▶ Apply the five primary movement patterns in exercise program design to enhance the performance of activities of daily living for older clients

▶ Use the ACE Integrated Fitness Training® (ACE IFT®) Model as a guideline for programming postural stability and kinetic chain mobility, balance, movement patterns, muscular training, and cardiorespiratory exercise for older adults of all fitness levels

▶ Implement exercise modifications, progressions, and regressions that are suitable for older adults

In Chapter 6, an overview of the components and phases of the ACE Integrated Fitness Training (ACE IFT) Model was presented. This chapter explores each phase of the ACE IFT Model as it relates to safe and effective exercise programming. Specifically, the programming focus is on the successful facilitation of physical activity in older clients as they initiate exercise programs and advance through the function–health–fitness–performance continuum (see Chapter 6).

Warm-up and Cool-down Techniques

Adequate warm-up and cool-down periods are especially important for older adults because, with age, sudden vigorous work or abrupt cessation of strenuous exercise may put undue stress on the cardiovascular system. Warm-up and post-conditioning cool-down periods (including stretching) of approximately 10 to 15 minutes are recommended for healthy participants. Beginners and persons with conditions such as **arthritis** or cardiovascular problems generally need longer warm-up and cool-down periods.

In addition to gradually increasing circulation and heart rate (HR), the warm-up should prepare the body for movements that will be required during the workout. As a general principle, the harder the conditioning phase of the workout and/or the older the exerciser, the more extensive the warm-up should be. Furthermore, all the major joints and muscle groups should be gently engaged by performing the five primary movement patterns (see Figure 6-3, page 171). The warm-up should primarily be devoted to continuous rhythmic movements, whereas intensive **static stretching** should be saved for the cool-down. A thorough warm-up should be completed whether the training to follow is cardiorespiratory, muscular, stretching, or some combination of the various forms of exercise. Keep in mind that the warm-up should adequately prepare clients for the exercise session, but it should not lead to undue fatigue that will affect the quality of their physical performance or diminish their ability to focus their attention.

Treadmill and stationary cycle warm-ups can be augmented by a few minutes of rhythmic movements targeting the whole body. The warm-up can be performed in a seated or standing position or in a swimming pool. Most standing or land-based warm-ups can be adapted to the chair or pool.

The cool-down period following cardiorespiratory exercise should be of approximately the same intensity and duration as the warm-up and feature activities that allow the HR to gradually decrease. Cutting short the cool-down can cause the blood to pool in the extremities, which may cause dizziness or even fainting. Many antihypertension medications may exacerbate this condition, as they cause **vasodilation.** Low- to moderate-intensity activity should be continued until respiration and/or the rating of perceived exertion (RPE) return to near pre-exercise levels. As with cardiorespiratory exercise, the cool-down period following intensive muscular training should include a few minutes of gentle cool-down activity (e.g., walking or slow cycling) prior to sustained static stretching to give the cardiorespiratory system a transition period after strenuous activity. The final cool-down period is also a good time to include relaxation activities.

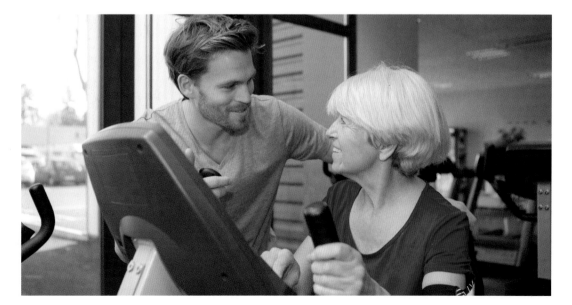

APPLY WHAT YOU KNOW

Chair-seated Exercise Techniques

Chair-seated exercises are particularly well-suited for older individuals who cannot tolerate standing for lengthy durations, such as in an hour-long workout session, due to balance, mobility, or endurance problems. However, exercise professionals should avoid training people in chairs without a good reason for doing so. Weight-bearing activities and movements in active functional positions are generally more productive than chair-seated work.

Most chair exercises are best performed with chairs that do not have armrests. This increases the potential range of movement and allows a broader variety of exercises. However, if armchairs are the only option available, the exercise professional must be able to work with these types of chairs as well. In addition, many chair-seated exercisers use wheelchairs. Therefore, it is important to develop the ability to work effectively using armchairs. During chair exercise, support may need to be provided for the participant's back, perhaps by utilizing a pillow, pad, or rolled towel, if necessary. It is also important that the participant's feet contact the floor fully, which can be accomplished by using a book, stool, or other type of platform.

Chair exercise offers wide training intensity options. A chair-exercise workout might include optional standing work using the back of the chair for balance support. It might feature energetic seated cardiorespiratory activity involving all the limbs in broad-ranging movement patterns, like chair marching. The chair also provides a secure position for the use of resistive exercise accessories such as dumbbells, elastic resistance bands, and ankle weights. On the other hand, chair classes can serve participants with restricted mobility who will benefit from performing limited exercises comprised of gentle stretching, posture, and breathing activities.

Muscular Training Based on the ACE IFT Model

The Functional and Movement Training phases of the Muscular Training component of the ACE IFT Model focus on **kinetic chain** mobility and postural stability. These phases are especially important for older clients, as declines in joint mobility and **proprioception** are commonplace due to declines in the function of the balance sensory systems (i.e., **visual system, vestibular system,** and **somatosensory system**). Good joint alignment facilitates effective muscle action and joint movement, serving as the foundation upon which good exercise technique is built.

In this section, programming concepts for Muscular Training are expanded to include progressions for each phase of training. Recall that the Muscular Training component provides a systematic approach for helping clients progress from establishing postural stability and kinetic chain mobility to general fitness, strength, and athletic performance. The Muscular Training component of the ACE IFT Model is divided into three phases, each with a title that defines its training focus (Figure 8-1 and Table 8-1).

FIGURE 8-1
ACE IFT Model
Muscular Training
phases

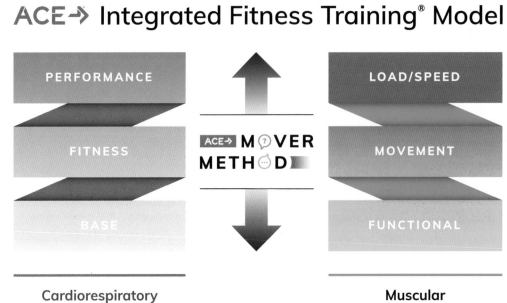

ACE→ Integrated Fitness Training® Model

TABLE 8-1	

Muscular Training

Functional Training	▸ Focus on establishing/reestablishing postural stability and kinetic chain mobility. ▸ Exercise programs should improve muscular endurance, flexibility, core function, and static and dynamic balance. ▸ Progress exercise volume and challenge as function improves.
Movement Training	▸ Focus on developing good movement patterns without compromising postural or joint stability. ▸ Programs should include exercises for all five primary movement patterns in varied planes of motion. ▸ Integrate Functional Training exercises to help clients maintain and improve postural stability and kinetic chain mobility.
Load/Speed Training	▸ Focus on application of external loads to movements to create increased force production to meet desired goals. ▸ Integrate the five primary movement patterns through exercises that load them in different planes of motion and combinations. ▸ Integrate Functional Training exercises to enhance postural stability and kinetic chain mobility to support increased workloads. ▸ Programs should focus on adequate resistance-training loads to help clients reach muscular strength, endurance, and hypertrophy goals. ▸ Clients with goals for athletic performance will integrate exercises and drills to build speed, agility, quickness, and power.

FUNCTIONAL TRAINING

Decreasing levels of activity and a propensity toward poor posture and muscle imbalance are commonly seen in older clients. Accordingly, poor posture and muscle imbalance change joint loading and movement mechanics, triggering compensations in the way people exercise and perform their daily activities. Thus, exercise professionals need to be aware of postural and movement deviations and be able to program exercises to reestablish appropriate levels of stability and mobility, which ultimately can result in more efficient movement and a decreased likelihood for musculoskeletal pain and structural imbalances.

Programming for Improved Posture

A static postural assessment is an excellent test for observing a client's joints and how they relate to each other, and for viewing how those joints maintain their positions against gravity in a relaxed, standing position (see pages 203–207) (Figure 8-2). Individuals who exhibit good posture generally demonstrate an appropriate relationship between stability and mobility throughout the kinetic chain (Figure 8-3). On the other hand, individuals who exhibit poor posture (Figure 8-4) typically lack the mobility required for normal joint movement, the stability to maintain good posture, or both. Tables 8-2 through 8-5 list common muscle imbalances [i.e., chronically shortened/facilitated (**hypertonic**) muscles and lengthened (inhibited) muscles] associated with **lordosis** posture, **kyphosis** posture, flat-back posture, and sway-back posture, respectively.

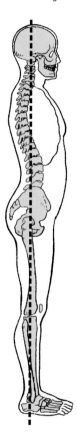

FIGURE 8-2

Neutral spine alignment with slight anterior (lordotic) curves at the neck and low back and a posterior (kyphotic) curve in the thoracic region

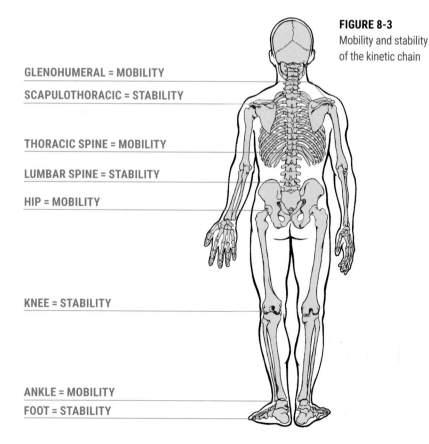

FIGURE 8-3

Mobility and stability of the kinetic chain

GLENOHUMERAL = MOBILITY

SCAPULOTHORACIC = STABILITY

THORACIC SPINE = MOBILITY

LUMBAR SPINE = STABILITY

HIP = MOBILITY

KNEE = STABILITY

ANKLE = MOBILITY

FOOT = STABILITY

FIGURE 8-4
Postural deviations

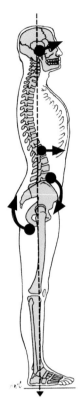
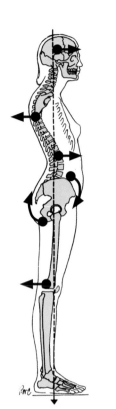
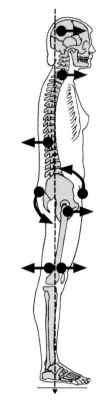
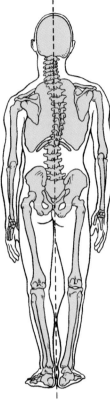

a. Lordosis: Increased anterior lumbar curve from neutral

b. Kyphosis: Increased posterior thoracic curve from neutral

c. Flat back: Decreased anterior lumbar curve

d. Sway back: Decreased anterior lumbar curve and increased posterior thoracic curve from neutral

e. Scoliosis: Lateral spinal curvature often accompanied by vertebral rotation

TABLE 8-2

Muscle Imbalances Associated with Lordosis Posture

Facilitated/Hypertonic (Shortened)	Inhibited (Lengthened)
Hip flexors	Hip extensors
Lumbar extensors	External obliques
	Rectus abdominis

TABLE 8-3

Muscle Imbalances Associated with Kyphosis Posture

Facilitated/Hypertonic (Shortened)	Inhibited (Lengthened)
Anterior chest/shoulders	Upper-back extensors
Latissimus dorsi	Scapular stabilizers
Neck extensors	Neck flexors

TABLE 8-4

Muscle Imbalances Associated with Flat-back Posture

Facilitated/Hypertonic (Shortened)	Inhibited (Lengthened)
Rectus abdominis	Iliacus/psoas major
Upper-back extensors	Internal obliques
Neck extensors	Lumbar extensors
Ankle plantar flexors	Neck flexors

TABLE 8-5

Muscle Imbalances Associated with Sway-back Posture

Facilitated/Hypertonic (Shortened)	Inhibited (Lengthened)
Hamstrings	Iliacus/psoas major
Upper fibers of posterior obliques	Rectus femoris
Lumbar extensors	External oblique
Neck extensors	Upper-back extensors
	Neck flexors

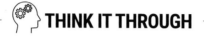 **THINK IT THROUGH**

Postural Deviations

Carefully read through the information presented in Tables 8-2 through 8-5. Because the postures depicted are common deviations, you are likely to observe an older client with one or more of these variants. Think about methods you would employ as an exercise professional to help clients with these muscle imbalances. Can you come up with at least one stretch for each shortened muscle group and one strengthening exercise for each lengthened muscle group?

If a client exhibits one of the five postural abnormalities depicted in Figure 8-4 and reports pain in the spine, the exercise professional should refer them to a physician for an evaluation to address the issue causing the pain. However, if a client can come close to adopting an ideal, "neutral" spine position through verbal coaching, they are probably suffering from muscle imbalances that can be helped through a program of appropriate stretching and strengthening of the affected muscle groups. That is, shortened muscle groups should be treated in ways that enhance mobility [e.g., **self–myofascial release (SMR)** and static stretching] and lengthened muscle groups should be treated in ways that promote stability (e.g., isometric holds and high-repetition, low-resistance movements).

It is important to note that it is rare for any person, especially an older adult, to present with a perfectly ideal posture. As long as the client does not report musculoskeletal pain, they should be able to begin stability and mobility exercises. The notable exceptions are clients with severe **scoliosis** or **osteoporosis** (osteoporosis is not only associated with excessive kyphosis, but also with brittle/fragile bones). These conditions warrant an evaluation and recommendations from the client's healthcare provider.

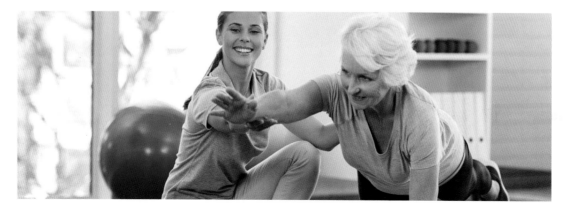

📖 APPLY WHAT YOU KNOW

Addressing Muscle Imbalances: Kyphosis–Lordosis Posture

Kyphosis of the thoracic spine related to poor posture or muscle imbalance often appears with lumbar lordosis. The lumbar spine curves more in the opposite (anterior) direction to compensate for the increased posterior thoracic curvature. The following sample routine is an example of Functional Training exercises that could be effective for an older adult who exhibits a slight kyphosis–lordosis posture (Table 8-6). Prior to working with an individual who has a postural deviation, be sure they can adopt a close-to-ideal posture when verbally coached (thus, indicating that the deviation is soft tissue–related versus a structural abnormality) and that there is no pain present. If pain is present, the client should be referred to their healthcare provider for evaluation. The proper sequence is to perform the exercises in each row from left to right before moving onto the next row (e.g., SMR for the hip flexors, seated 90–90° stretch, and glute bridge, then SMR for the lumbar extensors and so on).

Equipment:

▶ Foam roll or similar device

▶ Mat

▶ Chair or bench

▶ Towel or dowel

This approach mobilizes the hypertonic (facilitated) muscles first with SMR, then immediately lengthens those same hypertonic muscles through static stretching and finishes with a muscle-activation exercise for the antagonistic muscle group, which is typically inhibited in postural deviations. This routine can be performed immediately prior to a dynamic movement-pattern warm-up that prepares the body for more intense conditioning, or it can stand alone as an exercise routine that introduces the client to Functional Training.

TABLE 8-6

Stability/Mobility Warm-up for Kyphosis–Lordosis Posture (10 minutes)

Facilitated Muscles (Shortened)	SMR	Static Stretch (60 seconds)	Inhibited Muscles (Lengthened)	Isometric Exercise (5 repetitions x 10- to 15-second hold)
Hip flexors	Roll, ball, or Stick (Figure 8-5)	Seated 90-90° (Figure 8-6)	Hip extensors	Glute bridge (Figure 8-7)
Lumbar extensors	Roll or ball (Figure 8-8)	Extended child's pose with lateral flexion (Figure 8-9)	External obliques	Seated hip hinge (Figure 8-10)
Chest/anterior shoulders	Ball (Figure 8-11)	Anterior shoulder and chest wall stretch (Figure 8-12)	Upper-back extensors	Prone trunk lift with extension and external rotation of the shoulders (Figure 8-13)
Latissimus dorsi	Roll or ball (Figure 8-14)	Overhead dowel side bend (Figure 8-15)	Scapular stabilizers	Seated or standing wall angels (Figure 8-16)
Neck extensors	Roll or ball (Figure 8-17)	Chin to chest (Figure 8-18) and chin to armpit (Figure 8-19)	Neck flexors	Ab prep with chin rock (Figure 8-20)

Note: SMR = Self–myofascial release

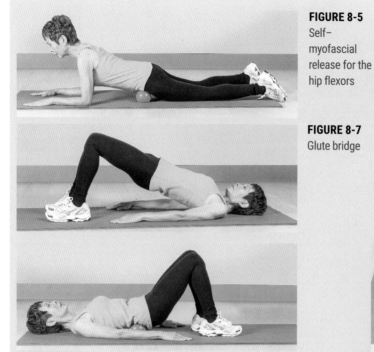

FIGURE 8-5
Self–myofascial release for the hip flexors

FIGURE 8-6
Seated 90–90°

FIGURE 8-7
Glute bridge

FIGURE 8-8
Self–myofascial release for the lumbar extensors

FIGURE 8-9
Extended child's pose with lateral flexion

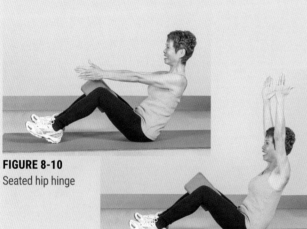

FIGURE 8-10
Seated hip hinge

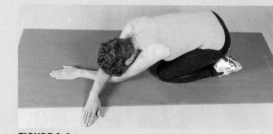

FIGURE 8-11
Self–myofascial release for the chest and anterior shoulder

FIGURE 8-12
Anterior shoulder and chest wall stretch

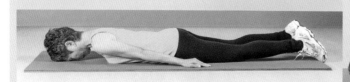

FIGURE 8-13
Prone trunk lift with extension and external rotation of shoulders

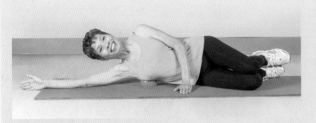

FIGURE 8-14
Self–myofascial release for the latissimus dorsi

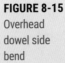

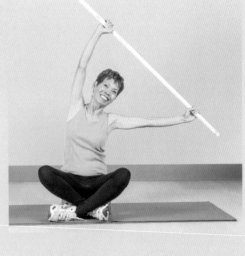

FIGURE 8-15
Overhead dowel side bend

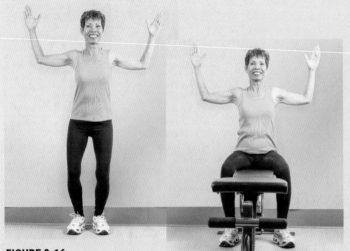

FIGURE 8-16
Standing or seated wall angels

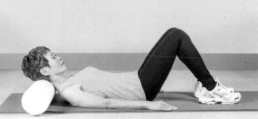

FIGURE 8-17
Self–myofascial release for the neck extensors

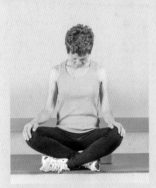

FIGURE 8-18
Chin to chest

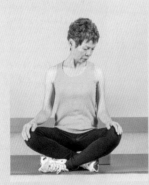

FIGURE 8-19
Chin to armpit (to the left and then to right)

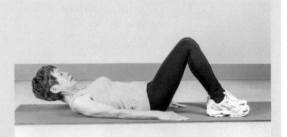

FIGURE 8-20
Ab prep with chin rock

Improving Muscle Condition to Enhance Stability

Strengthening muscles to improve posture should initially focus on having the client adopt positions of good posture and begin with a series of low-grade isometric contractions [<50% of maximal effort or **maximal voluntary contraction (MVC)**], with the client completing two to four repetitions of five- to 10-second holds. The goal is to condition the postural (tonic) muscles, which typically contain greater concentrations of **type I muscle fibers,** with volume as opposed to intensity. Higher intensities that require greater amounts of force will generally evoke faulty recruitment patterns. The exercise volume can be gradually increased (overload) to improve strength and endurance, and to reestablish muscle balance at the joints.

Many older clients may lack the ability to stabilize joints throughout the kinetic chain. For these individuals, an initial emphasis should be placed on muscle isolation using supportive surfaces and devices (e.g., floor, wall, or chair backrest) prior to introducing integrated (whole-body, unsupported) strengthening exercises. For example, to help a client strengthen weak posterior deltoids and rhomboids, which are associated with forward-rounded shoulders, an exercise professional could start by having the client perform reverse flys in a supine position, isometrically pressing the backs of the arms into the floor, rather than sets of dynamic back rows using external resistance. The use of support offers the additional benefit of kinesthetic and visual feedback, which is critical to helping clients understand the alignment of specific joints (e.g., when lying on the floor or positioned against a wall, the individual can feel and see the contact points when joints are placed in ideal postural positions). The strengthening exercises should ultimately progress to dynamic movement, initially controlling the range of motion (ROM) to avoid excessive muscle lengthening before introducing full-ROM movement patterns. An important concept to keep in mind is that while a muscle may be strong in a lengthened position, strength must be developed at a normal, healthy resting length. For example, to strengthen the rhomboids using more dynamic movements, the client should hold the scapulae in a good postural position and avoid scapular protraction and retraction during the movement. Dynamic strengthening exercises for good posture do not involve heavy loads, but rather volume training to condition the type I fibers. Consequently, exercise professionals should plan on one to three sets of 12 to 15 repetitions when introducing dynamic strengthening exercises. Performing movements in front of a mirror can also enhance postural awareness.

To summarize, the strengthening of weakened muscles follows a progressive model beginning with two to four repetitions of isometric muscle contractions, each held for five to 10 seconds at less than 50% of MVC in a supported, more isolated environment. The next progression is to dynamic, controlled ROM exercises incorporating one to three sets of 12 to 15 repetitions.

Improving Core Function for Enhanced Stability

Given the importance of balance and the condition of the core musculature to fitness and overall quality of life, baseline assessments should be collected to evaluate the need for comprehensive balance training and core conditioning during the early stages of a conditioning program. Exercise professionals should feel comfortable evaluating proprioceptive challenges using the Fullerton Advanced Balance Scale (see page 216). Core-function assessments should be performed by older adults who are interested in completing the core assessment battery and who are free from back pain.

Older adults with demonstrated deficiencies in core-muscle assessments, such as McGill's torso muscular endurance test battery (see page 234), may wish to include these same activities during exercise programming as part of their foundational exercises. The goal is to create ratios consistent with McGill's recommendations. Muscular endurance, more so than muscular strength or even ROM, has been shown to be an accurate predictor of back health (McGill, 2016). Low-back stabilization exercises have the most benefit when performed daily. When working with clients with low-back dysfunction, it is prudent to include daily stabilization exercises in their home exercise plans. Though clients' training objectives can vary from post-rehabilitation or prevention of low-back pain to optimizing health and fitness or maximizing athletic performance, all clients will benefit from exercises targeting core stability.

📖 APPLY WHAT YOU KNOW

Daily Routine for Enhancing Low-back Health

While there is a common belief that exercise sessions should be performed at least three times per week, it appears that low-back exercises have the most beneficial effect when performed daily. When selecting exercises for low-back strength and stability, more repetitions of less demanding exercises will assist in the enhancement of postural endurance and strength (McGill, 2016). Given that increasing muscular endurance of the slow-twitch postural muscles has a protective value, strength gains should not be overemphasized at the expense of endurance.

The following exercises are a simple daily routine that can be recommended to a client to strengthen the stabilizing musculature of the spine and enhance motor control to ensure that spine stability is maintained in all activities. These exercises may be included when training within the Functional Training phase of the Muscular Training component of the ACE IFT Model. Keep in mind that these are only examples of well-designed exercises and may not be for everyone; the initial challenge may or may not be appropriate for every individual, nor will the graded progression be the same for all clients. These are simply examples of exercises that challenge the muscles of the torso, improving fluidity of movement and postural stabilization.

CAT-COW

The routine begins with the cat-cow exercise (spine flexion-extension cycles) to improve flexibility and warm the tissue with rhythmic motion (Figure 8-21). Note that the cat-cow is intended as a motion exercise—not a stretch—so the emphasis is on motion rather than "pushing" at the end ranges of flexion and extension. As the client moves into the cat position, they should slowly exhale; as the client moves into the cow position, they should inhale. The neutral spine, or center point of the movement, is the time to transition the breathing.

FIGURE 8-21
Cat-cow

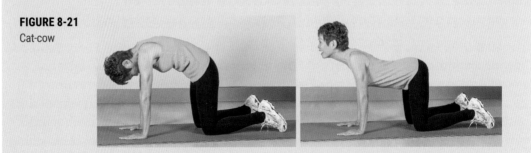

MODIFIED CURL-UP

The cat-cow motion exercise is followed by anterior abdominal exercises, in this case the modified curl-up (Figure 8-22). The hands or a rolled towel are placed under the lumbar spine to preserve a neutral spine posture. Do not allow the client to flatten the back to the floor, as doing so flexes the lumbar spine, violates the neutral spine principle, and increases the loads on the discs and ligaments. One knee is flexed but the other leg is straight to lock the pelvis–lumbar spine and minimize the loss of a neutral lumbar posture. Have clients alternate the bent leg (right to left) midway through the repetitions.

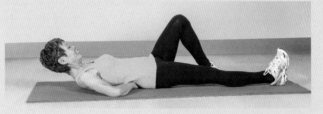

FIGURE 8-22
Modified curl-up

BIRD DOG

The extensor component of the program consists of the bird dog exercise (Figure 8-23). Starting with the client's hands placed directly under the shoulders and the knees directly under the hips, the exercise professional should instruct the client in finding a neutral spine position. Stabilization through the abdominal musculature is needed to ensure consistent neutral spine position while the opposite arm and leg are lifted in unison. If a client is not ready to stabilize this load, they can start with one arm or one leg and progress to the full exercise. Holding the position for 5 to 8 seconds for each repetition is recommended to improve muscular endurance before alternating sides (McGill, 2016).

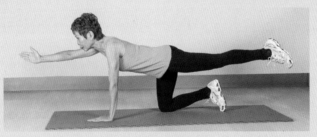

FIGURE 8-23
Bird dog

SIDE BRIDGE

The lateral muscles of the torso (i.e., quadratus lumborum and abdominal obliques) are important for optimal stability and are targeted with the side bridge exercise. The beginner level of this exercise involves bridging the torso between the elbow and the knees (Figure 8-24a). Once this is mastered and well-tolerated, the challenge is increased by bridging using the elbow and the feet (Figure 8-24b). It is important when performing the side bridge exercise to maintain a neutral neck and spine position. Holding the position for 5 to

8 seconds for each repetition before alternating sides is recommended to improve muscular endurance (McGill, 2016).

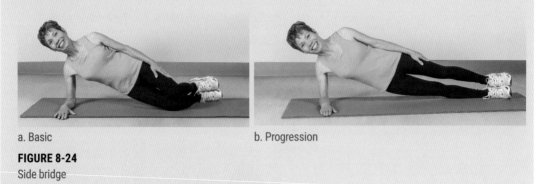

a. Basic

b. Progression

FIGURE 8-24
Side bridge

Programming should begin by first promoting stability of the lumbar region through the action and function of the core. Once an individual demonstrates the ability to stabilize this region, the program should then progress to the more **distal** segments. An example of an exercise progression that addresses **proximal** stability first and then advances the challenge with upper and lower extremity movement is shown in Figure 8-25 and Table 8-7.

FIGURE 8-25
Adopt a quadruped position with the knees under the hips and the hands beneath the shoulders. Maintain a neutral spine throughout all movements.

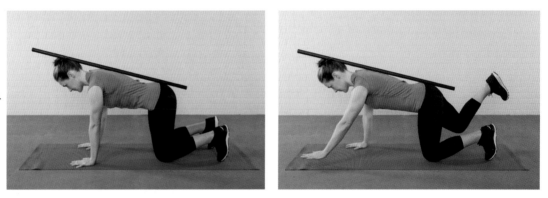

Adjacent to the lumbar spine are the hips and thoracic spine, both of which are primarily mobile. As thoracic spine mobility is restored, the program can target stability of the scapulothoracic region. An example of an exercise that promotes thoracic spine mobility is the cat-cow (see Figure 8-21) and an exercise for scapulothoracic stability is the rocking quadruped (Figure 8-26). Finally, once stability and mobility of the lumbopelvic, thoracic, and shoulder regions have been established, the program can then shift to enhancing mobility and stability of the distal extremities. Attempting to improve mobility within distal joints without developing more proximal stability only serves to compromise any existing stability within these segments. When a joint lacks stability, many of the muscles that normally mobilize that joint may need to alter their true functions to assist in providing stability. For example, if an individual lacks stability in the scapulothoracic joint, the deltoids, which are normally responsible for many glenohumeral movements, may need to compromise some of their force-generating capacity and assist in stabilizing scapulothoracic movement. This altered deltoid function decreases force output and may increase the potential for dysfunctional movement and injury.

TABLE 8-7

Exercise Progression for Core Stabilization

Action	Volume
1. Raise one arm 0.5 to 1 inch (1.25 to 2.5 cm) off the floor and perform the sequence of controlled shoulder movements: ▸ 6–12 inch (15–30 cm) sagittal plane shoulder movements (flexion/extension) ▸ 6–12 inch (15–30 cm) frontal plane shoulder movements (abduction/adduction) ▸ 6–12 inch (15–30 cm) multiplanar shoulder movements (circles or circumduction)	Perform 1–2 sets x 10 repetitions with a 2-second tempo, use 10–15 second rest intervals between sets
2. Raise one knee 0.5 to 1 inch (1.25 to 2.5 cm) off the floor and perform the sequence of controlled hip movements: ▸ 6–12 inch (15–30 cm) sagittal plane hip movements (flexion/extension) ▸ 6–12 inch (15–30 cm) frontal plane hip movements (abduction/adduction) ▸ 6–12 inch (15–30 cm) multiplanar hip movements (circles)	Perform 1–2 sets x 10 repetitions with a 2-second tempo, use 10–15 second rest intervals between sets
3. Raise contralateral limbs (i.e., one arm and the opposite knee) 0.5 to 1 inch (1.25 to 2.5 cm) off the floor and perform the sequence of movements: ▸ Repeat the above movements in matching planes (i.e., simultaneous movement in the same plane with both limbs) or alternating planes (i.e., mixing the planes between the two limbs). ▸ This contralateral movement pattern mimics the muscle-activation patterns used during the push-off phase portion of walking and is an effective exercise to train this pattern.	Perform 1–2 sets x 10 repetitions with a 2-second tempo, use 10–15 second rest intervals between sets

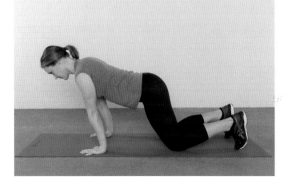 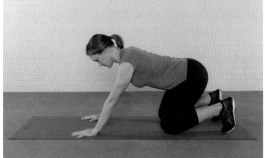

FIGURE 8-26
Rocking quadruped

Improving Range of Motion for Enhanced Mobility

Mobility can be thought of in two general aspects: (1) locally, as in ROM at a specific joint, and (2) globally, as in movement within the entire kinetic chain. Both aspects include the interplay of anatomical structures that surround the joints combined with motor control as influenced by the nervous system. If inadequate ROM is found at specific joints or if discrepancies are observed between the right and left sides of the body, a program of focused mobility for the areas in question should be initiated. There are several options to choose from when it comes to improving ROM and thus mobility. SMR and static stretching are good options to

FIGURE 8-27
Static stretch of the hamstrings

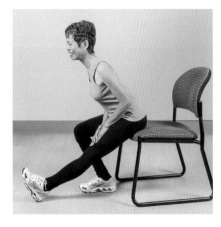

consider for the older adult population because both can be self-administered, which can be helpful when recommending to clients that they perform daily mobility exercises.

Static stretches involve moving a muscle/tendon group to where the targeted muscles reach a point of tension (Figure 8-27). Ideally, older adult clients should perform a total of 60 seconds of flexibility exercise per stretch, holding each repetition for 30 to 60 seconds [American College of Sports Medicine (ACSM), 2018].

EXPAND YOUR KNOWLEDGE

Understanding Self-myofascial Release

Understanding the concept behind SMR requires an understanding of the fascial system itself. **Fascia** is a densely woven, specialized system of connective tissue that covers and unites all of the body's compartments. The result is a system where each part is connected to the other parts through this web of tissue. Essentially, the purpose of the fascia is to surround and support the bodily structures, which provides stability as well as a cohesive direction for the line of pull of muscle groups. For example, the fascia surrounding the quadriceps keeps this muscle group contained in the anterior compartment of the thigh (stability) and orients the muscle fibers in a vertical direction so that the line of pull is more effective at extending the knee. In a normal healthy state, fascia has a relaxed and wavy configuration. It has the ability to stretch and move without restriction. However, with physical trauma, scarring, or inflammation, fascia may lose its pliability.

SMR is a technique that applies pressure to tight, restricted areas of fascia and underlying muscle in an attempt to relieve tension and improve flexibility. It is thought that applying direct sustained pressure to a tight area can inhibit the tension in a muscle. Tightness in soft tissue may be diminished through the application of pressure (e.g., SMR) followed by static stretching.

The practical application of myofascial release in the fitness setting is commonly done through the use of a foam roller, where the client controls their own intensity and duration of pressure. A common technique is to instruct clients to perform small, continuous, back-and-forth movements on a foam roller, covering an area of 2 to 6 inches (5 to 15 cm) over the tender region for 30 to 60 seconds (Figure 8-28). Because exerting pressure on

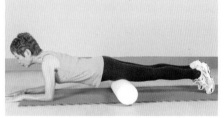

Myofascial release for gluteals/external rotators

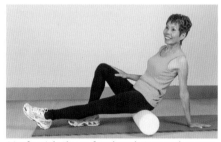

Myofascial release for the quadriceps

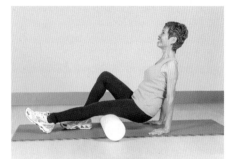

Myofascial release for the hamstrings

FIGURE 8-28
Myofascial release using a foam roller

an already tender area requires a certain level of pain tolerance, the intensity of the application of pressure determines the duration for which the client can withstand the discomfort. Exercise professionals should always be cognizant of the pain tolerance for rolling of their clients.

Evidence is lacking on the mechanisms and benefits of performing self-myofascial release, with some experts disparaging the use of the word "release" as an accurate depiction of what actually occurs. Exercise professionals who encourage the use of this technique to improve flexibility with clients should make every effort to stay current with research as it becomes available in this area.

Older adults might find using a foam roller (even one made from low-density foam) too hard to use, resulting in a painful experience that makes it difficult to promote successful realignment of tight muscles. Instead, exercise professionals should consider modifying the practice with small balls that are softer. Furthermore, some foam roller exercises require a greater level of upper-body and core strength than is possessed by many older adults. Using a small ball or smaller (half) foam roll can alleviate this problem in many cases. Another option is an apparatus like the Stick, which involves

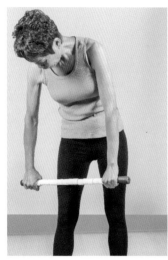

FIGURE 8-29
Use of the Stick involves self-myofascial release created by the pressure applied by rolling a stick with handles (resembling a rolling pin) over the target area.

SMR using the pressure applied by rolling a stick with handles (resembling a rolling pin) over the area (Figure 8-29). Aptly named, the original Stick is a 24-inch flexible plastic baton outfitted with a series of hard plastic rollers that works well for hard-to-access areas like the lower legs, quadriceps, anterior hip, and neck.

Improving Balance for Enhanced Stability

Balance is a foundational element of all exercise programming and should be emphasized early in the training program once core function is established and an individual shows improvements in postural stability and kinetic chain mobility. Balance not only enhances physical performance, but also contributes to increased balance confidence and **self-efficacy,** which can decrease fear of falling, risk of future falls, and behavior avoidance, and provide better functional outcomes (Landers et al., 2016). Balance is subdivided into static balance, or the ability to maintain an upright posture and keep the body's **line of gravity (LOG)** within its **base of support (BOS),** and dynamic balance, or the ability to maintain stability while shifting weight or changing the BOS (Dunsky, Zeev, & Netz, 2017).

Center of mass (COM), also known as the center of gravity (COG), represents the point around which all weight in the body or an object is balanced. It is generally located about 2 inches (5 cm) anterior to the spine in the location of the first and second sacral joints (S1 and S2), but varies in individuals according to body shape, size, and sex, being slightly higher in males due to greater quantities of musculature in the upper body (Figure 8-30). A person's COM constantly shifts as they change position, move, or add external resistance. BOS is defined as the two-dimensional distance between and including the body's points of contact with a surface.

FIGURE 8-30
Center of gravity

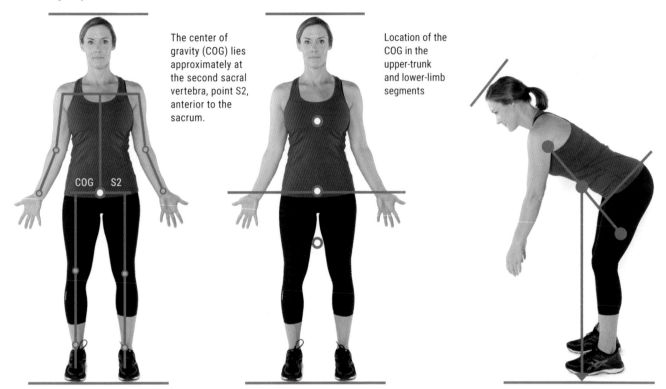

The center of gravity (COG) lies approximately at the second sacral vertebra, point S2, anterior to the sacrum.

Location of the COG in the upper-trunk and lower-limb segments

BALANCE-CONTROL STRATEGIES

An attempt to control standing balance when a person is perturbed (e.g., pushed from behind) is accomplished by a hierarchy of three automatic processes—the ankle, hip, and step strategies (Figure 8-31). For example, during a slight perturbation when a person is pushed gently from behind, the ankle strategy is used as a quick response to maintain balance. The upper and lower body move in the same direction and the COM is restored to a position of stability through movement centered at the ankles (see Figure 8-31a). Due to the relatively weak force that can be generated by the muscles of the ankle, individuals normally use this strategy to control balance when they are standing in an upright position or swaying through a very small ROM. Use of the ankle strategy requires adequate ROM (especially **dorsiflexion**) in the ankles, as well as plantar flexor strength. Therefore, a client who has difficulty keeping the heels in contact with the floor during a bend-and-lift movement pattern (e.g., squat) may have a lack of dorsiflexion ROM and will likely have balance problems, especially in advanced movement patterns. A firm, broad surface below the feet and an adequate level of sensation in the feet and ankles are also required for effective use of the ankle strategy. As such, those with foot **neuropathy,** which is common in people with advanced **diabetes,** may have balance issues.

If a greater perturbation is experienced, as in a more forceful push from behind, a person will use the hip strategy, which involves activation of the larger hip muscles and is used when the COM must be moved more quickly back over the BOS to restore stability (see Figure 8-31b). An individual who uses the hip strategy moves the upper and lower body in opposite directions by hinging at the hip. Therefore, a client who has difficulty maintaining appropriate

FIGURE 8-30 *(continued)*

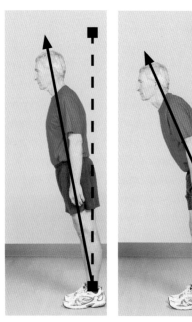

The added weight of the duffel bag to the shoulder girdle causes the COG to shift up and to the right. The person leans laterally to the left to bring the line of gravity back to the middle of their base of support.

spinal stability during bend-and-lift movement patterns (especially the hip hinge and deadlift movements) will most likely experience balance problems. Situations that require this strategy include responses to faster balance disturbances, standing on a relatively unstable support surface, and standing on a support surface that is smaller than the feet (e.g., balance beam). Effective use of the hip strategy requires an adequate amount of core function, muscle strength in the hip extensors, and ROM in the hip region.

An even greater perturbation (e.g., being shoved from behind or stumbling on an uneven surface) causes an individual to control balance using the step strategy (see Figure 8-31c). When the COM is displaced beyond stability limits or when the speed of perturbation is so fast that a hip strategy is no longer effective, the step strategy is utilized. To prevent a fall during these conditions, an individual must take one or more steps to establish a new BOS. A client who has difficulty performing exercises that mimic gait, such as single-leg movement patterns (e.g., single-leg stance and lunges), will probably have balance challenges as well. Lower-limb strength and the speed with which it can be generated (i.e., **power**) are two important characteristics of an effective step strategy. In other words, the ability of an individual to use muscular power of the legs, hips, and thighs to move rapidly during step initiation determines the success of this strategy. Furthermore, normal lower-body ROM

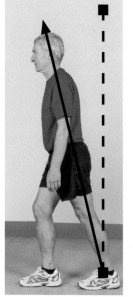

a. Ankle   b. Hip   c. Step

FIGURE 8-31
Three postural control strategies used to control balance

and adequate nervous system reaction speed are required for an effective step strategy. Although the three postural control strategies exist along a distinct continuum, various combinations of these strategies can occur when attempting to manage balance.

STATIC BALANCE TRAINING

After the client performs exercises to reestablish core function, static balance training, beginning with segmental or sectional stabilization training, can be introduced. This entails the use of specific static-balance exercises performed over a fixed BOS that impose small balance challenges to the body's core. Clients who are deconditioned may adopt an unsupported seated position that engages the core musculature. By following the training guidelines and manipulating the variables listed in Table 8-8, exercise professionals can gradually progress exercises by increasing the balance challenge until the client experiences difficulty in maintaining postural control, yet does not stumble or fall. The objective with these progressions is to increase the exercise challenge until a threshold of balance or postural control becomes evident, and then continue gradually from that point by manipulating any of the variables.

TABLE 8-8

Training Guidelines for Static Balance

Training Variables	Training Conditions
2–3 times per week	Narrow BOS (e.g., wide to narrow)
Perform exercises toward the beginning of workouts before the onset of fatigue (which decreases concentration)	Raise COM (e.g., raising arms overhead)
	Shift LOG (e.g., raising arms unilaterally, or leaning or rotating the trunk)
	Sensory alteration [e.g., shifting focal point to a finger 12 inches (30 cm) in front of one's face, performing slow hand-eye tracking, or performing slow head movements such as looking up and down]
Perform 1 set of 2–4 repetitions, each for 5–10 seconds	Sensory removal (e.g., closing eyes)

Note: BOS = Base of support; COM = Center of mass; LOG = Line of gravity

The natural progression from performing seated exercises is to performing standing exercises, thereby integrating the entire kinetic chain, which represents more function and mimics many activities of daily living (ADL). During integrated movements, the effects of external loads, gravity, and reactive forces all increase, thereby necessitating a greater need to stabilize the spine. McGill (2017) introduced the concept of **bracing,** explaining how it improves spinal stability by activating the muscles of the abdominal wall and the spinal extensors to form a girdle around the torso and creating a total stiffness greater than the sum of each muscle individually. To teach a client how to brace, an exercise professional can have them first practice simultaneous activation of flexors and extensors at other joints such as the elbow to better understand what is expected at the torso. Next, they can stand in a relaxed position and engage the core muscles while having the fingers pushed into the lateral obliques. A good cue to offer is to stiffen and push the fingers out to the sides. The client can then imagine a person standing in front of them who is about to deliver a quick jab to the stomach. In anticipation of the jab, the individual should stiffen up the trunk region by co-contracting both layers of muscles. This represents bracing, which, unlike centering (or drawing in the navel) that acts reflexively, is a conscious contraction used for short time periods during external loading on the spine (e.g., when performing a weighted squat or picking up a box).

The exercise professional should introduce standing static-balance training on stable surfaces before progressing to unstable surfaces (e.g., air disc, foam pad, or BOSU). Both of which gradually increase the balance challenge. Both forms of training are important to developing efficiency within the proprioceptive, vestibular, and visual systems, but the decision regarding which training surfaces to use depends primarily on the client's needs, capabilities, and goals. Regardless, all balance exercises should ultimately incorporate some form of dynamic balance training on stable surfaces (e.g., movement on the ground) to mimic ADL. When designing static balance–training programs, exercise professionals should follow the stance-position progressions illustrated in Figure 8-32. The exercise professional should identify which stance position challenges the client's balance threshold and then repeat the exercises with progressions outlined in Table 8-9.

FIGURE 8-32
Stance-position progressions

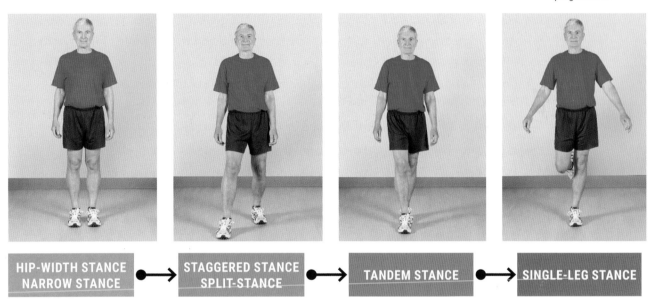

HIP-WIDTH STANCE
NARROW STANCE → STAGGERED STANCE
SPLIT-STANCE → TANDEM STANCE → SINGLE-LEG STANCE

TABLE 8-9

Balance Exercises and Training Variations

Position	Balance Exercise
Seated	▸ Sit upright and complete the following progressions. ▸ Perform leg activities while seated (heel raises, toe raises, or single-leg raises; marching).
Standing	▸ Clock: Balance on one leg (non-support leg knee flexed at 45 or 90° angle); the exercise professional calls out a time and the client moves the non-support leg to the time called (e.g., 5 o'clock or 9 o'clock); alternate legs ▸ Perform various leg activities while standing [heel raises, toe raises, or single-leg raises (non-support leg knee flexed at 45 or 90° angle); marching] ▸ Spelling: Balance on one leg (non-support leg knee flexed at 45 or 90° angle); the exercise professional asks the client to spell a word using the non-support leg (e.g., the client's name, day of the week, or a favorite food); alternate legs

Continued on the next page

TABLE 8-9 *(continued)*

Position	Balance Exercise
Moving	▸ Heel-to-toe walking along a 15-foot line on the floor (first with and then without the support of the exercise professional) ▸ Excursion: Alternating legs, lunge over a space separated by two lines of tape; progress to hopping or jumping (using single-leg or double-leg actions) back and forth across the space ▸ Dribble a basketball around cones that require the client to change direction multiple times

Note: Number of repetitions per exercise and rest intervals will be dependent on client conditioning and functional status.

Exercise professionals also can introduce more challenging variables, but only if they are considered appropriate and consistent with the client's goals:

▸ *Arm progressions:* Use a surface for support, hands on thighs, hands folded across the chest

▸ *Base-of-support progressions:* Reduce the points of contact (e.g., move from balancing on two feet to one foot)

▸ *Surface progressions:* Chair, balance disks, foam pad, stability ball

▸ *Visual progressions:* Open eyes, sunglasses or dim room lighting, closed eyes

▸ *Movement progressions:* Add directional changes (e.g., walking around cones that require a change in direction like forward and back, side-to-side, or diagonal)

▸ *Tasking progressions:* Single tasking, multitasking (e.g., balance exercise plus pass/catch a ball)

Each of these challenges should be introduced separately, gradually increasing the exercise difficulty by manipulating the variables provided in Table 8-9 under this new challenge. Next, exercise professionals can introduce an additional challenge in a similar manner (e.g., move to one foot and reintroduce the variables listed before implementing additional unstable surfaces, which should be introduced with two feet). Figure 8-33 presents sample exercise progressions.

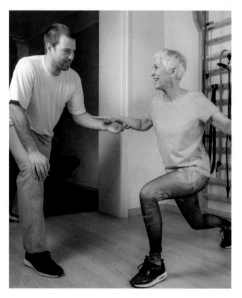

DYNAMIC BALANCE TRAINING

Once an older client demonstrates the ability to effectively stand on one leg, the exercise professional can introduce dynamic movements of the upper and lower extremity over a static BOS (Table 8-10). Next, various forms of resistance (e.g., medicine balls, cables, or elastic bands) that increase the stabilization demands and the potential need for bracing during movement can be introduced. This is where the exercise professional's creativity in programming becomes important—this will also heighten the fun factor. Programming can be creative but should always be progressed with common sense to keep the drills and exercises skill- and conditioning-level appropriate.

FIGURE 8-33
Sample progressions of balance exercises

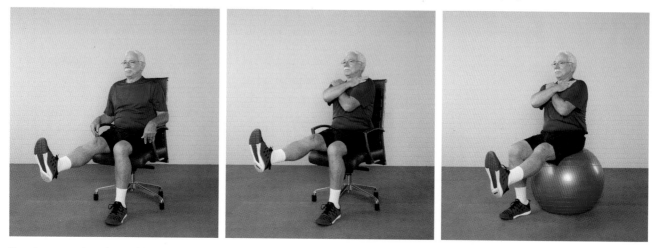

Sample progression of seated balance exercises (closed eyes, arms crossed, stability ball)

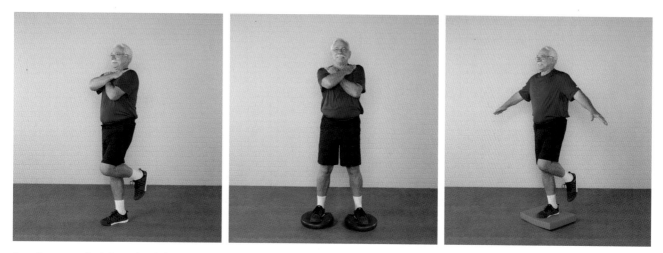

Sample progression of standing balance exercises (arms crossed, balance disks, foam pad)

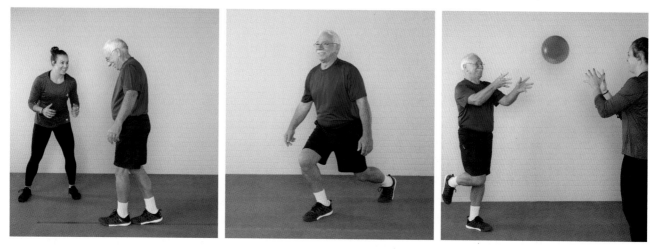

Sample progression of in-motion balance exercises (heel-to-toe, excursion, multitasking)

TABLE 8-10

Dynamic Movement Patterns Over a Static Base of Support

Action	Volume
Introduce upper-extremity movements ▶ Movements: ▪ Arms can move unilaterally (one arm at a time) ▪ Arms can move bilaterally (both arms move together) ▪ Arms can move reciprocally (alternating arm directions) ▪ Position the feet in any stance indicated in Figure 8-32 (except single-leg stance) ▶ Directions: ▪ Move arm(s) in the sagittal plane (flexion/extension) ▪ Move arm(s) in the frontal plane (abduction and adduction from an overhead position) ▪ Move arm(s) in the transverse plane (rotation from the shoulder-height position with a bent elbow)	Perform the following: ▶ 1–2 sets of 10–20 repetitions per side ▶ Slow, controlled tempos (avoid bouncing at the end-ROM) ▶ Less than 30-second rest intervals between sets
Introduce lower-extremity movements ▶ Movements: ▪ Stand on one leg ▪ Start by swinging the leg forward and backward, touching the toes to the floor at each end-ROM, then progress to unsupported leg swings ▶ Directions: ▪ Move the leg in the sagittal plane (flexion/extension) ▪ Move the leg in the frontal plane (abduction/adduction) ▪ Move the leg in the transverse plane (rotation in front or behind the stance leg)	Perform the following: ▶ 1–2 sets of 10–20 repetitions per side ▶ Slow, controlled tempos (avoid bouncing at the end-ROM) ▶ Less than 30-second rest intervals between sets
Integrate upper- and lower-extremity movements ▶ Move limbs ipsilaterally (same side) or contralaterally (opposite side) ▶ Move limbs "in synch"—moving in the same direction (e.g., the leg and arm move forward together) ▶ Move limbs "out of synch"—moving in opposite directions	Perform the following: ▶ 1–2 sets of 10–20 repetitions per side ▶ Slow, controlled tempos (avoid bouncing at the end-ROM) ▶ Less than 30-second rest intervals between sets

Note: ROM = Range of motion

Progression for the single-leg stance involves adding external resistance and increasing the balance challenge (Figures 8-34 and 8-35). Holding a medicine ball or dumbbell, or introducing partial single-leg squats, adds resistance to the kinetic chain and increases the balance challenge. As resistance (load) increases, the number of repetitions per set, and possibly the total number of sets, should be reduced and longer rest intervals should be introduced between sets (e.g., 30 to 60 seconds). For additional detailed explanations of exercises and programming guidelines for Functional Training, refer to *The Exercise Professional's Guide to Personal Training* (ACE, 2020).

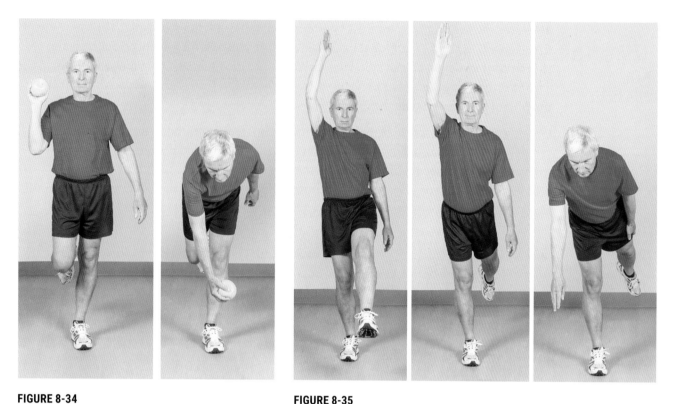

FIGURE 8-34
Single-leg reaches and touches

FIGURE 8-35
Single-leg sagittal plane movement with arm drivers

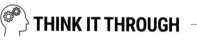 **THINK IT THROUGH**

Balance Training

Balance training, when implemented and progressed appropriately, can offer significant benefits for senior clients. However, it can also cause older clients to feel unstable and unsure of their abilities to avoid a fall during the training process. For example, even for clients who present with good balance, standing on one foot to perform an exercise can promote feelings of anxiety about falling. Thus, the exercise professional should set up balance-training exercises in such a way that the client feels safe (e.g., have the client stand next to a chair so that they can grab ahold of it if balance starts to become compromised). What measures will you take to ensure that your senior clients feel confident that they will not suffer a fall while performing balance-training exercises?

MOVEMENT TRAINING

Exercise professionals must stress the importance of learning how to perform the basic movements that encompass virtually all ADL:

▸ Bend-and-lift (e.g., deadlift and squatting)

▸ Single-leg (e.g., single-leg stance and lunging)

▸ Push (primarily in the vertical/horizontal planes)

▸ Pull (primarily in the vertical/horizontal planes)

▸ Rotation (spiral)

These are the five primary movement patterns that represent the foundation to all movement (see Figure 6-3, page 171). Proper execution of these movements enhances the potential to promote movement efficiency, as well as long-term maintenance and integrity of the joint structures, muscles, and connective tissues, as well as the central nervous system and **peripheral nervous system.**

Once the functional aspects of movement have been adequately addressed, clients can progress to muscular training with increasing loads. As discussed in Chapter 6, resistance-training exercise is an important component of an older adult's comprehensive exercise program and should be encouraged. Strength training improves the older client's fitness level by placing emphasis on muscle force production, which is crucial for facilitating improved performance of ADL.

Movement Training requires adequate postural stability and kinetic chain mobility (i.e., the ability to control the body's kinetic chain appropriately during static and dynamic situations), as described in the previous section. Once a client has successfully demonstrated the requisite stability and mobility, core function, and balance through progressive conditioning during Functional Training, they should begin to train the primary movement patterns.

Observing movement is an effective method to determine the contribution that muscle imbalances and poor posture have on neural control, and also helps identify movement compensations. Conducting movement assessments (see Chapter 7) allows exercise professionals to observe compensations that occur during a client's performance of the five primary movement patterns. If altered movement patterns are present, it is usually indicative of some form of adjusted neural action, which normally manifests itself as muscle tightness or an imbalance between muscles acting at the joint.

Once stability and mobility have been achieved, the training focus shifts to establishing efficient movement through a healthy ROM in all three **planes of motion** without compromising joint or postural stability. It is also important to encourage clients to breathe normally during exercise and avoid the **Valsalva maneuver** (exhalation against a closed glottis).

Exercise performed during Movement Training should emphasize proper sequencing and control of the body's COG throughout the individual's normal ROM. During this phase of training, it is also important to continually integrate Functional Training exercises to maintain kinetic chain mobility and postural stability. These functional exercises are often incorporated into the warm-up segment of the exercise session to prepare the body for the more rigorous movements that may follow.

In this phase, body-weight exercises are initially used, and external resistance is gradually added while the emphasis remains on the client's ability to control the movement being performed. Before adding an external load, the client should be able to perform the movement pattern with proper stability and mobility, postural control, proper form, controlled speed, and balance to decrease the risk of injury that can result from loading poorly executed movements. Adding a light external load [e.g., up to 50 to 60% of **one-repetition maximum (1-RM)**] to exercises that comprise the primary movement patterns is a safe and effective way to challenge clients' muscular capabilities after they have demonstrated they can perform the five primary movement patterns well and before they progress to even heavier resistances or more rapid movements in the Load/Speed Training phase. It is essential that the external loads are increased gradually so that correct movement patterns are not altered during the performance of the exercises. During this phase of training, exercise repetition should be emphasized over exercise intensity.

Moving more efficiently and eventually improving the functioning of the muscles involved in the five primary movement patterns will improve the client's ability to perform daily activities.

Bend-and-Lift Movements

The bend-and-lift movement associated with the squat is perhaps one of the most prevalent activities used in strength training and throughout most individuals' ADL (e.g., sitting and standing). Faulty movement patterns associated with poor technique could be linked to balance problems and will disrupt muscle function and joint loading, compromising performance and ultimately leading to overload and potential injury. Proper technique is therefore essential to performing bend-and-lift movements safely and effectively.

The bend-and-lift maneuver begins with a solid platform of good posture and bracing of the abdominal region (especially when using external loads). As the exercises in this training phase utilize body weight as the primary form of resistance, bracing might not be as critical, but clients should be encouraged to practice this skill, as they will need it when lifting external loads.

From a standpoint of functionality, people normally bend down to lift objects with their hands by their sides, so exercise professionals should teach these variations beginning with the most simplistic position (i.e., arms at the sides) prior to moving into high-arm positions (e.g., front squat, back squat, or overhead positions). Keep in mind that these high-arm positions require a greater degree of thoracic mobility, which many older clients may lack. Thus, clients should be taught the bend-and-lift in the deadlift position first (i.e., arms at sides), before being introduced to the front-squat position and then the back and overhead positions.

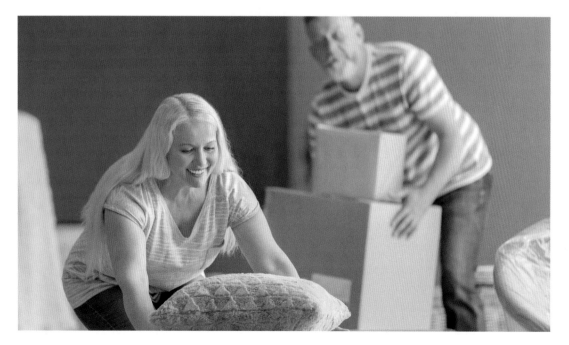

Single-leg Movements

A primary single-leg pattern involves teaching clients how to lunge effectively, a movement pattern that is often performed poorly in any plane. Although lunge mechanics are similar to bend-and-lift mechanics as far as spinal stability is concerned, many older clients may deviate from basic movement principles because of the increased balance challenge of a reduced BOS during single-leg movement patterns. For those having trouble with lunges, an appropriate exercise regression includes walking on a line taped to the floor, which reduces the BOS. Adding obstacles (e.g., walking around cones that require directional changes, like forward and back, side-to-side, or diagonal) will also enhance dynamic balance.

As with squats, people often find themselves performing variations to the traditional lunge during their daily activities (e.g., bending down and returning to standing after tying a shoe or ascending and descending stairs), workouts (e.g., side lunges), or even during sports (e.g., cutting and sidestepping). These variations involve directional lunges, foot-position variations, and movements with the upper extremities in all three planes of movement. Considering these variations represent daily movements, clients should be trained functionally to mimic these patterns. Once a client demonstrates proficiency with the standard lunge pattern, the exercise professional can progress the exercise to include directional changes, different foot positions, and upper-extremity movements. Bear in mind that high-arm positions require a greater degree of thoracic and hip mobility, which a client may lack. Therefore, clients should begin by driving the arms in the low position prior to incorporating the high-arm-position movements.

When working with older adults, exercise professionals should consider incorporating exercises that require lower-extremity muscular power. Single-leg movement patterns are a good option for introducing power, as they can progress to jumps, hops, or bounds. However, individuals should never begin jumping, bounding, or hopping activities until they can effectively demonstrate correct landing technique and the ability to decelerate the impact forces of landing (see page 320). Also, those with certain musculoskeletal conditions (e.g., **osteoarthritis**) should avoid high-impact movements.

Pushing Movements

Clients whose scapular stability is compromised, such as those who exhibit forward-rounded shoulders, abducted scapulae, or winging of the scapulae, should perform both pushing and pulling exercises—at least initially—from a position of scapular stability with very little resistance (external load). This means that the scapulae are in the set, or "packed," position and they do not move as the glenohumeral joint acts in extension or flexion. Figure 8-36 presents a sequence for teaching clients how to set their scapulae. Once the client has demonstrated that they are able to maintain the scapular set position for various pushing and pulling movements, scapular retraction and adduction can be added to the exercises to ensure that the scapulothoracic and glenohumeral joints have the opportunity to move as they should during normal daily activities.

During shoulder flexion (e.g., front raise exercise or pushing open a door) and overhead presses (e.g., shoulder press or putting luggage into an overhead compartment on an airplane), movement to 180 degrees is achieved by the collaborative effort of the scapulae rotating against the rib cage and the humerus rotating within the glenoid fossa. The

FIGURE 8-36
Shoulder packing

Objective: To kinesthetically improve awareness of good scapular position, improving flexibility and strength of key parascapular muscles

Preparation and position:

▸ Stand with the back against a wall, feeling the scapulae, pelvis, and rib cage in contact with the wall.

▸ Position the arms at the sides of the trunk with the palms facing away from the wall.

▸ Engage the core muscles to stabilize the lumbar spine in the neutral position. Maintain this position throughout the exercise (a).

Exercise:

▸ Exhale and perform two to four repetitions of each of the following, holding each contraction for five to 10 seconds (b):

  ▪ Scapular depression

  ▪ Scapular retraction

▸ Using passive assistance from the opposite arm, gently push down on the shoulder (posterior tilt on scapula) without losing lumbar stability. Hold this position for 15 to 60 seconds.

▸ Relax and repeat two to four times on each shoulder.

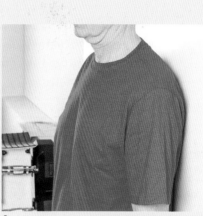

a.

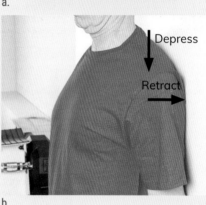

b.

movement generally requires approximately 60 degrees of scapular rotation and 120 degrees of glenohumeral rotation (Figure 8-37). While the scapulae require some degree of mobility to perform the various movements of the arm, they fundamentally need to remain stable to promote normal mobility within the glenohumeral joint. During these movements, insufficient, premature, or excessive activation of specific scapular muscles (e.g., dominant rhomboids resisting upward scapular rotation or overactive upper trapezius forcing excessive scapular elevation) will compromise scapular stability, which in turn affects the ability of the muscles around the glenohumeral joint to execute their function effectively. For example, if the scapulae cannot sink slightly while the arms extend overhead, this may interfere with scapular rotation and scapular stability. This illustrates the importance of setting or packing the scapulae prior to shoulder flexion or abduction movements.

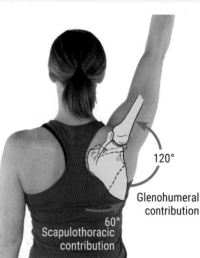

FIGURE 8-37
Scapulohumeral rhythm

The movement of the arm is accompanied by movement of the scapula—a ratio of approximately 2° of arm movement for every 1° of scapular movement occurs during shoulder abduction and flexion.

In everyday activities, pushing movements are pervasive, as they require movement of the arms in front of the body or over the head. If the shoulder joint and shoulder girdle muscles work together properly, pushing actions can be performed effectively with minimal stress to the upper-extremity joints. When altered joint mechanics are present, such as the case when muscles have become adaptively shortened or lengthened due to repetitive use or poor posture, the risk for injury increases.

Pushing exercises can progress beyond stability and shift toward integrating whole-body movement patterns. Exercises can begin with more traditional pushing and pulling movements that primarily target the shoulder girdle in a bilateral or unilateral fashion, using supported backrests, but should then progress to becoming unsupported (e.g., standing in a normal or split-stance position), which better mimics most ADL.

Pulling Movements

The common actions of pulling open a door and lifting objects to hold them close to the body (e.g., picking up a grandchild) are examples of how people use pulling movements in their everyday activities. Similar to the body mechanics of pushing, when the shoulder and shoulder girdle are functioning within their ideal ROM, pulling movements are effective actions that transfer minimal stress to the joints. However, when muscles do not provide the appropriate strength or stability in the upper extremity—especially those muscles that have attachments on the scapulae, rib cage, and humerus—can end up adding excess wear on the joints, as they cannot effectively transfer mechanical forces.

Exercises to promote effective pulling can begin with more traditional movements that primarily target the shoulder girdle in a bilateral or unilateral fashion, using supported backrests, then progress to performing unsupported actions (e.g., standing in a normal, split-stance, or lunge position) that mimic most ADL.

Rotational Movements

Rotational movements represent the last of the primary movements and are perhaps some of the most complex, given how many follow spiral or diagonal patterns throughout the body. These movements generally incorporate movement into multiple planes simultaneously (e.g., a golf backswing requires **transverse plane** rotation, thoracic and lumbar extension, and some lateral flexion). Many of these movements increase the forces placed along the vertebrae, so exercise professionals must use care when teaching these movements and only do so after the client has conditioned the core effectively.

Two key movements involving diagonal or spiral patterns of movement within the arms, shoulders, trunks, hips, and legs are the wood chop and the hay baler:

▸ *Wood chop:* This exercise involves a pulling action to initiate the movement down across the front of the body, followed by a pushing action in the upper extremity as the arms move away from the body (Figure 8-38). In addition, it requires stabilization of the trunk in all three planes (i.e., during flexion, rotation, and side-bending), and weight transference through the hips and between the legs to gain leverage and maintain balance. Concentric muscle action during the downward chop is achieved by using a high anchor point (e.g., high cable pulley or band).

FIGURE 8-38
Wood-chop spiral patterns

Note: Given the complexity of the wood-chop movement, the individual should first learn basic spiral patterns without placing excessive loads upon the spine.

Objective: To introduce basic spiral patterns with small, controlled forces placed along the spine

Preparation and position:

▸ While holding a dowel, assume a seated half-kneeling position, placing the rear knee directly under the hips. This position engages both the hip flexors and extensors to help stabilize the spine.

▸ Pack both shoulders (see Figure 8-36) and brace the core, holding these positions throughout the exercise.

▸ Raise the dowel toward the shoulder on the same side as the leading leg, keeping both hands close to the body (a).

▸ The hips and torso (chest) should remain aligned forward.

Exercise:

▸ Exhale and slowly perform a downward movement across the front of the body, moving the dowel toward the opposite hip (b) and keeping both arms close to the body to shorten the length of the lever (called the moment arm) (c).

▸ The hips and torso (chest) should remain aligned forward.

▸ Return to the starting position and repeat.

▸ Perform one or two sets of 12 to 15 repetitions in each direction, alternating the knee position with each directional change.

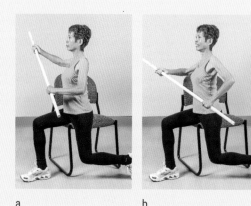
a.   b.

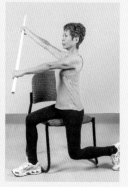
c.   d.

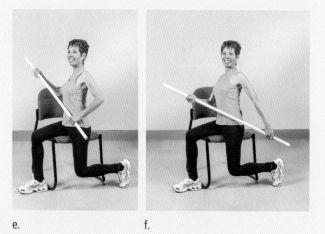
e.   f.

Progression—Long moment arm: Repeat the same movement but extend the arms (acting as a driver) to increase the ROM and leverage, but keep both arms close the body during the movement (d, e, & f). The hips and torso (chest) should remain aligned forward.

Progression—Standing short moment arm: Assume a split-stance position, placing the leg on the same side as the chop start position forward. Bend both elbows and raise the dowel toward the shoulder on the same side as the leading leg, keeping both hands close to the body. Repeat the same chopping movement with bent elbows. The hips and torso (chest) should remain aligned forward.

Progression—Standing long moment arm: Assume the same split-stance position and repeat the same chopping movement but extend the arms. The hips and torso (chest) should remain aligned forward.

▸ *Hay baler:* This exercise involves a pulling action to initiate the movement up across the front of the body, followed by a pushing action in the upper extremity as the arms move away from the body (Figure 8-39). In addition, it requires stabilization of the trunk in all three planes (extension in the **sagittal plane,** rotation in the transverse plane, and side-bending in the **frontal plane**), and weight transference through the hips and between the legs to gain leverage and maintain balance.

The need for thoracic mobility is greater during these movements than with the pushes and pulls, given the three-dimensional nature of the movement patterns. Performing these exercises without thoracic mobility or lumbar stability may compromise the shoulders and hips and increase the likelihood for injury. The thoracic spine offers greater mobility than the lumbar spine. Therefore, lumbar stability and control of lumbar rotation should be emphasized while promoting movement within the thoracic spine. Exercise professionals should use caution when implementing rotational movements for clients with, or at risk for, osteoporosis and avoid excessive twisting of the spine.

Exercise Guidelines for Enhancing Movement Patterns

The basic programming guideline in the Movement Training phase is to give clients exercises to help them develop proper control and adequate ROM while performing the five basic movement patterns. The timeframe for movement training could be two weeks to several months, depending on each client's initial level of movement ability and their rate of progression. The FIRST acronym can be used to guide exercise program design: frequency, intensity, repetitions, sets, and type.

FREQUENCY

Two to three days per week is adequate for the beginning stages of a Movement Training program. Considering that many older clients who are deconditioned will also be engaging in regular cardiorespiratory training, a frequency of two days per week may be a more appropriate recommendation.

INTENSITY

Initially, the goal in this phase is to focus on coordination and muscular conditioning for the basic movement patterns. Thus, clients should not use any external load while learning

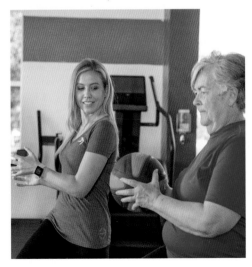

to perform the movement-pattern exercises properly. After the client has shown appropriate control along the kinetic chain during movement-pattern training, the intensity can be progressed to include added resistance. The rate at which an older client will progress is dependent on each individual's current level of fitness and ability to learn new motor skills (e.g., one client might be ready to add resistance to movement-pattern training after two exercise sessions, whereas another client might need two weeks of consistent exercise training before they are ready to increase the intensity by adding load). When adding load to movement-pattern training,

FIGURE 8-39
Hay baler

Objective: To introduce the full multiplanar hay-baler movement pattern while controlling forces placed along the spine

Preparation and position:

▸ Assume a staggered position, placing the forward leg 6 to 12 inches (15 to 30 cm) forward.

▸ Pack both shoulders (see Figure 8-36) and brace the core, holding these positions throughout the exercise.

▸ Sweep the arms in a diagonal direction (a & b).

▸ Load 60 to 70% of the body weight onto the back leg.

Exercise:

▸ Exhale and rotate through the chest and shoulders to bring the arms across the body and over the opposite shoulder while transferring the body weight from the back to the front leg.

▸ While the hips rotate, the chest and shoulders should remain aligned over the pubis (center of the pelvis).

▸ Return to the starting position and repeat.

▸ Perform one or two sets of 12 to 15 repetitions in each direction, alternating the stance position with each directional change.

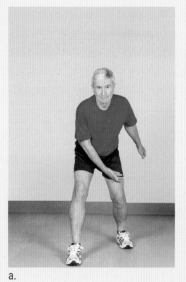
a.

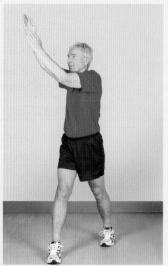
b.

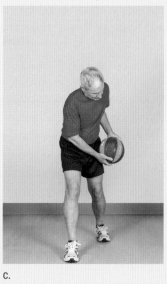
c.

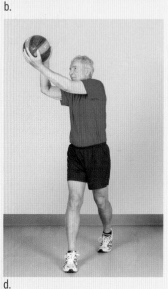
d.

Progression—Long moment arm: Repeat the same movement but extend the elbows (the use of a dowel might prove useful). A wide, extended grip concentrates force-generation from the hips and not from the shoulder or arms. Repeat the movement and, while the hips rotate, the chest and shoulders should remain aligned over the pubis (center of the pelvis).

Progression (c & d): Add external resistance in the form of a medicine ball, kettle bell, cable, or elastic tubing.

start with a light resistance (40 to 50% 1-RM) that allows clients to learn proper movement techniques and then over time progress to as high as 60 to 80% of 1-RM.

REPETITIONS

Initially, when a client is learning a new movement pattern and using only body weight as the training load, an appropriate repetition range is 12 to 20. The number of repetitions performed varies inversely with the intensity of the exercise set. That is, fewer repetitions can be performed with a higher resistance and more repetitions can be completed with a lower resistance. During the Movement Training phase, the lower training intensity permits more repetitions in each exercise set. It is therefore recommended that Movement Training exercises first be performed with no or light resistance that allows for proper movement patterns to be learned, and then progressed to heavier weightloads. Generally, if the resistance does not permit at least 12 repetitions, it should be reduced. When 16 repetitions can be properly performed, the resistance should be increased.

SETS

Ultimately, a range of one to three sets is appropriate for each Movement Training exercise. However, studies have demonstrated that one set of resistance exercise may be as effective as multiple training sets (Fragala et al., 2019), especially for beginning exercisers. For Movement Training workouts, one set of each exercise is certainly a good starting point, as increases in muscle strength do not seem to be dependent on the number of sets performed. However, as training progresses, a greater number of sets per session is associated with larger increases in lean body mass (Fragala et al., 2019). Single-set programs are an effective way to help previously physically inactive older adults become comfortable with the challenges of resistance training. When the client demonstrates consistent adherence and initial adaptations to a single-set program, the volume of sets can increase.

TYPE

Exercise selection should focus on the five basic movement patterns: deadlifts/squats, lunges, pushes (both in the horizontal plane and overhead), pulls, and rotational movements. The exercises should be selected to help the client learn and improve movement patterns with respect to their muscular fitness and strength-training experience. Clients with less strength-training experience should begin with basic exercises performed without external resistance and relatively stable conditions. In some cases, especially for older adults who are deconditioned, exercise selection can begin with selectorized weight machines, which utilize the basic movement patterns of exercise but provide stability and control the path of motion. Once a client demonstrates progress with motor control and muscular strength, they can begin performing ground-based standing exercises that emphasize muscle integration. Traditional selectorized machines are good for isolating a working muscle, but do not promote functional movement. Therefore, the goal is to move clients away from seated and supported machines to more functional strength activities.

Such exercises include dumbbell squats, overhead dumbbell presses, standing cable rows, and standing cable presses. As strength increases, emphasis may be placed on multiplanar

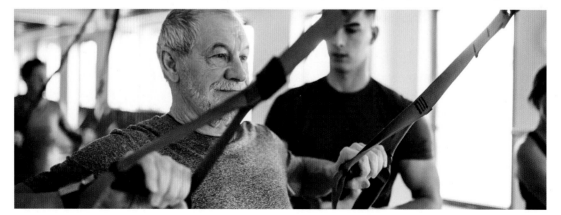

movements that require higher levels of muscle integration. Movements may be performed from unsupported postures, with closed- and open-kinetic-chain exercises for the upper- and lower-body muscles.

Appropriate Rates of Progression for Deconditioned Clients

The standard progression is a 5% resistance increase whenever the end-range number of repetitions can be completed. However, during the early stages of resistance training, the motor-learning effect enhances strength gains by facilitating muscle-fiber recruitment and contraction efficiency. Therefore, during the Movement Training phase, resistance increases may be more than 5% if the exerciser experiences a relatively fast rate of progression. For example, if a client has a goal repetition range of 12 to 16 and initially performs 12 repetitions of an exercise with 10 pounds (4.55 kg), the weight load may be increased up to 12 pounds (5.45 kg) (20% increase) after 16 repetitions are achieved, as long as proper body mechanics are maintained and at least 12 repetitions can be performed with the heavier resistance. Once the exercises can be executed with correct movement patterns while maintaining neutral posture, a stable COG, and controlled movement speed, clients may naturally progress to Load/Speed Training as they gain experience and become more efficient at controlling the body's COG throughout the normal ROM with both body weight and light external loads. For additional detailed explanations of exercises and programming guidelines for Movement Training, refer to *The Exercise Professional's Guide to Personal Training* (ACE, 2020).

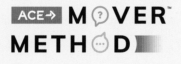

Is Lifting Weights Right for Me?

For the past six months, you have been working with a 69-year-old client, Patricia. She currently trains with you three times per week following the ACE IFT Model for Muscular Training. Patricia began her journey with goals to move better, improve balance and posture, and increase stability and mobility in her joints. Patricia has progressed from performing primarily Functional Training movements focusing on core and balance exercises to Movement Training. Here, the emphasis has been on continuing to develop what was accomplished during Functional Training and the development of good control when completing the five primary movement patterns. At this point in her training, Patricia will continue to include exercises specific to the Functional and Movement Training phases of the Muscular Training component of the ACE IFT Model, while gradually adding weight to the primary movement patterns. During a training session, you attempt to introduce 5-pound (2.3-kg) kettlebells to a bend-and-lift movement pattern and you sense that Patricia is uncomfortable with this change to her regularly performed body-weight squats. Patricia's body language and facial expressions shift, and it is clear she is not happy about something. It is important for exercise professionals to be aware of both verbal and nonverbal forms of communication, as the interpretation of both is important for understanding how a client is truly feeling.

The following example demonstrates how the ACE ABC Approach™ can be used to explore unique situations that may arise during training sessions.

ACE→ ABC APPROACH

Ask: Ask open-ended questions to uncover what may have occurred that led to a change in Patricia's demeanor.

Exercise Professional: When I mentioned adding weight to the squat exercise, you seemed to hesitate and it looked like you were not too sure about this progression. What caused your hesitation?

Client: I'm happy with the way things are going, and I'm not sure why I need to lift weights when I don't want to be a bodybuilder. The idea of using weights makes me nervous, and I'm not sure I'm ready or that it is even necessary.

Exercise Professional: You enjoy the program as it is, and you don't feel adding weight to your movement training is important because you don't want to be a bodybuilder. Is that correct?

Client: That's correct. I'm a 69-year-old woman and I don't want to have big bulky muscles. I just want to move better with improved balance and posture.

Break down barriers: Asking more open-ended questions will enable you to learn about the client's beliefs and hesitations.

Exercise Professional: What are your beliefs and understanding about muscular training and getting bulky and how it may impact your ability to move better?

Client: Well, it seems to me that all the people I see lifting weights get big and muscular, and that is not my goal. Are there other reasons why people lift weights? Why do you think it is important for me?

Exercise Professional: Great questions! There are a lot of reasons why people lift weights. One of those reasons may be to get bigger muscles or more defined musculature. Other people might lift weights to increase strength for the activities they do. Some might do it to improve their endurance so they can use their muscles effectively over a long period, or even to maintain or increase muscular power. Weight training is a vital component of slowing the loss of muscle mass that occurs with aging, which can be up to 5 pounds (2.3 kg) of muscle per decade. Other reasons to lift weights would be to increase or maintain **bone mineral density** to help prevent or combat osteoporosis. You could also reduce your risk of injury by becoming stronger through lifting weights. I know this is a lot of information. I don't want to make you feel like it is something you must do. It is up to you to decide if you want to incorporate resistance into your muscular-training program. Part of my job is to make sure you have all the information you need to make your decision. What else might you want to know about this topic?

Client: I had no idea there was so much to consider. I just thought lifting weights meant you got big. I didn't realize that you lost muscle as you got older! Won't I get bulky if I lift weights?

Exercise Professional: Under natural training conditions, women can enhance muscular strength and size, but they will rarely develop large, muscular physiques. Women naturally have lower levels of **anabolic** (muscle building) hormones and less muscle tissue and it is even harder to develop large muscles as you age. Just like in our current program, we would work together, one step at a time, to make sure what we are doing is working. If adding weights to your routine gives you undesired results, we can always modify your program at any time. Do you have any other questions related to this topic?

Client: I am starting to see how there are other reasons to lift weights, but how will this change to my program help me to move better?

Exercise Professional: Another great question, Patricia! Already in your program we have been working together to improve your postural stability and make certain parts of your body more mobile, and most recently we have been focusing on our five primary movement patterns. All this work so far has led to efficient movement. The other aspect of moving better is making sure you have the strength, power, and endurance to support the movements you do throughout the day. This is where the addition of appropriate load comes in. Often, when we do these primary movements we are lifting or lowering an object. Some examples would be lifting groceries and putting them away, carrying a laundry basket, and picking up a heavy cat litter box, as you had mentioned six months ago. Adding a load in a controlled environment will allow you to meet your goals as you become stronger in those activities and generally move more efficiently and safely.

Client: That makes sense! I'm still skeptical, but I'm willing to give it a try, as long as we can stop at any point if I don't like the way it makes me look or feel.

Collaborate: Work together with the client to determine next steps by partnering with her to decide how she would like to move forward with the introduction of weight to her existing training program.

Exercise Professional: You have my word; you are in control here. I would be doing you a disservice if I didn't give you all the information you need to make the best decision. How would you like to move forward today?

Client: Let's try what you have planned for today and check in at the beginning of our next session to reassess the addition of weight training to my existing program.

Exercise Professional: Great! Let's begin by introducing 5-pound (2.3-kg) kettlebells to your next set and see how the movement feels and how your body handles the added weight. We will communicate throughout the workout so we can make changes as needed.

The ACE ABC Approach may be used at any point, even during training sessions. Listening to, and partnering with, your client as soon as a situation arises can add significant value to the client's experience. As a result, the client will understand that their needs and wants are not only heard but also matter as they relate to goal accomplishment, thereby enhancing self-efficacy.

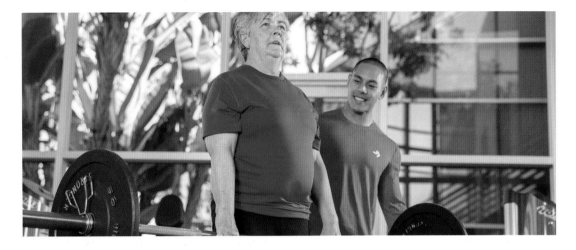

LOAD/SPEED TRAINING

Exercise professionals are often wary of encouraging older clients to take their neuromotor, flexibility, and muscle conditioning to an appropriate level to focus on force and/or speed production with goals of improving muscular fitness, **hypertrophy,** and body composition. However, as discussed in Chapters 3, 6, and 7, strength losses are one of the most debilitating consequences of physical inactivity combined with aging. Furthermore, strength is a factor in the ability to produce muscular power, which benefits older adults in their ability to avoid a fall. Thus, improving an older client's overall muscular strength through an appropriately designed and progressive resistance-training program should be a primary goal of exercise professionals who work with an older adult population.

📖 APPLY WHAT YOU KNOW

Using Movement-pattern Exercises in the Warm-up

Clients who are ready to progress to Load/Speed Training have demonstrated the ability to move efficiently with proper body mechanics. However, their movement-pattern training should not end once they progress to Load/Speed Training. In fact, regardless of age, continual practice of the five primary movement patterns should be a part of every client's training program. An effective method for ensuring continual movement-pattern training is to include these exercises in the client's dynamic warm-up. The 10 minutes devoted to movement-pattern exercise at the beginning of a workout will prepare the body for the more intense demands that will be required during the conditioning portion of the session.

The routine presented in Figure 8-40 includes an example of a whole-body movement-pattern warm-up that can be used with older adults to prepare for an exercise session, whether the focus is cardiorespiratory or muscular training. Note that exercise professionals can use the ACE IFT Model Exercise Programming Template to develop and progress exercise programs for their clients. Refer to *The Exercise Professional's Guide to Personal Training* (ACE, 2020) for more information on how to use the template, as well as case studies that provide examples of how an exercise professional can use this tool when working with a variety of clients.

Client Name: _____

Client Goals: To improve muscular fitness to be more active with their family during a six-week summer vacation

Client-centered Considerations: Wants to have fun during exercise sessions, enjoys tracking progress, and likes to try new exercises and discuss how they are helping to achieve goals

Frequency (active and rest days): Total-body Muscular Training three days per week with one rest day between workouts

FIGURE 8-40

Sample exercise session for a client in the Load/Speed Training phase of the Muscular Training component of the ACE IFT Model

Cardiorespiratory Training Phase:

☐ **Base Training**
  Focus on moderate-intensity exercise below the talk test threshold

☐ **Fitness Training**
  Build on Base Training through the introduction of zone 2 intervals performed from VT1 to just below VT2

☐ **Performance Training**
  Build on Fitness Training and introduce zone 3 intervals performed at and above VT2

Muscular Training Phase:

☐ **Functional Training**
  Focus on establishing postural stability and kinetic chain mobility

☐ **Movement Training**
  Focus on training the five primary movement patterns while incorporating Functional Training exercises in the warm-up and cool-down

☒ **Load/Speed Training**
  Focus on load and speed goals while including Functional Training exercises in the warm-up and cool-down and loading primary movement patterns

Exercise Goal*	Exercise/Exercise Mode	Intensity†	Volume‡
Warm-up: Prepare the muscles and joints for muscular and cardiorespiratory training			
Bend-and-lift movement pattern	Squat	1 to 2 pounds (~0.5 to 1 kg)	1 set x 12–16 repetitions

Continued on the next page

Exercise Goal*	Exercise/Exercise Mode	Intensity†	Volume†
Bend-and-lift movement pattern with shoulder flexion	Vertical wood chop	1 to 2 pounds (~0.5 to 1 kg)	1 set x 12–16 repetitions
Single-leg movement pattern	Forward lunge (alternating)	1 to 2 pounds (~0.5 to 1 kg)	1 set x 6–8 repetitions (each leg)
Single-leg movement pattern	Lateral lunge (alternating)	1 to 2 pounds (~0.5 to 1 kg)	1 set x 6–8 repetitions (each leg)

American Council on Exercise

Exercise Goal*	Exercise/Exercise Mode	Intensity†	Volume‡
Combined single-leg and rotational movement pattern	Forward lunge with rotation (alternating)	1 to 2 pounds (~0.5 to 1 kg)	1 set x 6–8 repetitions (each leg)

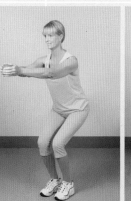

Combined bend-and-lift, pushing, and rotational movement patterns	Squat with 1-arm overhead spiral (right and left)	1 to 2 pounds (~0.5 to 1 kg)	1 set x 12–16 repetitions

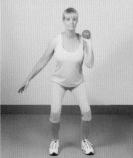
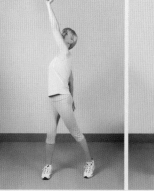

Combined pulling and bend-and-lift movement patterns	Narrow squat hip hinge with alternating arm row	1 to 2 pounds (~0.5 to 1 kg)	1 set x 6–8 repetitions (each leg)

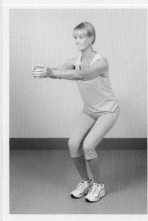
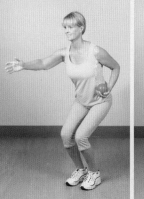
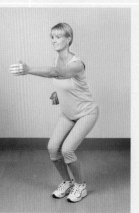

Continued on the next page

Exercise Goal*	Exercise/Exercise Mode	Intensity†	Volume‡
Conditioning: Load/Speed Training focused on increasing muscular strength through the five primary movement patterns			
Bend-and-lift	Squat with dumbbells	Dumbbells: 10 pounds (~4.5 kg)	1 set x 6–12 repetitions

Single-leg	Lunge	Dumbbells: 10 pounds (~4.5 kg)	1 set x 6–12 repetitions

Pushing	Bench press	Dumbbells: 10 pounds (~4.5 kg)	1 set x 6–12 repetitions

Exercise Goal*	Exercise/Exercise Mode	Intensity†	Volume‡
Pushing	Shoulder press	Dumbbells: 10 pounds (~4.5 kg)	1 set x 6–12 repetitions

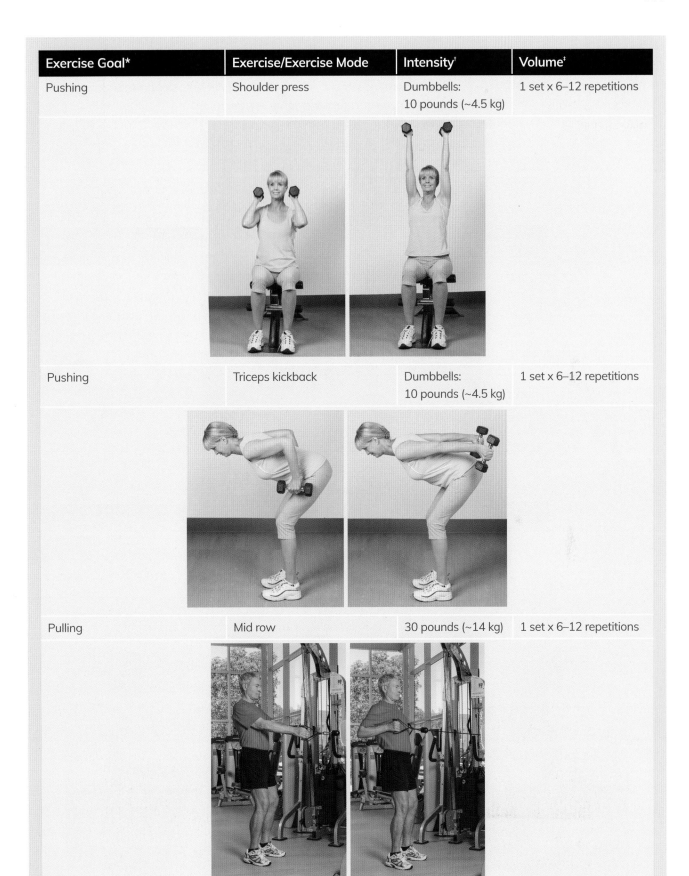

Pushing	Triceps kickback	Dumbbells: 10 pounds (~4.5 kg)	1 set x 6–12 repetitions
Pulling	Mid row	30 pounds (~14 kg)	1 set x 6–12 repetitions

Continued on the next page

Exercise Goal*	Exercise/Exercise Mode	Intensity†	Volume‡
Pulling	Lat pull-down	30 pounds (~14 kg)	1 set x 6–12 repetitions
Pulling	Pull-up	Body weight	1 set x 6–12 repetitions
Single-leg and rotational movement patterns	Split stance with cross-body rotation (right and left)	1 to 2 pounds (~0.5 to 1 kg)	1 set x 6–8 repetitions (each leg)

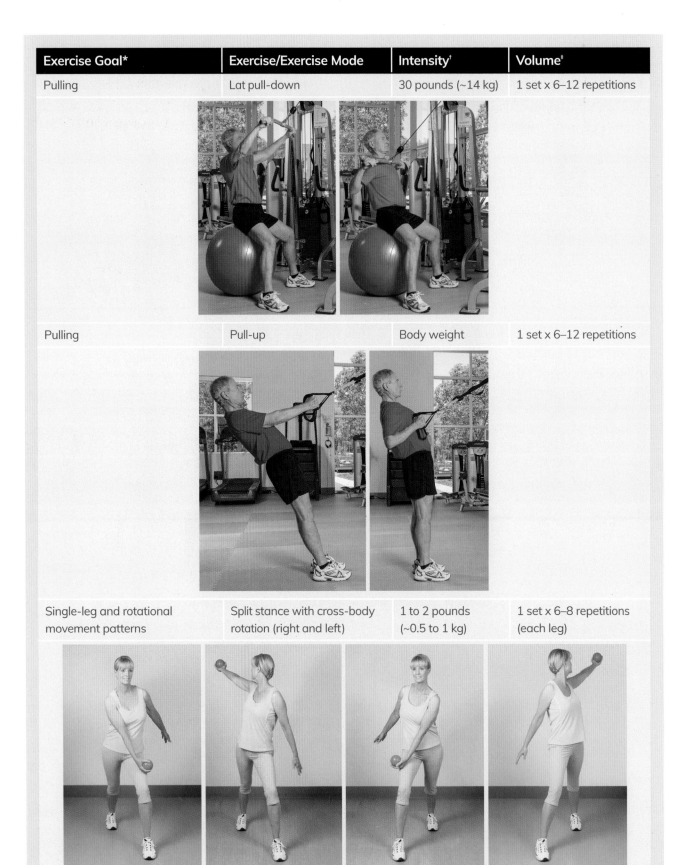

Exercise Goal*	Exercise/Exercise Mode	Intensity†	Volume‡
Cool-down: Include a few minutes of low-intensity walking or cycling prior to stretching to allow for an adequate transition period following strenuous activity; perform below exercises during every workout			
Shoulder mobility/range of motion	Anterior shoulder and chest wall stretch	Body weight	1 repetition x 30–60 seconds (each side)
Shoulder stability	Standing wall angel	Body weight	1 repetition x 30–60 seconds
Hip mobility/ROM	Seated hamstrings stretch	Body weight	1 repetition x 30–60 seconds (each side)

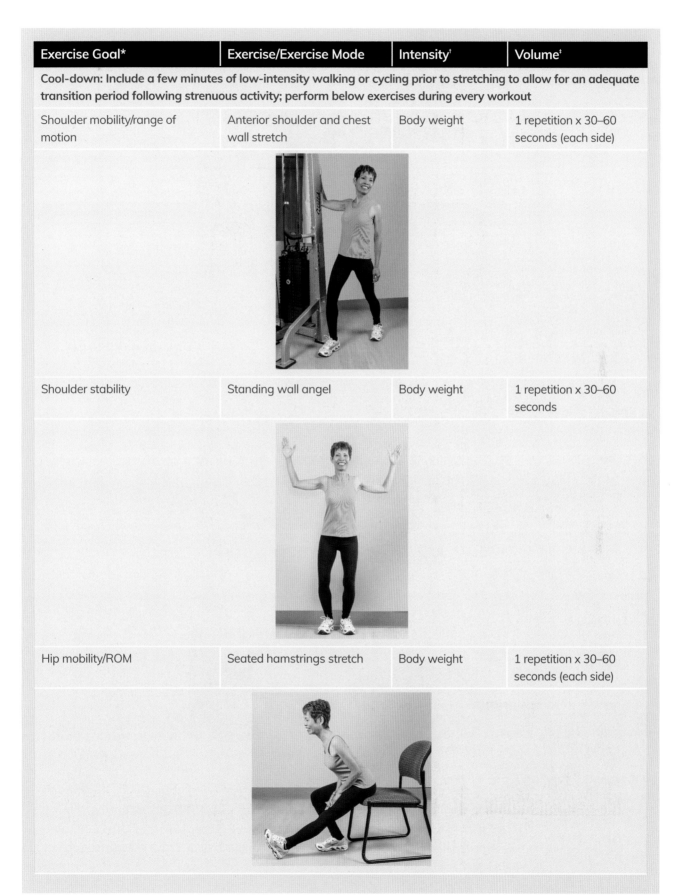

Continued on the next page

Exercise Goal*	Exercise/Exercise Mode	Intensity†	Volume‡
Hip mobility/range of motion	Seated 90-90° stretch	Body weight	1 repetition x 30–60 seconds (each side)

Spinal mobility	Overhead dowel side bend	Dowel	1 repetition x 30–60 seconds (each side)

Spinal mobility	Extended child's pose with lateral flexion	Body weight	1 repetition x 30–60 seconds (each side)

* = Movement pattern, technique, skill, recovery, etc.

† = Weight, load, speed, zone, etc.

‡ = Sets, repetitions, duration, rest, etc.

Programming Notes:

Note: VT1 = First ventilatory threshold; VT2 = Second ventilatory threshold; ROM = Range of motion

Exercise Guidelines for Improving Muscular Strength

Muscular strength is a measure of the maximal force that can be produced by one or more muscle groups and is typically assessed by the 1-RM load of an exercise (e.g., leg press or bench press). Although increases in muscular strength are accompanied by increases in muscular endurance, preferred protocols for strength development place more emphasis on training intensity or load.

FREQUENCY

Older adults should perform muscle-strengthening activities for all major muscle groups on at least two days per week (Fragala et al., 2019; ACSM, 2018; U.S. Department of Health & Human Services, 2018). Consequently, clients who complete total-body workouts that target all major muscle groups should schedule two training sessions per week. Clients who prefer to perform split routines (working different muscle groups or movement patterns on different days) should take at least 72 hours between workouts for the same muscles. For example, clients who do pushing movements for the chest, shoulders, and triceps on Mondays and Thursdays, pulling movements for the upper back and biceps on Tuesdays and Fridays, and squat, lunge, and rotational movements for the legs and trunk on Wednesdays and Saturdays perform six weekly workouts, but experience at least 72 hours of recovery time between exercises for the same muscle groups.

INTENSITY

Older adults may benefit from both increased muscular strength and increased muscular power. Initial stages of muscular training may be successfully conducted with a range of loads from light intensity (e.g., 40 to 50% of 1-RM) and gradually progress to moderate-to-vigorous intensity (80 to 85% of 1-RM). However, for optimal strength development, loads between 70 and 85% of 1-RM are required. To optimize muscular power, exercise should be performed at higher velocities during the concentric phase with moderate intensities of 40 to 60% of 1-RM. Another consideration when it comes to intensity is that similar functional and neuromuscular adaptations may be achieved at low, moderate, and high intensities if explosive training is used (Fragala et al., 2019), as there is an inverse relationship between the speed of a movement and load, which gives exercise professionals another variable to consider when designing an effective exercise program. Concurrent training, or the combining of endurance, power, and strength training, may be the most effective strategy for counteracting declines in strength, neuromuscular function, muscle mass, **functional capacity,** and cardiorespiratory fitness in older adults (Fragala et al., 2019). It is also important to keep in mind that intensity ranges may ultimately be determined by client comfort, and an individualized intensity range that minimizes joint stress should be utilized.

REPETITIONS

The number of repetitions performed is influenced by the amount of resistance, and a lower number of repetitions performed at a higher training intensity may lead to greater strength gains. Research suggests that exercise with relatively high loads performed for seven to nine repetitions is associated with the greatest effects on muscle strength and morphology. However, an overall repetition range of six to 12 represents the ideal for optimal strength and muscle size gains (Fragala et al., 2019). It is also recommended that older adults new to Muscular Training and those with frailty or other special considerations (e.g., osteoporosis and **cardiovascular disease**) use relatively lighter weight to perform 8 to 15 repetitions per set, beginning at a resistance that is well tolerated and using progressively heavier loads to decrease the number of repetitions completed. Consideration should also be given to research suggesting that performing repetitions to failure is not associated with increased physiological and neuromuscular adaptations. In addition, avoiding sets performed to concentric failure optimizes power output and prevents muscular fatigue. Ultimately, Muscular Training programs should be individualized to older adults' tolerance and ability levels, especially in the presence of osteoporosis, arthritis, and pain.

⚙ EXPAND YOUR KNOWLEDGE

Should Older Adults Lifts Heavy Weights?

In Chapter 3, the concept of the physical-function continuum for older adults was presented (see Figure 3-1, page 70). The continuum illustrates the various segments of physical function among seniors, with physically elite older adults making up the smallest percentage (i.e., 5%). These highly fit seniors require exercise programming that helps them maintain their fitness levels and provides conditioning for improved performance in competition or in strenuous vocational or recreational activities. Programming should include conditioning for muscular strength and endurance, flexibility, agility, and cardiovascular endurance. It also may include sport- or activity-specific training.

Although physically elite seniors are a small group in relation to others along the continuum, exercise professionals should be aware that older clients in this category can tolerate vigorous exercise programming and, in fact, need to perform strenuous activity in order to maintain their current levels of fitness or reach performance-related goals. Thus, while it may be uncommon to see older adults perform heavy resistance-training programs (e.g., those with loads corresponding to 80 to 90% of 1-RM for four to eight repetitions per set), exercise professionals should not assume that all clients over 50 years of age should avoid this activity. As such, supplying physically elite seniors with information concerning the adverse effects of overtraining and the need for appropriate recovery periods between workouts will give them the tools to prevent injury while training and competing.

SETS

Research and guidelines suggest that muscular training is effective for older adults when performed as either single- or multiple-set training for each major muscle group, with multiple sets potentially being more effective (Fragala et al., 2019; ACSM, 2018; U.S. Department of Health & Human Services, 2018). It may be prudent to start older adults who are new to muscular training and those with frailty with one challenging set of each exercise (after performing progressively challenging warm-up sets) and increase the number of stimulus sets in accordance with clients' interests and abilities. Generally, muscular-strength programs do not exceed three to four sets for each training exercise. To perform repeated exercise sets with relatively heavy loads, clients may need longer recovery periods between successive sets. Unlike muscular-endurance training, which features rest periods of 30 seconds or less between sets, muscular-strength training generally features two- to five-minute recovery periods between sets of the same exercise. The longer rests lead to longer workouts for muscular-strength training programs. The many variables discussed in this section can be adjusted to meet the time constraints of the client. Additionally, sessions lasting 30 minutes or more have been associated with less difficulty performing ADL (Fragala et al., 2019).

Fortunately, single-set training programs can effectively increase muscular strength in much shorter exercise sessions. For example, a single set of 10 exercises would require about 20 to 30 minutes for completion, and the inclusion of a warm-up set for each exercise would make the workout about 45 minutes in duration on the high end.

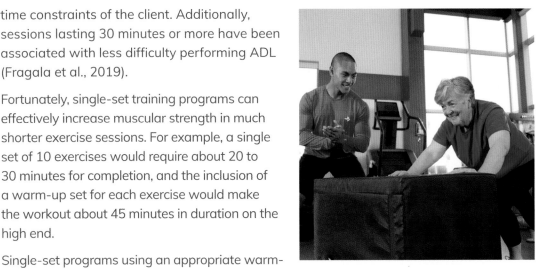

Single-set programs using an appropriate warm-up and a challenging training intensity are effective for helping most older adults clients achieve muscular-training improvements and maintain adherence to their programs when they have other demands for their time.

TYPE

Strength training may be performed with many types of resistance equipment, should be progressive in nature, can include weight-bearing calisthenics, and may include activities such as stair climbing. Generally, a combination of multijoint exercises targeting all major muscle groups (i.e., legs, hips, chest, back, abdomen, shoulders, and arms) utilized in the basic movements of daily living are the preferred method for increasing total-body strength. These exercises include the following patterns:

- *Bend-and-lift:* Squats, deadlifts, and leg presses
- *Single-leg:* Step-ups and lunges
- *Push:* Bench presses, incline presses, overhead presses, and bar dips
- *Pull:* Seated rows, lat pull-downs, and pull-ups
- *Rotate:* Wood chops and hay balers

Exercises that isolate specific muscle groups (e.g., leg extensions, leg curls, hip adductions, hip abductions, lateral raises, chest crosses, pull-overs, arm extensions, arm curls, trunk extensions, and trunk curls) can be included in strength-training workouts (especially for older adults who have strength deficits in specific areas), but these typically play a lesser role than the movement-based exercises that challenge multiple muscle groups at the same time while moving in a variety of planes of motion. Older adults with frailty, beginners, and those with functional limitations may benefit from isometric training or using resistance bands and selectorized weight or pneumatic exercise equipment, while others may achieve additional benefits from using free weights such as dumbbells, barbells, medicine balls, and kettlebells (Fragala et al., 2019). When appropriate, older adults may also benefit from the inclusion of variations to the BOS or body position during multijoint, complex, and dynamic functional movements. As described earlier in the chapter, exercises that mimic the five primary movement patterns should be included in any exercise program to promote optimal performance of ADL.

📖 APPLY WHAT YOU KNOW

Strength Training for Older Adults

The following exercise examples provide ideas for how to design a strength-training program for older adults (Figures 8-41 through 8-52). Refer to Figures 8-38 and 8-39 for rotational exercises. Notice that each figure presents an exercise that incorporates one or more of the five primary movement patterns, as strength can be developed by adding appropriate, progressive load to movements introduced in the Movement Training phase. For each exercise, an example of a foundational starting point is offered, followed by a sample progression. That is, the foundational exercise offers less of a stability and mobility challenge and could be considered part of a program for an older adult who is deconditioned and new to exercise, or who experiences balance problems and is therefore at a higher risk for falling. The sample progression exercise represents an option for the same muscle groups that is more appropriate for seniors who are competent in Functional and Movement Training and are ready to challenge their strength limits by lifting weights in a manner that requires whole-body stability and appropriate mobility.

FIGURE 8-41
Bend-and-lift: Squat

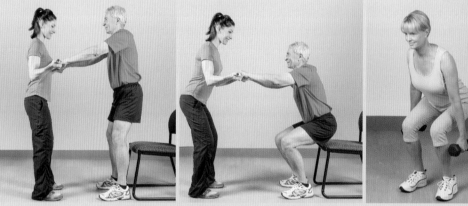
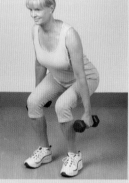

Foundational movement   Progression

FIGURE 8-42
Bend-and-lift: Deadlift

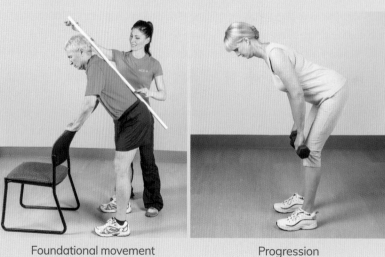

Foundational movement   Progression

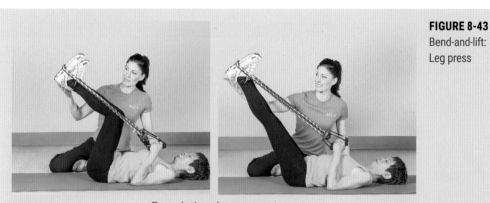

FIGURE 8-43
Bend-and-lift:
Leg press

Foundational movement

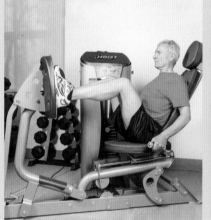

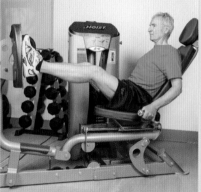

Progression

FIGURE 8-44
Single-leg: Step-up

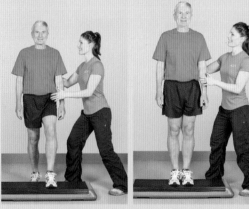

Foundational movement

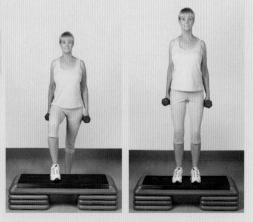

Progression

FIGURE 8-45
Single-leg: Lunge

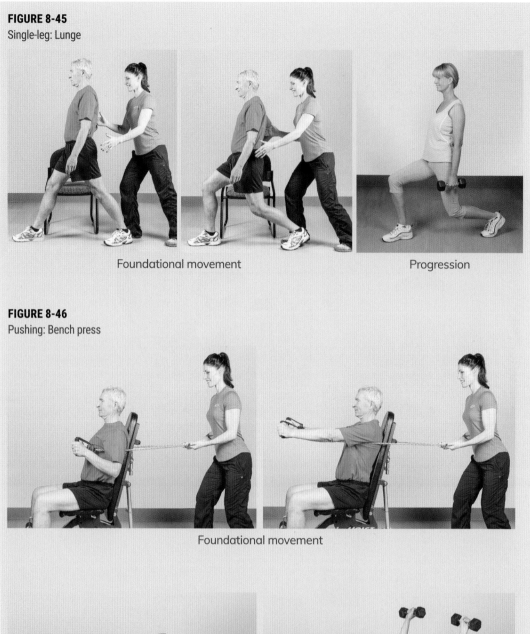

Foundational movement   Progression

FIGURE 8-46
Pushing: Bench press

Foundational movement

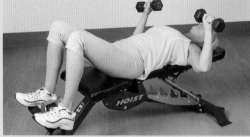 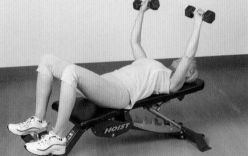

Progression

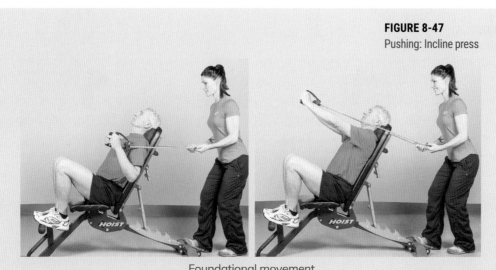

FIGURE 8-47
Pushing: Incline press

Foundational movement

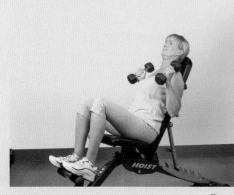

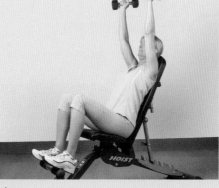

Progression

FIGURE 8-48
Pushing: Shoulder press

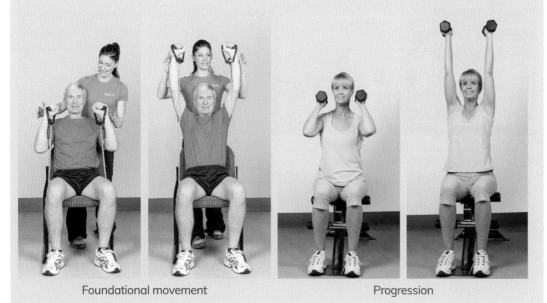

Foundational movement

Progression

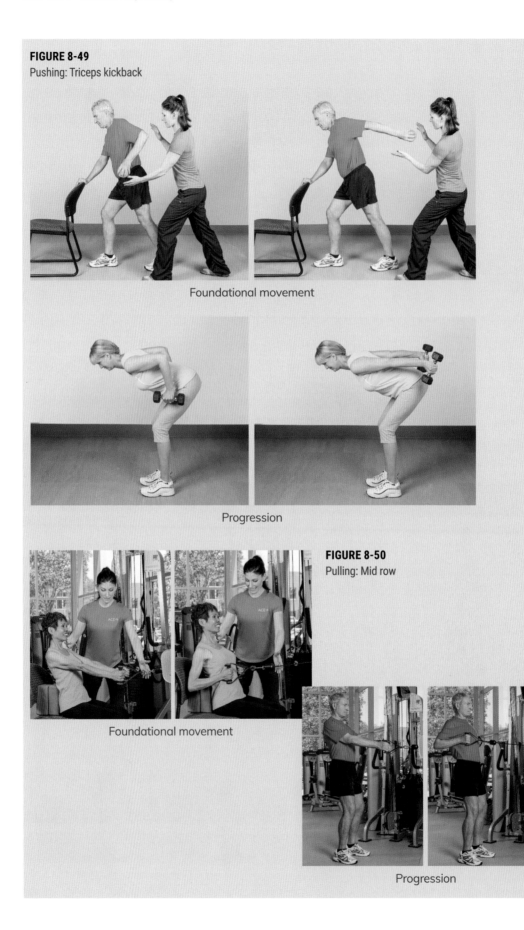

FIGURE 8-49
Pushing: Triceps kickback

Foundational movement

Progression

Foundational movement

FIGURE 8-50
Pulling: Mid row

Progression

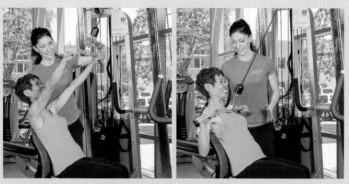

FIGURE 8-51
Pulling: Lat pull-down

Foundational movement

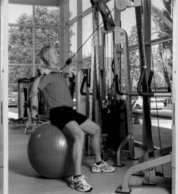

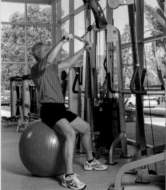

Progression

FIGURE 8-52
Pulling: Pull-up

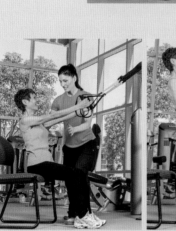

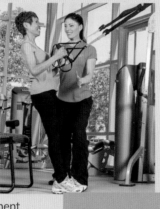

Foundational movement

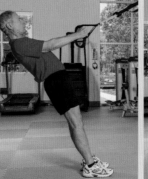

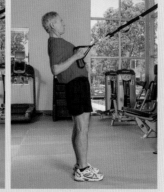

Progression

Appropriate Rates of Progression in Strength Training

The recommended method for improving muscular strength is the double-progressive training protocol. There are numerous factors that affect the rate of strength development, and progress varies considerably among individuals. Consequently, it is not practical to suggest weekly load increases, as some clients will progress more quickly and others will progress more slowly than the recommended resistance increments. To facilitate individual stimulus–response relationships and to reduce the risk of doing too much too soon, exercise professionals should factor both repetitions and resistance into the training progression.

First, the client's repetition range, such as six to 12 repetitions per set, must be established. Second, the client can continue training with the same exercise resistance until the terminal number of repetitions (e.g., up to 12) can be completed with proper technique. When this is accomplished, the exercise professional should increase the resistance by approximately 5%, which will reduce the number of repetitions the client can perform. The client should then continue with this resistance until they can again perform the terminal number of repetitions, at which point resistance can increase.

When progressing an exercise load, optimal recovery strategies and tolerance for the new load should be considered. In general, the progression in load for clients moves gradually from light intensity, where it is easier to learn and observe proper technique and movement patterns, to moderate and vigorous intensity and should be considered alongside other program progressions including increased sets, complexity of exercises, and type of equipment (Fragala et al., 2019). For more detailed explanations of exercises and programming guidelines for Load/Speed Training, as well as information on various methods for progressing Muscular Training programs through **periodization,** refer to *The Exercise Professional's Guide to Personal Training* (ACE, 2020).

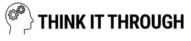 **THINK IT THROUGH**

Delayed-onset Muscle Soreness

Resistance training often results in **delayed-onset muscle soreness (DOMS),** which is soreness that typically occurs 24 to 48 hours after strenuous exercise. Senior clients who experience DOMS might interpret the discomfort as a sign of injury. How will you describe to your older clientele the differences between a **strain** or **sprain** injury versus DOMS? What approaches will you take to ensure that your senior clients are progressed appropriately in their strength-training programs so that the risk of overtraining is minimized?

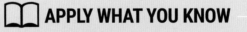 **APPLY WHAT YOU KNOW**

Training for Athletic Performance in the Load/Speed Phase

As noted earlier, only 5% of older adults make up the fit/elite population on the physical-function continuum, but exercise professionals should be prepared to work with these clients. For older clientele, the term athletic performance can take on two different meanings. In the traditional sense, performance goals are targeted by athletically oriented clients who want to progress in preparation for a specific athletic event or competition. In this instance, Load/Speed Training would progress to enhancing athletic skills for sports through the application of power exercises that emphasize the speed of force production, and the performance of specific drills that improve speed, agility, and quickness. Clients who progress to this level of training should have successfully completed both the Functional and Movement Training phases. They should demonstrate good postural stability, kinetic chain mobility, proper movement patterns, and relatively high levels of muscular strength to produce and control the forces needed for athletic performance training. To maintain the gains achieved during Functional and Movement Training, these exercises can be incorporated in dynamic warm-up activities prior to performing workouts to build speed, agility, quickness, and power.

The second meaning of athletic performance training, and the one that will apply to a large number of older clients, focuses on enhancing the skill-related components of fitness (e.g., power, speed, agility, and quickness) as they relate to performance of ADL. An effective way to promote these skills in older adults is to layer them into their existing exercise programs such that they perform a primary movement but modify them to introduce one or more of the skill-related components. For example, once a client has mastered the squat technique with load, they could perform body-weight squat jumps (Figure 8-53), or a variety of jumping

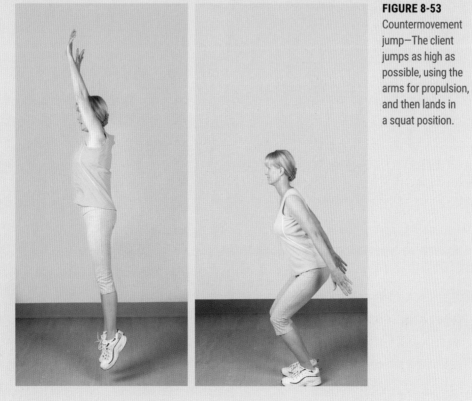

FIGURE 8-53
Countermovement jump—The client jumps as high as possible, using the arms for propulsion, and then lands in a squat position.

exercises (Figures 8-54 through 8-59), which introduce power and reactivity. Another example includes encouraging a client who has mastered weighted lunges to perform them more quickly using only body weight or to add small bounds from one foot to the other in various directions, introducing speed and agility, as well as a higher balance challenge, to a basic lunge (Figure 8-60). For more information on athletic performance training during the Load/Speed Training phase, refer to *The Exercise Professional's Guide to Personal Training* (ACE, 2020).

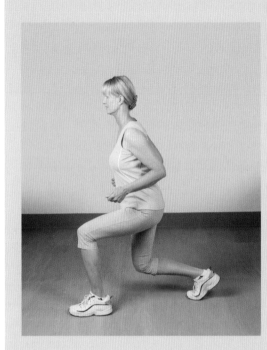

FIGURE 8-54
Stride jump—Starting from a front lunge position, the client drives the hips upward and lands with the opposite leg forward, again in a lunge position.

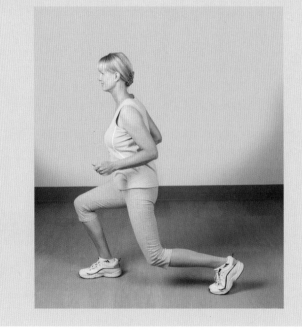

FIGURE 8-55

Split jump—Starting from a standing straddle position, the client jumps up, quickly brings the legs together, and lands in the same standing straddle position.

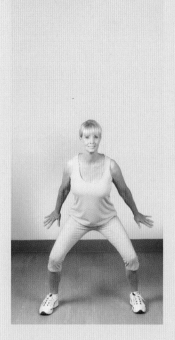 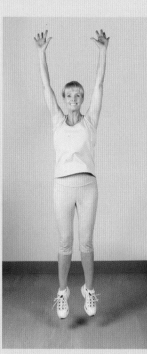 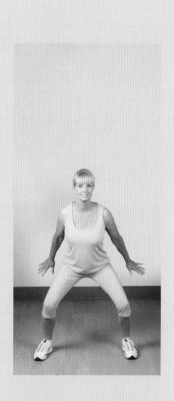

FIGURE 8-56

Double-leg butt kicks—From a standing position, the client jumps with both legs, kicks the buttocks, and lands on both feet, emphasizing maximal distance.

FIGURE 8-57

Ankle hops or hop progressions—The client performs basic, small, double-leg hops as quickly as possible.

FIGURE 8-58

Cone or hurdle hops—The client performs large, high, two-footed hops over barriers such as cones or low hurdles. The goal is to minimize the time spent on the ground.

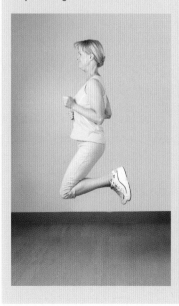 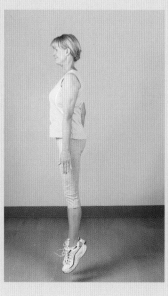 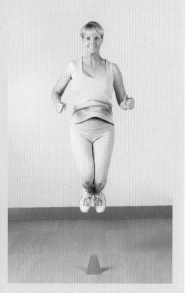

FIGURE 8-59

Box jump progression—Using several 4- to 8-inch steps (group fitness benches work well) spaced two to three feet apart, the client jumps onto and off of the succession of steps, spending as little time on the floor as possible. Pauses, if any, should be made on top of the bench rather than on the floor.

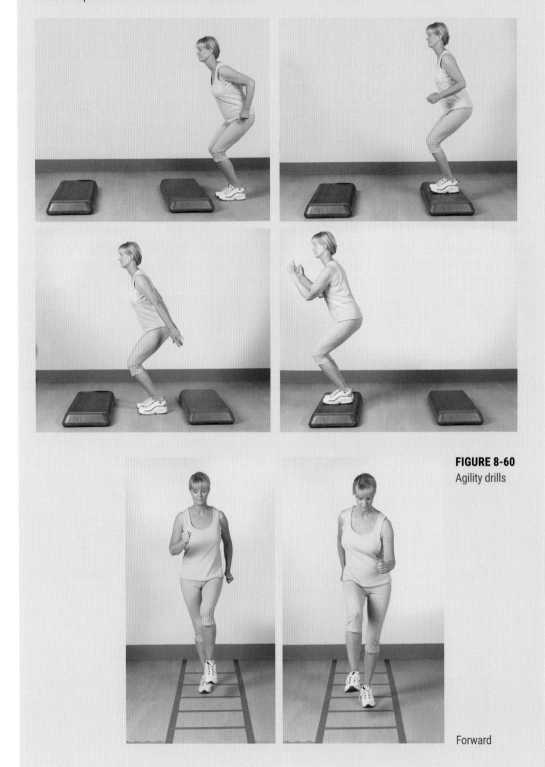

FIGURE 8-60
Agility drills

Forward

FIGURE 8-60 *(continued)*

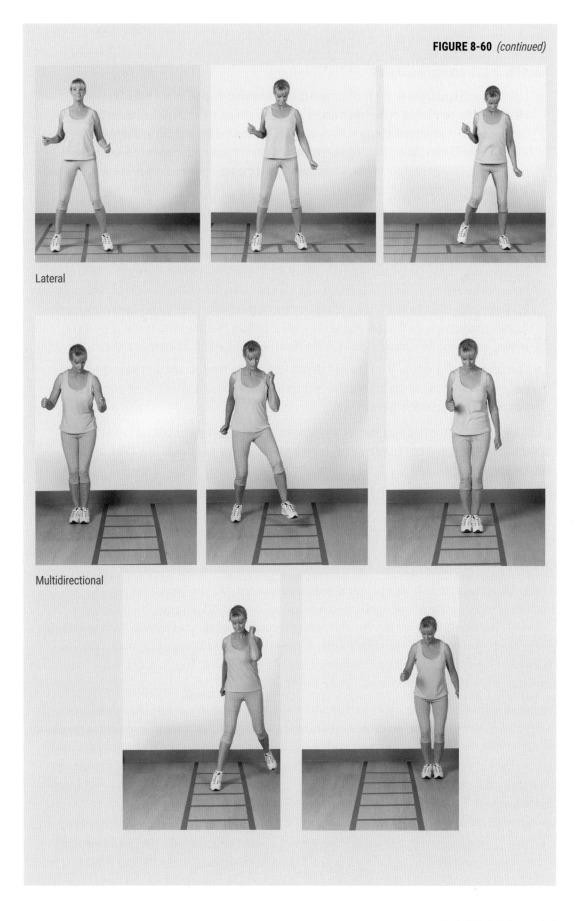

Lateral

Multidirectional

⋯ EXPAND YOUR KNOWLEDGE ⋯

Jumping and Hopping Techniques

▸ Clients should land softly on the midfoot, and then roll forward to push off the ball of the foot. Landing on the heel or ball of the foot must be avoided, as these errors increase impact forces. Landing on the midfoot also shortens the time between the eccentric and concentric actions (i.e., the **amortization phase**), thus increasing the potential for power development if another jump follows. Ensure alignment of the hips, knees, ankles, and toes due to the potential for injury, especially in women.

▸ Encourage clients to drop the hips to absorb the impact forces and develop gluteal dominance.

▸ Clients must avoid locking out the knees upon landing, which leads to the development of quadriceps dominance (see page 243). Poor landing technique can increase the risk of knee injuries. Proper hip mechanics during flexion and extension, along with the requisite muscular strength, is extremely important for developing lower-body power, which is why it is recommended that clients go through both the Functional and Movement Training phases before progressing to Load/Speed Training exercises. Instruct clients to engage the core musculature, which stiffens the torso, protects the spine during landing, and allows for increased force transfer during the subsequent concentric contraction (or jump).

▸ Clients should land with the trunk inclined slightly forward, the head up, and the torso rigid. Exercise professionals can cue clients to keep their "chests over their knees" and their "nose over their toes" during the landing phase of jumps.

CAUTION: THESE ACTIVITIES MAY NOT BE APPROPRIATE FOR THOSE WITH CERTAIN HEALTH CONDITIONS, INCLUDING OSTEOARTHRITIS, OSTEOPOROSIS, LOW-BACK DYSFUNCTION, AND FOOT NEUROPATHY.

Cardiorespiratory Training Based on the ACE IFT Model

Similar to the Muscular Training principles already discussed, the basic concept of cardiorespiratory program design is to create a routine with appropriate frequency, intensity, and duration to match the older client's current health and fitness, with adequate progressions to help the client safely achieve their goals. Choosing appropriate exercise modes is especially important for the senior population as well. The ACE IFT Model has three Cardiorespiratory Training phases (Figure 8-61).

Programming in each phase is based on the three-zone intensity model shown in Figure 8-62, using HR at the **first ventilatory threshold (VT1)** and the **second ventilatory threshold (VT2),** or more commonly in the older adult population the **talk test** or RPE (0 to 10 scale) to develop individualized programs based on each client's unique metabolic responses to exercise and perceived exertion (see Chapter 7). These markers provide a convenient way to divide intensity into training zones that are determined without any use of, or reference to, predicted or measured maximal heart rate (MHR):

▸ Zone 1 (Moderate intensity exercise) reflects heart rates below VT1 where clients can talk comfortably, but not sing, and rate their intensity at an RPE of 3 to 4 (0 to 10 scale).

ACE→ Integrated Fitness Training® Model

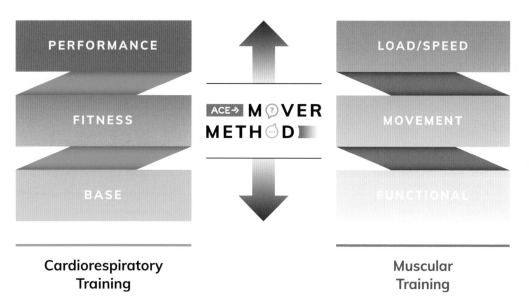

FIGURE 8-61
ACE IFT Model
Cardiorespiratory Training
phases

PERFORMANCE

FITNESS

BASE

ACE→ M?VER METH☺D▐

LOAD/SPEED

MOVEMENT

FUNCTIONAL

Cardiorespiratory Training

Muscular Training

▸ Zone 2 (Vigorous intensity exercise) reflects heart rates from VT1 to just below VT2 and clients are not sure if talking is comfortable and rate their intensity at an RPE of 5 to 6 (0 to 10 scale).

▸ Zone 3 (Near maximal/maximal intensity) reflects heart rates at and above VT2 and clients definitely cannot talk comfortably and rate their intensity at an RPE of 7 to 10 (0 to 10 scale).

Advanced age, along with taking certain medications, such as **beta blockers,** renders standard target **heart-rate reserve (HRR)** calculations inaccurate. Therefore, zone training is especially useful with these individuals.

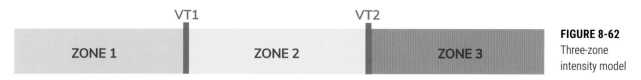

VT1   VT2

| ZONE 1 | ZONE 2 | ZONE 3 |

FIGURE 8-62
Three-zone
intensity model

Note: VT1 = First ventilatory threshold; VT2 = Second ventilatory threshold

Stated simply, if a client can talk comfortably, they are training in zone 1. If the client is not sure they can talk comfortably, they are working in zone 2. If the client definitely cannot talk comfortably while training, they are working in zone 3.

It is important to note that training principles in the ACE IFT Model's Cardiorespiratory Training phases can be implemented using various exercise intensity markers, including ones based on predicted values such as a percentage of HRR (%HRR) or a percentage of MHR (%MHR), but these measures of exercise intensity may not be as accurate for most older adult clients as actual measures of VT1 and VT2 (Table 8-11). It is for this reason that exercise intensity is most appropriately based on the ability to talk comfortably and the client's RPE.

TABLE 8-11

Three-zone Intensity Model Using Various Intensity Markers

Intensity Markers		Zone 1	Zone 2	Zone 3	Advantages/Limitations
Category terminology for exercise programming	Light	Moderate	Vigorous	Near maximal/ maximal	
Metabolic markers: VT1 and VT2* (HR relative to VT1 and VT2)*		Below VT1 (HR <VT1)	VT1 to just below VT2 (HR ≥VT1 to <VT2)	VT2 and above (HR ≥VT2)	▸ Based on measured VT1 and VT2 ▸ Ideally, VT1 and VT2 are measured in a lab with a metabolic cart and blood lactate ▸ Field assessments are relatively easy to administer, require minimal equipment, and provide accurate corresponding HRs at VT1 and VT2 ▸ Programming with metabolic markers allows for personalized programming
Talk test*		Can talk comfortably Can talk but not sing	Not sure if talking is comfortable Cannot say more than a few words without pausing for a breath	Definitely cannot talk comfortably	▸ Based on actual changes in ventilation due to physiological adaptations to increasing exercise intensities ▸ Very easy for practical measurement ▸ No equipment required ▸ Can easily be taught to clients ▸ Allows for personalized programming
RPE (terminology)*	Very, very weak to light	"Moderate" to "somewhat hard/strong"	"Hard/strong" to "very hard"	"Very strong to very, very hard/strong to maximal"	▸ Good subjective intensity marker ▸ Correlates well with talk test, metabolic markers, and measured %$\dot{V}O_2$max ▸ Easy to teach to clients
RPE (0 to 10 scale)*	0.5 to 2	3 to 4	5 to 6	7 to 10	▸ Good subjective intensity marker ▸ Correlates well with talk test, metabolic markers, and measured %$\dot{V}O_2$max ▸ 0 to 10 scale is easy to teach to clients
RPE (6 to 20 scale)	9 to 11	12 to 13	14 to 17	≥18	▸ Good subjective intensity marker ▸ Correlates well with talk test, metabolic markers, and measured %$\dot{V}O_2$max ▸ 6 to 20 scale is not as easy to teach to clients as the 0 to 10 scale ▸ Note: An RPE of 20 represents maximal effort and cannot be sustained as a training intensity.
%$\dot{V}O_2$R	30 to 39%	40 to 59%	60 to 89%	≥90%	▸ Requires measured $\dot{V}O_2$max for most accurate programming ▸ Impractical due to expensive equipment needed for assessment ▸ Increased error with use of predicted $\dot{V}O_2$max or predicted MHR ▸ Relative percentages for programming are population-based and not individually specific

TABLE 8-11 *(continued)*

Intensity Markers		Zone 1	Zone 2	Zone 3	Advantages/Limitations
%HRR	30 to 39%	40 to 59%	60 to 89%	≥90%	▸ Requires measured MHR and RHR for most accurate programming ▸ Measured MHR is impractical for the vast majority of trainers and clients ▸ Use of RHR increases individuality of programming vs. strict %MHR ▸ Use of predicted MHR introduces potentially large error; the magnitude of the error is dependent on the specific equation used ▸ Relative percentages for programming are population-based and not individually specific
%MHR	57 to 63%	64 to 76%	77 to 95%	≥96%	▸ Requires measured MHR for accuracy in programming ▸ Measured MHR is impractical for the vast majority of trainers and clients ▸ Use of predicted MHR introduces potentially large error; the magnitude of the error is dependent on the specific equation used ▸ Does not include RHR, as is used in %HRR ▸ Relative percentages for programming are population-based and not individually specific
METs	2 to 2.9	3 to 5.9	6 to 8.7	≥8.8	▸ Requires measured $\dot{V}O_2$max for most accurate programming ▸ Can use in programming more easily than other intensity markers based off $\dot{V}O_2$max ▸ Limited in programming by knowledge of METs for given activities and/or equipment that gives MET estimates ▸ Relative MET ranges for programming are population-based and not individually specific (e.g., a 5-MET activity might initially be perceived as vigorous by a previously sedentary client)
%$\dot{V}O_2$max	37 to 45%	46 to 63%	64 to 90%	≥91%	▸ Refer to %$\dot{V}O_2$R ▸ Actual measurement is individualized and not based on a prediction

Note: VT1 = First ventilatory threshold; VT2 = Second ventilatory threshold; HR = Heart rate; RPE = Rating of perceived exertion; $\dot{V}O_2$max = Maximal oxygen uptake; $\dot{V}O_2$R = Oxygen uptake reserve; HRR = Heart-rate reserve; MHR = Maximal heart rate; RHR = Resting heart rate; METs = Metabolic equivalents

*These are the preferred intensity markers to use with the three zone-intensity model when designing, implementing, and progressing cardiorespiratory training programs using the ACE Integrated Fitness Training Model.

Table 8-12 provides an overview of the Cardiorespiratory Training phases of the ACE IFT Model. This is followed by detailed descriptions that explain the training focus of each stage and strategies for implementing and progressing exercise programs to help clients reach their goals within each phase. It is important to note that not every client will start in Base Training, as some clients will already be regularly participating in cardiorespiratory exercise, and only clients with very specific performance or speed goals will move into Performance Training. In addition, no cardiorespiratory assessments are recommended for beginning in Base Training. VT1 and VT2 heart rates can be assessed using the submaximal talk test for VT1 (see page 229) prior to engaging in Fitness Training, whereas the VT2 threshold test (see page 231) can be used before moving on to Performance Training. However, determining these heart rates is not a requirement for programming cardiorespiratory exercise for older adults, as there are other ways to monitor intensity. The talk test and RPE, for example, may be used to gauge intensity. In Table 8-11, an RPE of 5 to 6 is equivalent to zone 2 training, so if the exercise plan included zone 2 intervals the client would need to achieve an RPE of 5 or 6 for the work portion of the interval. The same idea can be applied using the talk test such that clients should achieve an intensity that does not allow them to speak comfortably during zone 2 training.

TABLE 8-12

Cardiorespiratory Training

Base Training	▸ Focus on moderate-intensity cardiorespiratory exercise (RPE = 3 to 4), while keeping an emphasis on enjoyment. ▸ Keep intensities below the talk-test threshold (below VT1). ▸ Increase duration and frequency of exercise bouts. ▸ Progress to Fitness Training when the client can complete at least 20 minutes of cardiorespiratory exercise below the talk test threshold at least three times per week.
Fitness Training	▸ Progress cardiorespiratory exercise duration and frequency based on the client's goals and available time. ▸ Integrate vigorous-intensity (RPE = 5 to 6) cardiorespiratory exercise intervals with segments performed at intensities below, at, and above VT1 to just below VT2.
Performance Training	▸ Progress moderate- and vigorous-intensity cardiorespiratory exercise. ▸ Program sufficient volume for the client to achieve goals. ▸ Integrate near-maximal and maximal intensity (RPE = 7 to 10) intervals performed at and above VT2 to increase aerobic capacity, speed, and performance. ▸ Periodized training plans can be used to incorporate adequate training time below VT1, from VT1 to just below VT2, and at or above VT2.

Note: RPE = Rating of perceived exertion (0 to 10 scale); VT1 = First ventilatory threshold; VT2 = Second ventilatory threshold

BASE TRAINING

Base Training has a principal focus of getting older clients who are either physically inactive or have little cardiorespiratory fitness to begin engaging in regular cardiorespiratory exercise of low-to-moderate intensity with a primary goal of improving health and a secondary goal of building fitness. These clients may have long-term goals for fitness and possibly even sports performance, but they need to progress through Base Training first. The primary goal for the exercise professional during this phase should be to help the client have positive experiences with cardiorespiratory exercise and to empower them to adopt exercise as a regular habit. The intent of this phase is to develop a stable cardiorespiratory base upon which the client can achieve improvements in health, endurance, energy, mood, and caloric expenditure.

Once regularity of exercise habits is established, the duration of exercise is extended until the individual can perform 20 to 30 continuous minutes of cardiorespiratory exercise at least three days per week with little residual fatigue, at which point they can progress to Fitness Training. This approach to training ensures the safety of exercise, while at the same time promotes some of the potential physiologic adaptations and most of the health benefits. Within this general design is recognition that the benefit-to-risk ratio of moderate-intensity zone 1 training is very high for the beginning exerciser, with the possibility for very large gains in health and basic fitness and almost no risk of either cardiovascular or musculoskeletal injury. As the exerciser develops more ambitious goals, more demanding training (either longer or more intense) can be performed.

The primary goal of this phase is to help clients have positive experiences with exercise to facilitate program adherence and success. Cardiorespiratory fitness assessments are not necessary at the beginning of this phase, as they will only confirm low levels of fitness and potentially serve as negative reminders about why the physically inactive client with low levels of fitness may not have good self-efficacy regarding exercise. All cardiorespiratory exercise during this phase falls within zone 1 (below VT1), so the exercise professional can use the client's ability to talk comfortably as the upper exercise-intensity limit. The exercise professional can also teach the client to use the 0 to 10 category ratio scale, with the client exercising at an RPE of 3 to 4 (moderate to somewhat strong) (Figure 8-63).

As a general principle, exercise programs designed to improve the cardiorespiratory base begin with zone 1–intensity exercise below VT1 (RPE 3 to 4) performed for as little as 10 to 15 minutes two to three times each week. However, this should be progressed as rapidly as tolerated to 20 minutes or more at moderate intensity (zone 1; below the talk test threshold), performed three to five times each week. Changes in duration from one week to the next should not exceed a 10% increase versus the week prior. Once this level of exercise can be sustained on a regular basis, the primary adaptation of establishing a cardiorespiratory base will be complete. For additional detailed explanations of exercises and programming guidelines for Base Training, refer to *The Exercise Professional's Guide to Personal Training* (ACE, 2020).

FIGURE 8-63
Rating of perceived exertion: Category ratio scale

| 0 Nothing at all |
| 0.5 Very, very weak |
| 1 Very weak |
| 2 Weak |
| 3 Moderate |
| 4 Somewhat strong |— VT1 |
| 5 Strong |
| 6 |— VT2 |
| 7 Very strong |
| 8 |
| 9 |
| 10 Very, very strong |

Note: VT1 = First ventilatory threshold; VT2 = Second ventilatory threshold

FITNESS TRAINING

Fitness Training has a principal training focus of increasing the duration of cardiorespiratory exercise, increasing session frequency, and introducing higher-intensity intervals to improve fitness and health. However, it is important to understand that after a cardiorespiratory base has been achieved, additional gains in fitness will become progressively smaller, or require disproportionately large increases in training intensity, frequency, or duration. At this time, the exercise professional should collaborate with the client to adjust, reaffirm, or set new goals.

Fitness Training is the primary Cardiorespiratory Training phase for regular exercisers in a fitness facility who have goals for improving or maintaining fitness and/or health. Fitness

Training includes increasing the workload by modifying frequency, duration, and intensity. Intervals are introduced that push into zone 2 (e.g., vigorous intensity, RPE 5 to 6, and cannot say more than a few words without pausing for a breath) and eventually approach zone 3 intensities. The zone 2 intervals in this phase provide a stimulus that will eventually increase the exertion levels required to reach the **ventilatory threshold,** resulting in the client being able to exercise at a lower RPE for the same activity.

Clients performing Fitness Training who have a goal to complete an event, such as a 10K run, can reach their goal of completing the event within the training guidelines of this phase. Once a client begins working toward multiple endurance goals, trains to improve their competitive speed, or simply wants to take on the challenge of training like an athlete, the client should move on to Performance Training.

For the many clients who never develop competitive goals or the desire to train like an endurance athlete, training in Fitness Training will provide adequate challenges to help them improve and maintain cardiorespiratory fitness for life. The workouts in most nonathletically focused group exercise classes fall into this phase. Fitness Training covers the principles for building cardiorespiratory efficiency that are important for most clients and fitness enthusiasts.

When embarking on Fitness Training, the exercise professional should ensure that the client is skilled at identifying the point at which talking becomes uncomfortable and which intensity is associated with an RPE of 5 to 6, as these markers will be utilized for programming. Effort will need to be reassessed periodically as fitness improves to see if greater intensities can be reached before an RPE of 5 or 6 is achieved or talking becomes uncomfortable, and training intensities may need to be adjusted.

This phase of Cardiorespiratory Training is dedicated to enhancing the client's cardiorespiratory efficiency by progressing the program through increased duration of sessions, increased frequency of sessions when possible, and the introduction of zone 2 intervals. In the Fitness Training phase, the warm-up, cool-down, recovery intervals, and

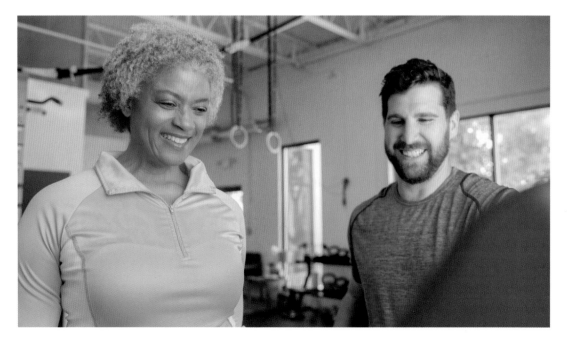

steady-state cardiorespiratory exercise segments are performed just below the VT1 at an RPE of 3 to 4 (0 to 10 scale) to continue advancing the client's cardiorespiratory base. Intervals are introduced at a level that is at or just above VT1, or an RPE of 5 to 6 (0 to 10 scale). The goal of these intervals is to improve cardiorespiratory efficiency by raising the intensity of exercise performed at VT1, improve the client's ability to utilize fat as a fuel source at intensities just below VT1, improve exercise efficiency at VT1, and add variety to the exercise program.

As a general principle, intervals should start out relatively brief (initially about 30 seconds), with an approximate hard-to-easy ratio of 1:3 (e.g., a 60-second work interval followed by a 180-second recovery interval), eventually progressing to a ratio of 1:2 and then 1:1. The duration of these intervals can be increased in regular increments, depending on the goals of the exerciser, but should be increased cautiously over several weeks depending on the client's fitness level.

Low zone 2 intervals should first be progressed by increasing the time of each interval and then moving to a 1:1 work-to-recovery (hard-to-easy) interval ratio. As the client progresses, intervals can progress into the upper end of zone 2 (RPE of 6) at a 1:3 work-to-recovery ratio, progressing first to longer intervals and then eventually moving to intervals with a 1:1 work-to-recovery ratio. Well-trained and motivated nonathletes can progress to where they are performing as much as 50% of their cardiorespiratory training in zone 2, while those with endurance performance-oriented goals will typically progress to Performance Training. For additional detailed explanations of exercises and programming guidelines for Fitness Training, refer to *The Exercise Professional's Guide to Personal Training* (ACE, 2020).

PERFORMANCE TRAINING

Performance Training is designed for clients who want to advance their endurance performance. Performance Training is appropriate for clients focused on achieving success in endurance sports and events such as setting a personal record, qualifying for a national event, or finishing top-five at a state or national championship. Training programs in this phase will progress beyond the parameters of fitness to target performance through increased speed, power, and endurance. Performance Training requires an appropriate training volume to initially prepare clients to comfortably complete events and eventually progress to intensity levels adequate to achieve success in goals that go far beyond simply finishing an event. However, clients do not need to be highly competitive athletes to move into Performance Training. They need only to be motivated, have one or more endurance-performance goals requiring specialized training, and the requisite cardiorespiratory efficiency from Fitness Training upon which to build.

In older clients who are already routinely exercising and who desire to move toward their optimal biological potential, most training (approximately 80%) should be performed at intensities where speech is comfortable (zone 1), and about 10% of training should be performed at intensities at and above VT2 (zone 3), where the physiological provocation to make large gains is present. As a client's total weekly training time increases, a greater percentage of their training time will typically be at moderate intensities to accommodate the increased training volume and to allow for recovery from higher-intensity interval-training sessions. Periodized training plans can be utilized to adjust the daily training focus between distance, speed, power, and recovery to help clients reach their unique performance goals.

With the increase in training load during Performance Training, consideration must also be given to the amount of recovery time between training sessions. Where a regular recreational exerciser in the Base Training phase can safely and comfortably perform essentially the same training bout every day, a competitive-level exerciser will need to use a periodized approach to training. Otherwise, they will be at risk for problems related to accumulating fatigue and loss of training benefit from the inability to maintain high-intensity training. In any case, even in the most seriously trained athlete, it is generally not productive to perform more than three to four workouts with zone 2 or 3 intervals during weeks where the goal is to increase the load.

Program design during this phase should be focused on helping the client enhance their cardiorespiratory efficiency to ensure completion of goal events, while building **anaerobic capacity** to achieve endurance-performance goals. Improved anaerobic capacity will help the client perform physical work at or near VT2 for an extended period, which will result in improved endurance, speed, and power to meet primary performance goals. Detailed information on VT2 threshold testing administration and program design based on VT2 assessment results can be found in Chapter 7.

If the client begins showing signs of overtraining (e.g., increased resting heart rate, disturbed sleep, decreased physical performance, reduced enthusiasm, or altered appetite on multiple days), the exercise professional should decrease the frequency and/or intensity of the client's intervals and provide more time for recovery. Also, if the client cannot reach the desired intensity during an interval, or is unable to reach the desired recovery intensity or HR during the recovery interval, the interval session should be stopped and the client should recover with cardiorespiratory exercise at an RPE of 3, and no more than 4, to prevent overtraining.

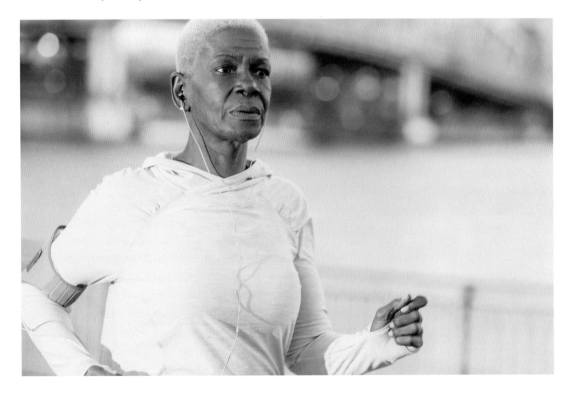

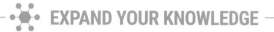

EXPAND YOUR KNOWLEDGE

High-intensity Interval Training and Older Adults

ACSM ranked **high-intensity interval training (HIIT)** as number two in its list of the top 10 worldwide fitness trends for 2020 (Thompson, 2019), which means that this form of exercise may be a topic of interest. By now, exercise professionals may be aware of the benefits of HIIT, but is this training method beneficial when appropriately used with an older adult population?

Research suggests that the degree of intensity during exercise is the variable most associated with health-related benefits such as cardiorespiratory fitness, which is a strong predictor of **morbidity** and premature mortality. Studies indicate few adverse events with brief higher intensity intervals, sprints, and resistance training, and show promising results for improved fitness, all components of **metabolic syndrome,** body composition, mitochondrial function, cardiometabolic health, and cognitive function and may delay the onset of morbidity and mortality (Winett & Ogletree, 2019). Also, performing high-intensity exercise does not have a compensatory effect on daily energy expenditure and total daily physical activity in older adults (Bruseghini et al., 2020). Bruseghini et al. (2020) observed that during eight weeks of HIIT, no negative significant changes in lifestyle habits occurred in older adults, including sleep and sedentary time, with levels of light physical activity remaining the same on training days. Another study conducted by the Mayo Clinic looked to observe improved metabolic and physical adaptations in young and older persons with different modes of training. The results of this study indicate that HIIT and resistance training performed for 12 weeks enhances **insulin sensitivity** and lean mass, while HIIT and combined training with HIIT and resistance training also may lead to improved muscular fitness and **aerobic capacity.** In addition, the group performing HIIT displayed a reversal of many age-related differences in expressed proteins at the cellular level that may protect the cells from aging (Robinson et al., 2017).

Even though there are many benefits to performing HIIT, this method of training may seem out of reach for many older clients, especially since walking is a preferred method for cardiorespiratory exercise. However, interval walking is a way to transform walking into a form of HIIT. Just like traditional HIIT, interval walking alternates between periods of low-intensity exercise and high-intensity exercise. This method of training, which may be a good introduction to higher-intensity training, decreases risk factors for lifestyle diseases and improves aerobic capacity and knee extension and flexion force production (Masuki, Morikawa, & Nose, 2017). These physiological benefits, combined with high adherence rates, make this form of walking effective for older adults.

SUMMARY

Like people of all ages, older adults benefit from comprehensive training that includes cardiorespiratory and muscular training. Exercise professionals can use the ACE IFT Model to program exercise selection, intensity, and duration to fit the needs and abilities of older clients. Although many older clients may never progress to training for power, speed, agility, and quickness, facilitating their efforts in these areas can have a significant impact on health and quality of life. It is important to note that client observation is especially vital when working with the senior exerciser. It is not uncommon for this population to have several health challenges that require a delicate balance of rest and activity. Therefore, the exercise professional should be prepared to adjust exercise programs accordingly. Helping older adults achieve enhanced health and fitness goals and maintain their functional independence is a worthwhile service that appropriately trained professionals can provide this unique population.

REFERENCES

American College of Sports Medicine (2018). *ACSM's Guidelines for Exercise Testing and Prescription* (10th ed.). Philadelphia: Wolters Kluwer.

American Council on Exercise (2020). *The Exercise Professional's Guide to Personal Training.* San Diego: American Council on Exercise.

Bruseghini, P. et al. (2020). High intensity interval training does not have compensatory effects on physical activity levels in older adults. *International Journal of Environmental Research and Public Health,* 17, 3, 1083.

Dunksy, A., Zeev, A, & Netz, Y. (2017). Balance performance is task specific in older adults. *BioMed Research International,* Article ID: 6987017.

Fragala, M.S. (2019). Resistance training for older adults: Position statement from the National Strength and Conditioning Association. *The Journal of Strength and Conditioning Research,* 33, 8, 2019–2052.

Landers, M.R. et al. (2016). Balance confidence and fear of falling avoidance behavior are most predictive of falling in older adults: Prospective analysis. *Physical Therapy,* 96, 4, 433–422.

Masuki, S., Morikawa, M., & Nose, H. (2017). Interval walking training can increase physical fitness in middle-aged and older people. *Exercise and Sport Science Reviews,* 45, 3, 154–162.

McGill, S.M. (2017). *Ultimate Back Fitness and Performance* (6th ed.). Ontario, Canada: Backfitpro Inc.

McGill, S.M. (2016). *Low Back Disorders: Evidence-Based Prevention and Rehabilitation* (3rd ed.). Champaign, Ill.: Human Kinetics.

Robinson, M.M. et al. (2017). Enhanced protein translation underlies improved metabolic and physical adaptations to different exercise training modes in young and old humans. *Cell Metabolism,* 25, 3, 581–592.

Thompson, W.R. (2019). Worldwide survey of fitness trends for 2020. ACSM's *Health & Fitness Journal,* 23, 6, 10–18.

U.S. Department of Health & Human Services (2018). *Physical Activity Guidelines for Americans* (2nd ed.). www.health.gov/paguidelines/

Winett, R.A. & Ogletree, A.M. (2019). Evidence-based, high-intensity exercise and physical activity for compressing morbidity in older adults: A narrative review. *Innovation in Aging,* 3, 2.

SUGGESTED READINGS

American College of Sports Medicine (2009). Position stand: Exercise and physical activity for older adults. *Medicine & Science in Sports & Exercise,* 41, 7, 1510–1530.

American Council on Exercise (2020). *The Exercise Professional's Guide to Personal Training.* San Diego: American Council on Exercise.

Rose, D.J. (2010). *FallProof!* (2nd ed.). Champaign, Ill.: Human Kinetics.

Signorile, J.F. (2011). *Bending the Aging Curve: The Complete Exercise Guide for Older Adults.* Champaign, Ill: Human Kinetics.

U.S. Department of Health & Human Services (2018). *Physical Activity Guidelines for Americans* (2nd ed.). www.health.gov/paguidelines/

CHAPTER 9

Common Health Challenges Faced by Older Adults

LEARNING OBJECTIVES

After reading this chapter, you will be able to:

▸ Recognize common health challenges faced by older adults in order to provide quality exercise programs for this clientele

▸ Determine the need for obtaining medical clearance and exercise guidelines and limitations for a client with a chronic health condition from their healthcare provider

▸ Incorporate general, recommended exercise guidelines for individuals with various chronic health issues related to cardiovascular, cerebrovascular, pulmonary, musculoskeletal, metabolic, neurological, and sensory disorders

▸ Provide practical solutions for older adults suffering from chronic illness that include modifications to cardiorespiratory and muscular-training exercise to decrease the risk for health complications during training that might result from inappropriate exercise intensity, balance problems, and musculoskeletal limitations

The fastest growing segment of adults older than 65 is composed of those older than 85 (Roberts et al., 2018). This remarkable extension of life brings with it the reality that most older adults will live for years, maybe even decades, with one or more chronic conditions (i.e., diseases with long duration and generally slow progression). However, though these conditions limit the ability of older adults to exercise, they should not be a deterrent to physical activity. Adults entering their seventh and eighth decades of life have heard for the last quarter century that exercise is one of the most important aspects of a healthy lifestyle. As a result, many are continuing to participate in physical activity well into their 70s, 80s, and 90s.

Clearly, despite the number of chronic health problems that an older person may acquire in later life, exercise can and should be an integral part of maintaining and, in some cases, improving functional mobility. Research demonstrates that older adults with chronic conditions such as **arthritis, diabetes,** or **cardiovascular disease (CVD)** can improve their health and physical function by engaging in regular physical activity (Kraus et al., 2019; Wang et al., 2018; Sveaas et al., 2017).

Given this demographic shift toward an older population, exercise professionals must understand the major types of chronic conditions that affect the elderly and be able to develop safe and effective exercise programs for this clientele. This chapter presents the chronic conditions most commonly experienced by older adults and discusses guidelines for developing safe and appropriate exercise programs that address them.

The Development of Health Problems in Older Adults

In older adults with chronic health conditions, disablement (i.e., the process of becoming physically challenged) is a clearly defined progression of deterioration that includes several rapid changes in an individual's life. A simple disablement model, adopted by both the Institute of Medicine (IOM) and the World Health Organization (WHO), describes the main pathway of the disablement process as four sequential and interrelated components that begin with (1) **pathology** (2) **impairments,** (3) **functional limitations,** and (4) **disability** (Whiteneck, 2006; WHO, 2001).

During the first stage, pathology, a person develops a disorder such as **rheumatoid arthritis** or **osteoporosis** that causes an impairment. Anatomical impairments can be classified as either structural in nature (e.g., bone loss) or functional (e.g., muscle **atrophy**), both of which can lead to a restriction in certain physical or mental tasks (e.g., difficulty walking). If the individual does not reverse this process through exercise and rehabilitation, the functional limitation usually worsens, resulting in a disability. During this final stage, the individual is unable to perform certain essential movements, such as dressing, walking, getting in and out of a bathtub or shower, and climbing steps, and depends more on others for care. The loss of physical mobility often sets off a spiral of **depression** and failing health.

Exercise professionals can play an important role in helping to prevent older adults with chronic health conditions from entering the impairment or functional limitation stages by guiding them to incorporate exercise into their lifestyles. Exercise can slow the decline

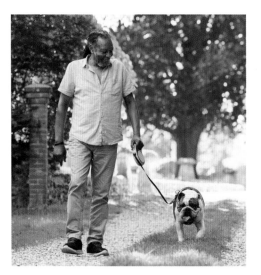

in physical function by preventing further deterioration and, in some instances, by improving the individual's functional mobility.

The goal of an exercise program for older persons with chronic health conditions is not to eliminate the disorder, but to increase their fitness level so they are able to maintain as much physical independence as possible. For example, an exercise program for a person with rheumatoid arthritis is not aimed at eliminating the condition, but rather at improving the ability to perform **basic activities of daily living** and **instrumental activities of daily living,** giving the client greater control over the environment.

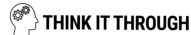 **THINK IT THROUGH**

Finding Your Niche

This chapter presents a number of chronic health conditions that commonly affect older adults. Is there a particular area in which you are more interested? For example, are you inclined to help older adults with balance-training programs to decrease their risk for falls? Perhaps you are more interested in finding unique ways to help senior clients enhance cardiorespiratory endurance to positively influence their cardiometabolic profiles. Spend some time thinking about the specific areas of health that you would like to focus on in your offerings for older clients. How will you further your education in these areas? How will you promote your specialties to potential senior clients?

Age-related medical conditions that affect the older adults can be divided into six categories: cardiovascular and cerebrovascular, pulmonary, musculoskeletal, metabolic, neurological, and sensory (Table 9-1).

TABLE 9-1

Chronic Conditions Often Experienced by Older Adults

Cardiovascular/Cerebrovascular	Pulmonary	Musculoskeletal
Coronary artery disease	Asthma	Arthritis
Peripheral artery disease	Bronchitis	Low-back pain
Hypertension	Emphysema	
Stroke		
Metabolic	**Neurological**	**Sensory**
Diabetes	Dementia	Visual disorders
Obesity	Alzheimer's disease	Auditory disorders
Osteoporosis	Parkinson's disease	
Menopause		

Cardiovascular and Cerebrovascular Disorders

Heart disease is the number one killer of Americans and the most common cause of death among older persons (Heron, 2019). While nearly every older adult has an element of heart disease, recent medical advances allow more and more individuals with this condition to live longer.

CORONARY ARTERY DISEASE

Coronary artery disease (CAD) is the primary type of heart disease experienced by older adults. As a person ages, fatty **plaque** forms inside the arterial walls and causes the **arteries** to become narrow or blocked. Consequently, blood flow to the **myocardium** (heart muscle) is reduced. This process is known as **atherosclerosis,** a condition that causes the artery walls to become narrow and brittle. When the arteries become almost completely blocked, or if an unstable arterial plaque ruptures, the person may experience a heart attack (**myocardial infarction**).

Other cardiovascular conditions include **hypertension** (high blood pressure), **congestive heart failure** (stiffness and/or weakness of the heart muscle rendering it ineffective as a forceful pump), cardiac arrhythmia (an irregular heart rhythm), heart valve problems, and **peripheral vascular disease** (atherosclerosis in the legs). Any of these conditions make the heart less effective in pumping blood to the working muscles and should be considered when developing exercise programs for older clients.

·:**:· EXPAND YOUR KNOWLEDGE

Automated External Defibrillation

While **cardiopulmonary resuscitation (CPR)** alone cannot change an abnormal heart rhythm, it is important to buy time before defibrillation. During cardiac arrest, the heart is beating erratically and ineffectively. The most common rhythm during cardiac arrest is **ventricular fibrillation (VF),** which is a spasmodic quivering of the heart that is too fast to allow the heart chambers to adequately fill and empty, so little or no blood is pushed out to the body or lungs. An **automated external defibrillator (AED)** is used to convert VF back to a normal rhythm by delivering an electric shock to the heart through two adhesive electrode pads on the person's chest. By keeping the tissues perfused with oxygenated blood, CPR preserves the heart and brain and can prevent VF from deteriorating into an unshockable rhythm while waiting for an AED to arrive.

The AED should be used as soon as it becomes available, ideally within the first three to five minutes. When a shock is provided within the first minute of cardiac arrest, victims with VF have survival rates as high as 90%. The number of AEDs in a fitness facility should depend on the size of the building and the time it takes to get the AED to any location in the facility. If a building has multiple floors, having one per floor is recommended. Defibrillation cannot treat all heart rhythms, and an AED will not shock a victim when a normal heart rhythm is found. The machine will first analyze the heart to determine if a shock is appropriate. When a shock is delivered, the heart's pacemaker (i.e., the **sinoatrial node**) is able to restart.

Many states, including California, Illinois, Indiana, Massachusetts, Michigan, New Jersey, New York, Pennsylvania, and Rhode Island, as well as the District of Columbia, have passed laws that require at least one AED in health clubs, and several other states are considering adopting similar legislation. Good Samaritan laws exist in most states that offer liability protection to the person who administers the AED. The federal government also passed the Cardiac Arrest Survival Act in 2000, which granted Good Samaritan protection for anyone in the U.S. who acquired an AED or who uses an AED in a medical emergency, except in cases of wanton misconduct or recklessness. This federal law does not override state policies but fills in the gaps for those states without these laws. This legal protection should allay any fears of liability for those organizations that want to offer a public-access defibrillation program, as well as the first responders who use them.

Symptoms

An early symptom of CAD is **angina pectoris** (chest pain or discomfort), but it is less common in older adults than in younger persons. More common symptoms of CAD in older individuals include **dyspnea** (difficulty breathing), diminished exercise tolerance, chronic fatigue, and disorders of the heart rhythm, which may cause **syncope** (faintness), **paresthesia** (tingling sensation), and confusion.

Developing a Safe Exercise Program

A cardiac rehabilitation program administered under the guidance of a physician, nurse, and/or medical exercise specialist is the safest exercise environment for a person with known CAD. However, there may come a point when both the client and physician decide that independent exercise at a fitness center or other location is acceptable. When working with older adults who have CAD, exercise professionals must be certain that the exercise regimen is safe for them. Request a specific **exercise prescription** from the client's physician and/or cardiopulmonary rehabilitation specialist, and do not alter the program without written approval. Adhere to the following safety concerns when working with clients with CAD.

▸ *Reduce physical exertion:* Be aware of the signs of heart distress as they relate to the individual client (e.g., chest pain, a change in heart rhythm associated with distress, difficulty breathing, pallor, and dizziness), and make sure the client does not exhibit any of these symptoms while exercising. If these symptoms do appear, stop the exercise immediately and notify the client's doctor. Always keep emergency telephone numbers on file in case a client needs immediate medical attention. Clients who are symptomatic during exercise should be referred to their physicians to discuss the need for an inpatient cardiac rehabilitation program where they will be closely monitored and supervised.

▸ *Avoid exposure to extreme heat or cold:* With advancing age, a person's body becomes more sensitive to heat and cold, and it is more difficult to retain or dissipate heat. Maintain a comfortable temperature and humidity level inside the exercise room and avoid extreme hot or cold temperatures. Frequent water breaks and adequate ventilation are two ways to avoid temperature-induced problems.

▸ *Mitigate emotional stress:* Emotional stress is a trigger for heart problems. If a client exhibits early signs of depression, or a personality change, there may be new sources of stress in their life. This could exacerbate a heart condition or predispose the client to new problems. The loss of a spouse or close friend, for example, can be a tremendous hardship. If a client is experiencing more stress than usual, consider reducing exercise intensity and/or duration. A couple of brief, friendly phone calls to check in with the client during these difficult times may enhance the client–professional relationship.

▸ *Discourage consumption of large meals before exercise:* Older adults should avoid exercise after eating a large meal. Consumption of a large meal (especially one that is high in fat and carbohydrate) could trigger a heart attack in clients with advanced CAD. Evidence suggests that postprandial spikes in levels of blood glucose and lipids stimulate immediate and proportional increases in oxidative stress, endothelial dysfunction,

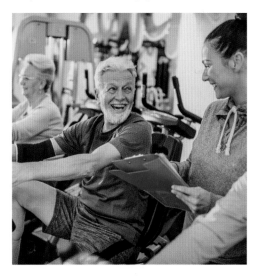

vasoconstriction, atherosclerosis, hypercoagulation, and **sympathetic nervous system** hyperactivity (O'Keefe, Carter, & Lavie, 2009). If combined with exercise, large meal consumption may put clients at an even higher risk. Suggest to older clients with CAD that they do not exercise sooner than one hour (ideally closer to two hours) after a meal.

Exercise Guidelines for Clients with Coronary Artery Disease

In addition to the guidelines summarized in Table 9-2, exercise professionals should adhere to the following:

▸ *Obtain medical clearance:* Medical clearance is needed for all symptomatic clients regardless of current participation in regular physical activity. For those clients with known CAD but who are asymptomatic, the need for medical clearance depends on current physical-activity levels and intensity. If clients are asymptomatic and currently do not participate in regular physical activity (i.e., at least 30 minutes on at least three days per week at a moderate intensity for the past three months), medical clearance is recommended. If clients have known CAD but currently participate in regular physical activity, medical clearance is recommended only before progressing to vigorous-intensity exercise. The medical clearance should specifically indicate that the client's heart condition will not be adversely affected by the exercise regimen. Adhere to the exercise prescription and do not alter it in any way unless written approval is provided by the client's physician.

▸ *Check the client's heart rate and blood pressure before, during, and after exercise:* Make sure that the client has appropriately taken all prescribed medications prior to beginning each exercise session and always check their heart rate (HR) and blood pressure (BP) before beginning activity. Contraindications for exercise in clients with CAD include uncontrolled hypertension [i.e., resting systolic blood pressure (SBP) >180 mmHg and/or diastolic blood pressure (DBP) >110 mmHg], orthostatic blood pressure decrease of greater than 20 mmHg with symptoms, and uncontrolled tachycardia >120 bpm [American College of Sports Medicine (ACSM), 2018]. Take BP readings before, during, and after exercise to ensure that there are no major cardiovascular changes occurring during the session.

▸ *Use perceived exertion to monitor intensity:* Use the rating of perceived exertion (RPE) scale to gauge exercise intensity in clients who are taking **beta blockers, calcium channel blockers,** and other heart medications that blunt the HR response to exercise. The client should be taught how to assess RPE to ensure accuracy (Figure 9-1).

▸ *Work with clients one-on-one whenever possible:* Personalized exercise programs are recommended for persons with CAD because group activities usually do not allow the attention that is required to monitor a client's vital signs (i.e., BP, HR, respiration, skin color, RPE, and general feelings). Though a physician-prescribed program is the safest method, a client may prefer group exercise. In this instance, the client should request written physician approval for a program that includes specific guidelines and recommended activities that can be performed within a specified intensity level.

TABLE 9-2
Exercise Guidelines Summary for Clients with Cardiovascular Disease

Cardiorespiratory Training	
Frequency	▶ At least 3, but preferably 5 or more, days of the week
	▶ Clients with limited exercise capacity can perform short, 1- to 10-minute sessions daily, as needed.
Intensity	▶ Moderate to vigorous intensity*
	▶ Intensity may be determined through the following methods:
	▪ With an exercise test, use 40–80% HRR or $\dot{V}O_2R$ or $\dot{V}O_2$ peak
	▪ Without an exercise test, use RPE of 3–6 (0–10 scale) or add 20–30 bpm to RHR
	▪ HR should remain at least 10 bpm below the HR associated with the ischemic threshold (if exercise ischemic threshold has been determined)
	▶ High-intensity interval training may be a safe and effective method for enhancing cardiorespiratory fitness for individuals with stable disease and a base level of conditioning.
Time	▶ Eventual goal of 20–60 minutes for cardiorespiratory training
	▶ Warm-up and cool-down activities lasting 5–10 minutes should be included in each exercise session.
Type	▶ Rhythmic, large-muscle-group exercise that emphasizes whole-body conditioning and utilizes multiple activities and pieces of equipment, such as:
	▪ Arm ergometer
	▪ Upright and recumbent cycle ergometer
	▪ Recumbent stepper
	▪ Rower
	▪ Elliptical
	▪ Treadmill for walking
Progression	▶ Progress following the ACE Integrated Fitness Training® Model based on client goals and availability.
	▶ Sessions may include continuous or intermittent exercise.
Muscular Training	
Frequency	▶ 2–3 days per week with a minimum of 48 hours separating exercise for the same muscle group
Intensity	▶ 40–60% 1-RM, or a load that can be lifted 10–15 repetitions without straining
	▶ RPE of 2–4 (0–10 scale)

Continued on the next page

TABLE 9-2 *(continued)*

Muscular Training

Time	▸ No specific session duration has been found to be most effective.

Type	▸ Various equipment can be used for resistance training, including:
	  ▪ Elastic resistance
	  ▪ Free weights
	  ▪ Pulleys
	  ▪ Selectorized machines
	▸ Each major muscle group should be trained initially with one set.
	▸ Multiple-set routines may be introduced later, as tolerated.

Progression	▸ Progress following the ACE Integrated Fitness Training Model based on client goals and availability. ▸ Progression can be introduced through increases in resistance, number of repetitions or sets, or decreasing rest periods between sets. ▸ Progression should be slow and dependent on tolerance. ▪ Volume can be increased 2–10% once clients comfortably complete 1–2 repetitions beyond the target range on two consecutive training sessions.

*Moderate intensity = Heart rates <VT1 where speech remains comfortable and is not affected by breathing; Vigorous intensity = Heart rates from ≥VT1 to <VT2 where clients feel unsure if speech is comfortable.

Note: HRR = Heart-rate reserve; $\dot{V}O_2R$ = Oxygen uptake reserve; RPE = Rating of perceived exertion; bpm = Beats per minute; HR = Heart rate; RHR = Resting heart rate; 1-RM = One-repetition maximum; VT1 = First ventilatory threshold; VT2 = Second ventilatory threshold

Source: American College of Sports Medicine (2018). *ACSM's Guidelines for Exercise Testing and Prescription* (10th ed.). Philadelphia: Wolters Kluwer.

FIGURE 9-1
Rating of perceived exertion: Category ratio scale

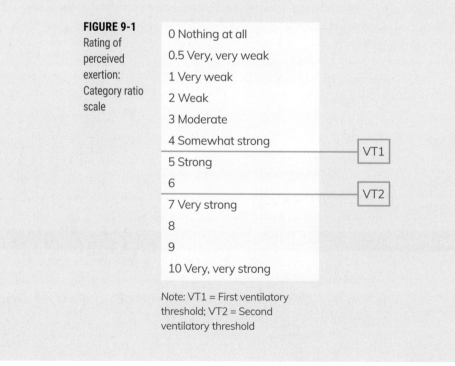

0 Nothing at all
0.5 Very, very weak
1 Very weak
2 Weak
3 Moderate
4 Somewhat strong — VT1
5 Strong
6 — VT2
7 Very strong
8
9
10 Very, very strong

Note: VT1 = First ventilatory threshold; VT2 = Second ventilatory threshold

PERIPHERAL ARTERY DISEASE

Peripheral artery disease (PAD) is characterized by the presence of significant narrowing of arteries in the periphery of the body, typically due to atherosclerosis, that most commonly affects the lower limbs. Because PAD is usually a manifestation of atherosclerosis, risk factors for both conditions are congruent and include smoking, diabetes, hypertension, high cholesterol, and systemic **inflammation** as detected by elevated **homocysteine** levels in the blood (Song et al., 2019). Thus, treatment of PAD aims to improve longer-term cardiovascular outcomes through risk-factor modification combined with antiplatelet and lipid-lowering primary medical therapy. **Intermittent claudication** is the hallmark symptom of PAD and is typically treated with pharmacological agents that dilate the vessels of the legs, or by endovascular (**percutaneous transluminal coronary angioplasty** and/or stenting) or surgical interventions (O'Donnell et al., 2011).

Symptoms

PAD is initially asymptomatic but can progress to the point where intermittent claudication is present. Intermittent claudication is lower-extremity muscular pain, cramping, fatigue, and reproducible aching brought on by exercise and relieved by short periods of rest. The pain is a result of the inability of the lower-limb vasculature to maintain adequate tissue perfusion and oxygenation during exertional activity (ACSM, 2018; Norgren et al., 2007). PAD is common in older adults, with a prevalence that rises steeply with age to nearly 25% of adults ≥80 years old in the U.S. (Benjamin et al., 2019).

Exercise Guidelines for Clients with Peripheral Artery Disease

The goals of exercise intervention for PAD are threefold: (1) to reduce limb symptoms; (2) to improve exercise capacity and prevent or lessen physical disability; and (3) to decrease the occurrence of cardiovascular events (Hamburg & Balady, 2011). In individuals with stable intermittent claudication, walking exercise is an integral part of treatment for PAD, as it improves both peripheral vascular and cardiovascular health. Exercise also improves gait patterns in nonsurgical patients.

In addition to the guidelines summarized in Table 9-3, exercise professionals should adhere to the following:

▸ *Asymptomatic individuals:* Clients without intermittent claudication should follow the same exercise guidelines as described for CAD. It should be noted that most individuals with PAD are asymptomatic (Treat-Jacobson et al., 2019).

▸ *Clients with intermittent claudication should be referred to their personal physicians for medical clearance before beginning an exercise program:* The recommendations for this population focus on pain management during exercise. For example, consider an individual who walks on a treadmill at a given work rate at which they experience the onset of claudication. The individual continues walking until they reach a moderate claudication pain score (2 on a 0 to 4 scale) and then stops until the pain completely subsides (ACSM, 2018) (Table 9-4). Then, the individual resumes exercise at a similar intensity and repeats the rest/exercise bouts. The individual is progressed to a higher work rate when they are able to walk for eight-minute bouts without the need to stop due to leg symptoms (Bronas et al., 2009).

TABLE 9-3

Exercise Guidelines Summary for Clients with Peripheral Artery Disease

Cardiorespiratory Training	
Frequency	▸ 3–5 days per week
Intensity	▸ Moderate intensity
	▸ Below VT1 HR; can talk comfortably; RPE of 3–4 (0–10 scale)
	▸ Walking speed and/or grade or workload that causes claudication pain within 2–6 minutes. Because the intensity is more closely associated with pain, use of HRR or $\dot{V}O_2R$ alone may not be appropriate.
	▸ Do not exceed 2 out of 4 on the claudication pain scale.
Time	▸ 30–45 minutes (excluding rest periods) for up to 12 weeks
	▸ May progress to 60 minutes
Type	▸ Weight-bearing
	▪ Walking
	▪ Intermittent exercise with seated rest when moderate pain (2 out of 4 on the claudication pain scale) is reached and resumption when pain dissipates
Progression	▸ Progress following the ACE Integrated Fitness Training Model based on client goals and availability.
Muscular Training	
Frequency	▸ At least 2 days per week performed on nonconsecutive days
Intensity	▸ 60–80% 1-RM
Time	▸ 2–3 sets of 8–12 repetitions
	▸ 6–8 exercises targeting all major muscle groups
Type	▸ Whole body, focusing on large muscle groups
	▸ Emphasize lower-limbs exercise if time is limited
Progression	▸ Progress following the ACE Integrated Fitness Training Model based on client goals and availability.

Note: VT1 = First ventilatory threshold; HR = Heart rate; RPE = Rating of perceived exertion; $\dot{V}O_2R$ = Oxygen uptake reserve; HRR = Heart-rate reserve; 1-RM = One-repetition maximum

Source: American College of Sports Medicine (2018). ACSM's Guidelines for Exercise Testing and Prescription (10th ed.). Philadelphia: Wolters Kluwer.

TABLE 9-4

Claudication Pain Scale

0 - No pain

1 - Definite discomfort or pain, but only at initial or modest levels (established, but minimal)

2 - Moderate discomfort or pain from which the individual's attention can be diverted (e.g., by conversation)

3 - Intense pain (short of grade 4) from which the individual's attention cannot be diverted

4 - Excruciating and unbearable pain

HYPERTENSION

Hypertension, as defined by Whelton et al. (2017), affects approximately 108 million Americans, or 46% of the population, with incidence increasing with age. It has been coined the silent killer because many people who have hypertension are unaware of it. A review of the literature suggests a strong evidence-based relationship between the causal role of high BP and CVD (Fuchs et al., 2012).

Hypertension is a SBP of 130 mmHg or greater or a DBP of 80 mmHg or greater (Whelton et al., 2017) (see Table 7-3, page 201). One of the more common hypertension conditions among older persons is isolated systolic hypertension, which is defined as an SBP of 160 mmHg or greater and a DBP 90 mmHg or lower (Whelton et al., 2017). Several clinical studies have shown that an elevated SBP may be a better predictor of cardiovascular complications in older adults than an elevated DBP (Aronow et al., 2011).

Symptoms

Most people with mild to moderate hypertension do not exhibit any symptoms, but those with severe hypertension may experience headaches, fatigue, dizziness, and heart palpitations.

Exercise Guidelines for Clients with Hypertension

In addition to the guidelines summarized in Table 9-5, exercise professionals should adhere to the following:

▸ *Obtain medical clearance:* ACSM (2018) recommends that individuals with a resting SBP ≥140 mmHg and/or DBP ≥90 mmHg should consult with their physician before starting an exercise program to determine if an exercise test is warranted.

▸ *Begin exercise after hypertension is under control:* Persons with resting SBP ≥160 mmHg and/or DBP ≥100 mmHg or with target organ disease (e.g., left ventricular **hypertrophy** or **retinopathy**) should not begin an exercise program, including exercise testing, prior to a medical evaluation and adequate BP management (ACSM, 2018).

▸ *Use perceived exertion to monitor intensity:* Use RPE to monitor exercise intensity, especially with clients taking medications that alter HR response, such as beta-blocking drugs. Consult with their physicians to determine the RPE value that should be targeted.

▸ *Check the client's BP before, during, and after exercise:* Pay special attention to clients' pre-exercise BP to ensure they have taken their antihypertensive medication (older persons who have forgotten to take their medication may have an elevated BP). It is suggested to maintain an SBP ≤220 mmHg and/or a DBP of ≤105 mmHg when exercising (ACSM, 2018).

▸ *Be aware of the potential for postexercise hypotension:* A single bout of mild to moderate exercise can lead to a postexercise decrease in BP (i.e., **postexercise hypotension**) in both **normotensive** and hypertensive individuals. In many cases, this is a positive effect of exercise training in that it helps to lower BP for up to 13 hours after physical activity (Carpio-Rivera et al., 2016). However, for some individuals on antihypertensive medication, BP can be drastically reduced after a bout of exercise, leading to syncope or pre-syncope symptoms. Exercise professionals should extend the duration of the cool-down period and stay with their older clients with hypertension for several minutes after the end of the cool-down to ensure that the clients have support if they do experience symptoms of syncope.

▶ *Be mindful of the client's breathing pattern:* Instruct all hypertensive individuals to maintain normal breathing patterns while performing muscular training, since breath holding can induce a **Valsalva effect,** causing an excessive, transient rise in BP.

▶ *Approach recommending high-intensity exercise with caution:* Traditionally, the recommendation has been that hypertensive individuals avoid high-intensity exercise. However, several studies suggest that **high-intensity interval training (HIIT)**, which consists of several bouts of high-intensity exercise (~85% to 95% of $\dot{V}O_2max$) lasting one to four minutes combined with intervals of rest or active recovery, is superior to continuous endurance exercise (e.g., moderate-intensity for 30 minutes) for improving cardiorespiratory fitness and cardiovascular function in patients with hypertension as well as individuals with normal BP (Ciolac, 2012). Furthermore, research supports HIIT as a viable solution for improving physical work capacity as well as desirable metabolic responses even in older adults with disease-imposed limitations (Whitehurst, 2012). Although the optimal dosage of HIIT still needs to be established, and as such exercise professionals should practice on the conservative side, this type of training for older adults with hypertension could result in better compliance with exercise because it decreases the time required pursuing increased fitness.

▶ *Focus on low resistance:* The BP response to resistance training is directly correlated to the training load (i.e., heavy training loads are associated with higher BP levels). A muscular-training program for clients with hypertension should generally emphasize a high number of repetitions at a low resistance (ACSM, 2018).

▶ *Manage body weight and dietary intake and quit smoking:* Along with the exercise program, encourage clients with hypertension to lose weight (if they have **overweight** or **obesity**); limit alcohol consumption, as even moderate drinking (seven to 13 drinks per week) increases risk (Aladin et al., 2019); reduce sodium intake; stop smoking; and reduce dietary **saturated fat** and cholesterol (ACSM, 2018).

TABLE 9-5

Exercise Guidelines Summary for Clients with Hypertension

Cardiorespiratory Training

Frequency	▶ Most, but preferably all, days of the week
Intensity	▶ Intensity may be determined through the following methods: • 40–59% HRR or $\dot{V}O_2R$ • RPE of 3–4 (0–10 scale) • Below VT1 HR; can talk comfortably
Time	▶ Eventual goal of at least 30 minutes of continuous or accumulated exercise ▶ Clients with limited exercise capacity can accumulate bouts of intermittent exercise (10 minutes) throughout the day.
Type	▶ Emphasis should be placed on rhythmic, large-muscle-group activities: • Walking • Jogging • Cycling • Swimming

TABLE 9-5 *(continued)*

Cardiorespiratory Training	
Progression	▸ Progress following the ACE Integrated Fitness Training Model based on client goals and availability.
	▸ Progression should be personalized dependent on tolerance and consideration of the following factors:
	▪ Recent changes in antihypertensive drug therapy
	▪ Medication-related adverse effects
	▪ The presence of target-organ disease and/or other comorbidities

Muscular Training	
Frequency	▸ 2–3 days per week with a minimum of 48 hours separating exercise for the same muscle group
Intensity	▸ 60–80% 1-RM
	▸ 40–50% 1-RM for older adults and novice exercisers
Time	▸ 2–4 sets of 8–12 repetitions
	▸ Each major muscle group should be trained.
Type	▸ Either machine weights or free weights should be used to supplement cardiorespiratory training.
	▸ Avoid the Valsalva maneuver during resistance training.
Progression	▸ Progress following the ACE Integrated Fitness Training Model based on client goals and availability.

Note: HRR = Heart-rate reserve; $\dot{V}O_2R$ = Oxygen uptake reserve; RPE = Rating of perceived exertion; VT1 = First ventilatory threshold; HR = Heart rate; 1-RM = One-repetition maximum

Source: American College of Sports Medicine (2018). ACSM's Guidelines for Exercise Testing and Prescription (10th ed.). Philadelphia: Wolters Kluwer.

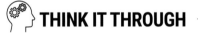 **THINK IT THROUGH**

Measuring Blood Pressure

Because hypertension is prevalent in the older population, exercise professionals who work with senior clients should have first-hand knowledge of proper technique for measuring BP. This includes having access to tools such as a sphygmomanometer and stethoscope. Do you feel comfortable training clients with hypertension? If not, consider advancing your education and practical skills in BP assessment. Also, practice measuring BP with family and friends until you feel very comfortable with the process.

STROKE

There are two types of **stroke**—ischemic and hemorrhagic. An **ischemic stroke** develops when a blood clot from an atherosclerotic lesion blocks a blood vessel in the brain. The clot may form in the blood vessel or travel from somewhere else in the bloodstream. About eight out of 10 strokes are ischemic strokes, and they are the most common type of stroke in older adults (Benjamin et al., 2019). A **hemorrhagic stroke** occurs when an artery in the brain leaks or bursts, which causes bleeding inside the brain or near the surface of the brain. Hemorrhagic strokes are less common but more deadly than ischemic strokes.

Annually, 795,000 people in the U.S. suffer a stroke (either ischemic or hemorrhagic), which equates to approximately 1 person every 40 seconds, and nearly one-quarter of these strokes are recurrent (Benjamin et al., 2019). Moreover, the incidence of stroke is likely to continue to escalate because of an expanding population of elderly Americans; increased prevalence of diabetes, obesity, and physical inactivity among the general population; and a greater number of heart failure patients. Ischemic stroke shares many of the same predisposing, potentially modifiable risk factors as CAD (i.e., hypertension, abnormal blood lipids and **lipoproteins,** cigarette smoking, physical inactivity, obesity, and diabetes), which highlights the prominent role lifestyle plays in the origin of stroke and CVD.

Improved short-term survival after a stroke has resulted in a population of close to 7 million stroke survivors in the U.S. (Benjamin et al., 2019). Stroke survivors are often deconditioned and predisposed to a sedentary lifestyle that limits performance of activities of daily living (ADL), increases the risk for falls, and may contribute to a heightened risk for recurrent stroke and CVD. Thus, stroke survivors can benefit from participation in physical activity and exercise training.

Symptoms

The brain controls various body functions, so symptoms of a stroke depend on what area of the brain is affected. Typical effects of a stroke include facial droop, weakness or paralysis of the body, vision problems, memory loss, and speech or language problems.

The exercise professional should be aware of the warning signs of a stroke:

- Sudden numbness or weakness of the face, arms, or legs
- Sudden confusion or trouble speaking or understanding others
- Sudden trouble seeing in one or both eyes
- Sudden walking problems, dizziness, or loss of balance and coordination
- Sudden severe headache with no known cause

The simple acronym FAST (facial drooping, arm weakness, speech difficulties, and time to call emergency services) serves as a mnemonic to help exercise professionals recognize and respond to the needs of a client having a stroke.

Individuals who experience any of these symptoms should contact their doctor immediately, even if the symptoms resolve quickly, because they may be indicative of a **transient ischemic attack (TIA),** sometimes called a mini-stroke. In about 12% of cases, a TIA is a warning that a full-blown stroke may happen soon (Benjamin et al., 2019). Getting early treatment for a TIA can help prevent a stroke.

Exercise Guidelines for Clients Recovering from a Stroke

There is a lack of straightforward exercise recommendations for people recovering from stroke because an individual's ability to exercise will vary with stroke type, residual disability, age, and comorbidity. Mobility impairment is a significant concern post-stroke. Thus, a primary goal of stroke rehabilitation is to improve mobility in the presence of motor, balance, and visual-spatial deficits. In addition to the guidelines summarized in Table 9-6, exercise professionals should adhere to the following general guidelines, which represent current trends in physical activity for stroke survivors.

▸ *Obtain medical clearance:* All stroke survivors should undergo a complete medical history and physical examination aimed at the identification of neurological complications and other medical conditions that require special consideration or constitute a contraindication to exercise. A client's physician and other healthcare providers should dictate exercise-programming guidelines for the post-rehabilitative phase of activity for stroke survivors.

▸ *Incorporate cardiorespiratory exercise as a primary mode of training:* Cardiorespiratory training has been shown to enhance physical fitness and reduce cardiovascular risk factors in stroke patients, who are generally less physically active than age-matched counterparts, and help reduce the risk of recurrent events. Exercise on a treadmill appears to be particularly effective for helping stroke survivors improve gait mechanics, if they have sufficient balance and ambulation. The recommended frequency of training is three to five days a week, with a duration of 20 to 60 minutes per day of continuous or accumulated exercise (e.g., 10-minute bouts), depending on the client's level of fitness (ACSM, 2018).

▸ *Include muscular training on two nonconsecutive days per week:* Although there are no accepted guidelines for determining when and how to initiate muscular training after a stroke, a whole-body program consisting of 8 to 15 repetitions (i.e., moderate to high repetitions with reduced loads) for each set of exercises might be prudent. Some studies suggest that such regimens may promote gains in strength and gait velocity and that eccentric training may be more suitable for stroke survivors than concentric training (Fernandez-Gonzalo et al., 2016).

▸ *Consider including circuit training:* Investigations into circuit-training programs for stroke survivors have yielded positive results. In one study, individuals with a mild to moderate stroke who had been discharged home completed eight mobility-related stations in small groups for 90 minutes twice weekly for 12 weeks. The author reported that this mode of training was as effective as individual therapy in improving mobility (e.g., balance, physical conditioning, and walking) and may be a more efficient way of delivering physical activity (Dean, 2012).

TABLE 9-6

Exercise Guidelines Summary for Clients Recovering from Stroke

Cardiorespiratory Training	
Frequency	▸ 3 to 5 days per week
Intensity	▸ Light, moderate, or vigorous intensity*
	▸ If HR data are available from recent GXT, use 40–70% HRR.
	▸ In the absence of GXT, or if atrial fibrillation is present, use RPE of 2–5 (0–10 scale).
Time	▸ Progressively increase from 20–60 minutes and consider multiple bouts of exercise throughout the day.
Type	▸ Considering functional and cognitive deficiencies, some use of equipment may need modifications.
	▪ Cycle ergometry
	▪ Recumbent seated steppers
	▪ Treadmill walking

Continued on the next page

TABLE 9-6 *(continued)*

Cardiorespiratory Training	
Progression	▸ Progress following the ACE Integrated Fitness Training Model based on client goals and availability.

Muscular Training	
Frequency	▸ 2 nonconsecutive days per week
Intensity	▸ 50–70% 1-RM
Time	▸ 1–3 sets of 8–15 repetitions
Type	▸ Use equipment and exercises that improve safety in those with deficits (e.g., machine versus free weights and seated versus standing)
Progression	▸ Progress following the ACE Integrated Fitness Training Model based on client goals and availability.

*Moderate intensity = Heart rates <VT1 where speech remains comfortable and is not affected by breathing; Vigorous intensity = Heart rates from ≥VT1 to <VT2 where clients feel unsure if speech is comfortable.

Note: HR = Heart rate; GXT = Graded exercise test; HRR = Heart-rate reserve; RPE = Rating of perceived exertion; 1-RM = One-repetition maximum; VT1 = First ventilatory threshold; VT2 = Second ventilatory threshold

Source: American College of Sports Medicine (2018). *ACSM's Guidelines for Exercise Testing and Prescription* (10th ed.). Philadelphia: Wolters Kluwer.

Pulmonary Disorders

The three most common pulmonary disorders in older adults are **asthma, bronchitis,** and **emphysema.** Bronchitis and emphysema usually occur together and are the two most common conditions that contribute to **chronic obstructive pulmonary disease (COPD),** which is a functional diagnosis referring to a group of diseases that cause breathing problems related to airflow blockage. Pulmonary disorders are ranked among the top 10 leading causes of death among older persons (Heron, 2019).

ASTHMA

Asthma, which comes from the Greek word meaning "to pant," is an inflammatory airway disease in which the airways become narrow, resulting in labored breathing (e.g., wheezing, coughing, and shortness of breath). Three pathological changes simultaneously occur during an asthma exacerbation, or "attack," making it extremely difficult for the person to breathe:

- ▸ The smooth muscles around the **bronchioles,** which are the small airway tubes in the lungs, go into spasm, contracting and squeezing the bronchial tubes and making it difficult for air to enter.

- ▸ Thick secretions of mucus accumulate inside the bronchial tubes, further deteriorating the lungs' ability to get oxygen into the blood.

- ▸ The lining of the bronchial tubes thickens and becomes engorged with blood.

Causes of Asthma

There are multiple causes of asthma, including everything from allergens (substances to which one can acquire a sensitivity) to physical and emotional stress. Asthma induced by exposure to chemical irritants (e.g., air pollution, cigarette smoke, and diesel exhaust particles), air temperature, acute illness, and exercise has also been reported (Global Initiative for Asthma, 2020).

▸ *Allergens:* Common allergens include pollen; animal dander; certain types of foods (e.g., strawberries, nuts, and chocolates); food additives (e.g., monosodium glutamate); feathers; certain medications (e.g., aspirin and penicillin); and dusts and molds.

▸ *Chemical irritants:* These include dust, paint, deodorants, perfumes, and cigarette smoke. For some, the chlorine found in swimming pools also may be a chemical irritant, and new carpeting may precipitate an asthma episode in others. Identify which clients have asthma and alert them to any irritants in the exercise facility that may trigger an attack.

▸ *Temperature:* Cold air is a primary trigger of asthma attacks. Many older individuals with asthma may not want to venture out of their homes during the cold winter months to get to a fitness center.

▸ *Psychological and nervous system stimuli:* Emotional outbursts of laughter, crying, or screaming can stimulate the vagus nerve, which causes the muscles in the bronchial lining of the lungs to tighten and trigger an attack.

▸ *Infection:* The increased mucus production caused by sinusitis or influenza further narrows the airways and increases the risk of an attack. Pay close attention to a client with asthma who is recovering from a respiratory infection.

▸ *Exercise:* **Exercise-induced bronchoconstriction (EIB)** occurs in individuals who do not have a history of asthma and who have bronchospasm associated with only exercise. EIB is associated with increased breathing through the mouth (versus the nose), which can be problematic because with this type of breathing the temperature in the respiratory passages is lowered and water vapor is removed. This causes a cooling and drying effect in the lungs, which may trigger an attack. For EIB, treatment usually consists of acute measures to reduce the symptoms (e.g., short-acting inhaled beta-adrenergic agonists) (Parsons et al., 2013).

Symptoms of Asthma

The following symptoms are common when a person's asthma is triggered and an exacerbation occurs:

▸ *Shortness of breath:* The major symptom of asthma is shortness of breath. This uncomfortable feeling has been described as trying to breathe through a pinched straw and can be an extremely scary experience for older adults.

▸ *Coughing:* Persons with asthma may experience a great deal of coughing, particularly during the winter months when cold air exacerbates their condition. The coughing sometimes is associated with an upper respiratory infection, which also can trigger an asthma attack.

▸ *Wheezing:* When the coughing sounds as if it originates in the lungs, and audible vibrations can be heard within the chest, the person is wheezing. The whistling noise that is heard when a person is wheezing is related to air being forced through the mucus-filled air passages in the lungs.

Medications Used to Treat Asthma

Exercise professionals who work with clients who suffer from asthma should familiarize themselves with the drugs most often used to treat asthma and their common side effects.

Medications for asthma are categorized into two general classes: long-term control medications used to achieve and maintain control of persistent asthma and quick-relief medications used to treat acute symptoms and exacerbations.

Commonly prescribed long-term-control medications include the following:

▸ *Corticosteroids (fluticasone and budesonide):* These are the most potent and effective anti-inflammatory medications currently available. Inhaled corticosteroids are used in the long-term control of asthma. Possible side effects include hoarseness, headache, and mouth infection. A short course of oral corticosteroids is used to gain prompt control of the disease when initiating long-term therapy. Long-term use of systemic steroids is used for severe persistent asthma. Short-term use of oral corticosteroids can cause weight gain, fluid retention, mood changes, and high BP, while long-term use can cause **hyperglycemia,** osteoporosis, cataracts, muscle weakness, and immune suppression.

▸ *Long-acting beta agonists (salmeterol and formoterol):* These are bronchodilators that relax or open airways in the lungs and that work for at least 12 hours. They are used in combination with inhaled corticosteroids for long-term control and prevention of symptoms in moderate or severe persistent asthma and are the preferred therapy in combination with inhaled corticosteroids for individuals over 12 years old. Possible cardiopulmonary side effects include tremor, rapid heartbeat, elevated BP, and upper airway irritation.

▸ *Cromolyn sodium and nedocromil:* These medications are used as an alternative, not preferred, medication for treatment of mild persistent asthma. They can also be used as preventive treatment prior to exercise or unavoidable exposure to known allergens. Dry cough is a possible side effect.

▸ *Immunomodulators (omalizumab):* These are used as an adjunctive therapy for individuals over 12 years old who have allergies and severe persistent asthma. Note that anaphylaxis may occur.

▸ *Leukotriene modifiers (montelukast, zafirlukast, 5-lipoxygenase inhibitor):* This is an alternative therapy for mild persistent asthma. Note that anaphylaxis may occur.

▸ *Methylxanthines (theophylline):* These are mild to moderate bronchodilators used as an alternative adjunctive therapy with inhaled corticosteroids.

Commonly prescribed quick-relief medications include the following:

▸ *Short-acting beta agonists (albuterol, levalbuterol, pirbuterol):* Short-acting beta agonists, or bronchodilators, relax or open airways in the lungs. They are the therapy of choice for relief of acute symptoms and prevention of EIB. Bronchodilators activate the sympathetic nervous system and may cause rapid heartbeat, tremors, **anxiety,** and nausea.

▸ *Anticholinergics (ipratropium bromide):* These medications reduce vagal tone of the airway, leading to dilation. They provide additive benefit to short-acting bronchodilators in moderate-to-severe asthma exacerbation. Possible side effects include dizziness, nausea, heartburn, and dry mouth.

▸ *Oral corticosteroids (prednisone and dexamethasone):* Though not short-acting, they can be used for moderate and severe exacerbations, in addition to short-acting bronchodilators, to speed recovery and prevent recurrence of exacerbation.

While it certainly is not the exercise professional's responsibility (or within scope of practice) to evaluate and manage a client's prescription drugs, it is worth noting that asthma medications may have increased adverse effects in senior patients (Reed, 2010). For example, airway response to bronchodilators may change with age. Older adults, especially those with preexisting ischemic heart disease, may be more sensitive to a short-acting beta agonist's side effects, including tremor and **tachycardia.** Also, systemic corticosteroids can provoke confusion, agitation, and changes in glucose metabolism in the elderly. Exercise professionals should be diligent about ensuring that their older clients who have asthma are complying with their prescribed medication use.

Exercise Guidelines for Clients with Asthma

Unfortunately, the senior population is underexplored in the research, though it has been reported that older people with asthma are less active than their non-affected peers, which may be the result of associated functional limitations and perceived barriers to physical activity (Dogra, Meisner, & Baker, 2008). Nonetheless, older adults with asthma have the ability to be active and exercise without severe limitations, provided they take necessary precautions. Furthermore, exercise professionals who assist older adults with asthma with accomplishing basic physical-activity and exercise goals may help them realize that their disease is not a disability, thereby increasing self-perceived health. The following exercise guidelines can help facilitate the process of getting older adults with asthma to become more physically active.

In addition to the guidelines summarized in Table 9-7, exercise professionals should adhere to the following:

▸ *Pay close attention to the exercising client:* Physically inactive older adults and those newly diagnosed with asthma need to be involved in safe, structured exercise programs. It is important to pay close attention to the client, particularly during the early stages of the program when the risk of an asthma episode is higher.

▸ *Start with shorter-duration bouts of activity:* Some older clients with asthma have difficulty exercising for extended periods of time; short, intermittent bouts of exercise may be more effective than one long bout. The exercise program should consist of five or six one- to two-minute exercise bouts, with a one-minute rest between each. Once the client becomes conditioned to the program and is able to tolerate longer periods of activity, progressively increase the duration of exercise.

▸ *Encourage frequent rest periods:* Clients with asthma should rest as often as necessary, particularly during group activities. If a client exhibits excessive shortness of breath, they should stop the activity and rest until they feel comfortable returning to the group. If the client prefers to do something while waiting to rejoin the group, have them perform **diaphragmatic breathing** or **pursed-lip breathing** exercises.

▸ *Start at a low intensity:* Older persons with asthma should always begin exercising at an intensity below the **first ventilatory threshold (VT1)** (RPE below 5 on the

0 to 10 scale). Watch for shortness of breath during the initial stages of the program. Once the client increases their conditioning level, gradually increase the intensity as long as there are no asthma symptoms.

▶ *Encourage a range of frequency:* The frequency of exercise can range from three to five days per week, depending on the client's interest, availability, and the severity of the asthma.

▶ *Encourage exercise in the water:* Swimming may be one of the best exercise modalities for clients with asthma. The temperature and humidity just above the water's surface allow airways to remain warm and moist, thus preventing an asthma episode. For older persons who do not like to swim or who are sensitive to the chemicals used to treat swimming pools (e.g., chlorine), short bouts of exercise using a stair stepper, stationary cycle, or rowing machine should be relatively safe. Jogging appears to be one of the biggest triggers for exercise-induced asthma and is only recommended for an individual who prefers no other modality. Walking and low-impact aerobic dance may be safe if not performed too strenuously.

▶ *Ask clients if they have taken their asthma medication:* Older adults with EIB should take their medications as prescribed by their medical provider prior to exercise to prevent the onset of an attack. In addition, clients should always carry an inhaler with them, as using it is the only way to reverse an attack. If symptoms arise during the early stages of the program, reduce the activity to a level that will not excessively elevate the client's heart or breathing rates.

▶ *Focus on warming up and cooling down:* Warm-ups and cool-downs are especially important for people with asthma. A 10- to 15-minute low-intensity warm-up (e.g., easy movements in the pool, walking, and riding a stationary bike) and the same type of cool-down can reduce the incidence of asthma during exercise.

▶ *Use a peak flow meter:* A small plastic device called a peak flow meter measures how quickly a person expires air from the lungs and is a reliable instrument for determining airflow obstruction before an asthma attack occurs. Many individuals have their own peak flow meter and know how to use it based on guidance from their physician or respiratory therapist. Exercise professionals should ask their clients with asthma if they have a peak flow meter. As such, clients should use their peak flow meter according to their own personal-action plan recommended by a healthcare professional. Measuring peak flow rate (Table 9-8) before a class or exercise session can help to determine whether the client can safely exercise on that day. Generally, the guidelines indicate that an exerciser with asthma can perform an activity if their peak flow rate is >80% of normal values. If the client's peak flow rate is <80%, the exercise program should be modified to avoid an asthma episode (National Asthma Education and Prevention Program, 2007). It is a good idea also to measure peak flow after exercise, so that the pre- and postexercise values may be compared.

▸ *Know the steps of managing an asthma attack:* It is crucial to know what to do when an older client has an asthma attack. Refer to Table 9-9 for specific recommendations.

TABLE 9-7

Exercise Guidelines Summary for Clients with Asthma

Cardiorespiratory Training	
Frequency	▸ 3–5 days per week
Intensity	▸ Initially, below VT1 ▸ 40–59% HRR or $\dot{V}O_2R$. If well tolerated, progress to 60–70% HRR or $\dot{V}O_2R$ after 1 month. ▸ RPE 3–4 (0–10 scale)
Time	▸ Progressively increase to at least 30–40 minutes per session
Type	▸ Rhythmic large-muscle-group exercise, such as: ▪ Walking ▪ Running ▪ Cycling ▪ Swimming in a nonchlorinated pool
Progression	▸ Progress following the ACE Integrated Fitness Training Model based on client goals and availability.

Muscular Training	
Frequency	▸ A minimum of 2, preferably 3, nonconsecutive days per week
Intensity	▸ 50–85% 1-RM (lower intensity to start)
Time	▸ 1–3 sets of 8–10 repetitions (10–15 repetitions to start)
Type	▸ All major muscle groups ▸ At least 8–10 exercises to near fatigue ▸ Resistance machines and free weights
Progression	▸ Progress following the ACE Integrated Fitness Training Model based on client goals and availability.

Note: VT1 = First ventilatory threshold; $\dot{V}O_2R$ = Oxygen uptake reserve; HRR = Heart-rate reserve; RPE = Rating of perceived exertion; 1-RM = One-repetition maximum

Source: American College of Sports Medicine (2018). *ACSM's Guidelines for Exercise Testing and Prescription* (10th ed.). Philadelphia: Wolters Kluwer.

TABLE 9-8

How to Measure Peak Flow Rate

▸ Have the client stand, take a deep breath, and place their lips around the cardboard mouthpiece that slides into the peak flow meter.

▸ The client should blow as fast and as hard as possible into the peak flow meter.

▸ Perform the peak flow measurement three times and record the highest score.

▸ Perform the peak flow measurement during the early stages of the program to obtain baseline values for the client.

TABLE 9-9

What to Do if a Client Is Having an Asthma Attack

▸ If episode occurs during exercise, reduce intensity, but avoid stopping the workout suddenly.

▸ Encourage the client to take their own rescue medication as prescribed.

▸ Encourage the person to breathe deeply and slowly (diaphragmatic breathing).

▸ A warm drink may help loosen mucus secretions. Do not allow the client to drink cold beverages, since this may cause further tightening of the chest.

▸ Seek medical attention if symptoms do not improve in a few minutes.

▸ After reducing exercise intensity to minimal, encourage the client to rest in a comfortable position (usually sitting down with the arms placed over a table or chair to "open" up the chest).

BRONCHITIS AND EMPHYSEMA

Two types of COPD commonly seen in the elderly are chronic bronchitis and emphysema. Chronic bronchitis is an inflammation of the **bronchi,** the larger airway tubes in the lungs. This condition causes an irritating and productive cough that lasts up to three months and recurs for at least two consecutive years. It is often linked to heavy cigarette smoking, passive cigarette smoke (i.e., "second-hand smoke"), and occupational/environmental exposure to toxins. Emphysema usually occurs in people between the ages of 60 and 70 years, and is characterized by progressive destruction of the **alveoli,** the sponge-like tissues in the lungs where the exchange of oxygen and carbon dioxide takes place. It also is linked to heavy cigarette smoking. It is important to note that clients with COPD may have emphysema along with other comorbidities. A review of the literature revealed that among the most common conditions associated with COPD are obesity, CAD, ischemic heart disease, osteoporosis, **osteoarthritis,** and depression (Reid et al., 2012). Accordingly, any exercise program developed for an older client with COPD should take into consideration the potential for these comorbidities.

Symptoms

The symptoms of these two chronic obstructive pulmonary diseases are similar, and include dyspnea, coughing, and increased mucus production that can be heard in the chest when coughing and wheezing.

Exercise Guidelines for Clients with Bronchitis and Emphysema

Exercise training for older adults with COPD should include cardiorespiratory exercise and muscular training, with a special focus on balance and functional training (Beauchamp et al., 2017). As with the general senior population, older adults with COPD have a high relative risk of falls. Thus, training an older client who suffers from COPD requires extra vigilance from the exercise professional, as this type of client is at a significantly greater risk for falling (Oliveira et al., 2015).

In addition to the guidelines summarized in Table 9-10, exercise professionals should adhere to the following:

▶ *Consult with the client's healthcare team:* Even though clients with COPD do not require medical clearance before beginning an exercise program, it is a good idea to consult with the client's physician and/or a respiratory therapist for ideas and tips on managing dyspnea during exercise. There is a good possibility that the client may already have undergone some kind of a rehabilitation program, and that there are written reports on the client's physical status that may help the exercise professional develop a safe and effective program.

▶ *Measure peak expiratory flow rate (see Table 9-8) before and after exercise:* This process will help determine the effects of the activity on breathing capacity. Some activities may produce better airflow readings than others. Those that cause the lowest amount of dyspnea should be used in the program.

▶ *Use the dyspnea rating scale:* A rating of dyspnea can be used to gauge the intensity of exercise in persons with COPD (ACSM, 2018). The dyspnea rating scale ranges from 0 to 4 (Table 9-11).

▶ *Emphasize interval-training techniques for clients exhibiting a high degree of dyspnea during exercise:* Providing short periods of rest (one to two minutes) between exercise bouts (one to five minutes in duration) should reduce dyspnea.

▶ *Avoid high-intensity exercise:* Exercises that do not produce huge fluctuations in oxygen cost are safer and more effective for this clientele. High-impact exercises or activities that result in dramatic increases in oxygen cost (e.g., running or walking briskly up a flight of stairs) may cause dyspnea.

▶ *Extend the warm-up:* Each exercise session should be preceded by a 10- to 15-minute warm-up that gradually elevates the client's HR and is similar to what the client will be doing during the conditioning portion of the workout. Walking outdoors or on a treadmill at a pace that allows the individual to comfortably carry on a conversation is an example of a good warm-up activity.

▶ *Focus on relaxation and breathing techniques in the cool-down:* End each exercise session with cool-down activities that include flexibility exercises, relaxation techniques, and breathing exercises. Diaphragmatic breathing and pursed-lip breathing are recommended for persons with COPD. These techniques have been shown to increase the amount of air taken in through the damaged tissues of the lungs and reduce the incidence of dyspnea.

▶ *Teach the client techniques to avoid hyperventilation:* Some clients with COPD have a tendency to hyperventilate during exercise. This causes further dyspnea since shallow breathing does not allow oxygen to reach the deepest layers of the lungs where gases are exchanged. If a client has a tendency to hyperventilate, teach them how to breathe correctly using diaphragmatic and pursed-lip breathing while walking, riding a stationary cycle, or using an upper-arm ergometer.

▶ *Encourage low-intensity resistance exercise and balance training movements:* For muscular endurance activities, incorporate high repetitions at a low resistance to avoid dyspnea. Emphasize smooth, coordinated movements that do not require tremendous variations in breathing rate, as would occur while doing push-ups or pull-ups.

▸ *Exercise programs may need to be modified during the winter months:* Respiratory infections and cold temperatures often worsen COPD, and many clients will have to severely curtail their activity levels during illness or when temperatures drop below freezing. Suggest that clients wear a scarf or surgical mask while traveling to the facility during the winter months. Breathing in cold air before exercise can precipitate dyspnea.

▸ *Encourage smoking cessation:* Some clients with COPD (or their spouses) continue to smoke, even though they have been diagnosed with a serious disease. Provide as much information as possible about smoking-cessation techniques and remind these clients that even second-hand smoke can exacerbate their condition.

▸ *Be familiar with the standard termination criteria for the cardiorespiratory complications:* If any of these signs (see page 210) appear during exercise, stop the activity and contact the client's physician for further advice.

▸ *Consider using an oximeter to record oxygen saturation:* This device ensures that the exercise program is not causing an oxygen saturation level that is too low, which could lead to respiratory complications. Most respiratory therapists recommend that oxygen saturation remain above 85% during exercise (at rest, oxygen saturation is around 97 to 98%). If oxygen saturation drops below 85%, exercise should be stopped and the client should rest and perform diaphragmatic and pursed-lip breathing before resuming the activity.

TABLE 9-10

Exercise Guidelines Summary for Clients with Chronic Bronchitis and Emphysema

Cardiorespiratory Training	
Frequency	▸ At least 3–5 days per week, ideally every day
Intensity	▸ Moderate to vigorous
	▸ Below, at, and above VT1 but below VT2 HR
	▸ 50–80% peak work rate*
	▸ RPE 4–6 (0–10 scale)
Time	▸ 20–60 minutes per session
	▸ Intermittent exercise (i.e., interval training) may be used during initial sessions until longer durations are achieved.
Type	▸ Walking or cycling, upper-body endurance activities to help improve activities of daily living
Progression	▸ Progress following the ACE Integrated Fitness Training Model based on client goals and availability.

Muscular Training	
Frequency	▸ 2–3 days per week
Intensity	▸ 60–70% of 1-RM for beginners' muscular strength
	▸ ≥80% of 1-RM for experienced weight trainers' muscular strength
	▸ <50% of 1-RM for muscular endurance

TABLE 9-10 *(continued)*

Muscular Training	
Time	▸ 2–4 sets of 8–12 repetitions for muscular strength
	▸ ≤2 sets of 15–20 repetitions for muscular endurance
Type	▸ Weight machines, free weights, or body-weight exercise
Progression	▸ Progress following the ACE Integrated Fitness Training Model based on client goals and availability.

*Peak work rate is measured in watts.

Note: VT1 = First ventilatory threshold; VT2 = Second ventilatory threshold; HR = Heart rate; RPE = Rating of perceived exertion; 1-RM = One-repetition maximum

Source: American College of Sports Medicine (2018). *ACSM's Guidelines for Exercise Testing and Prescription* (10th ed.). Philadelphia: Wolters Kluwer.

TABLE 9-11
Dyspnea Rating Scale

0 - No shortness of breath

1 - Light, barely noticeable

2 - Moderate, bothersome

3 - Moderately severe, very uncomfortable

4 - Most severe or intense dyspnea ever experienced

Musculoskeletal Conditions

It is rare to find an older person in their 70s or 80s who does not experience joint pain. Musculoskeletal disorders are common in older adults, with women typically reporting more pain and dysfunction than men (Fejer & Ruhe, 2012). Painful joints could be the result of a variety of musculoskeletal conditions, including one of the various forms of arthritis and problems associated with low-back dysfunction.

ARTHRITIS

The most common cause of joint pain is arthritis, which affects approximately 54.4 million Americans (22.7% of all adults) (Barbour et al., 2017). However, more recently adjusted estimates suggest that arthritis prevalence in the U.S. has been substantially underestimated when including patients who were doctor-diagnosed with arthritis, as well as people who reported joint symptoms consistent with a diagnosis of arthritis. The adjusted estimate suggests that potentially more than 91 million adults in the U.S. are living with arthritis (Jafarzadeh & Felson, 2018).

Although there are more than 100 different diseases or conditions referred to as arthritis, the two most common types are osteoarthritis and rheumatoid arthritis. Arthritis is the leading cause of disability in the U.S., with approximately 43% reporting activity limitations due to arthritis (Barbour et al., 2017). Almost half of all adults with heart disease (49.3%) or diabetes (47.1%) and almost one-third (30.6%) of those who have obesity also have arthritis (Barbour et al., 2017). In general, arthritis prevalence is significantly higher among women (23.5%) than among men (18.1%) and lower among individuals meeting physical-activity recommendations (18.1%) versus those who reported insufficient activity (23.1%) or were almost completely inactive (23.6%) (Barbour et al., 2017).

Osteoarthritis

Osteoarthritis is sometimes referred to as **degenerative joint disease** or **osteoarthrosis.** Osteoarthrosis means an abnormal condition of the joint, which some experts say is a more accurate term than arthritis, which means an inflammation of the joint. There is usually little joint inflammation with osteoarthritis. Most of the pain is due to the progressive deterioration of **articular cartilage,** which covers the ends of the bones inside diarthrodial joints. The joints most often affected by osteoarthritis are the cervical and lumbar spine, hip, knee, and distal joints of the hand (the joints closest to the ends of the fingers).

Osteoarthritis is caused by a deterioration in articular cartilage, normally smooth tissue that allows the ends of the bones to glide without friction. During deterioration, the water content of this cartilage increases, indicating that the collagen that provides its structure is breaking up. The cartilage loses its ability to withstand compressive forces and starts to fray and develop fissures (clefts) that extend into the bone. These bone fragments are called **osteophytes,** or bone spurs. The deteriorating articular cartilage and the accompanying osteophytes create a great deal of pain for millions of older adults.

⚛ EXPAND YOUR KNOWLEDGE

Osteoarthritis of the Knee

The knee is the most often studied joint affected by osteoarthritis. Researchers have determined that body weight is one of the most important modifiable risk factors associated with osteoarthritis of the knee. In older adults, approximately 25% of the onset of knee pain with osteoarthritis could be related to overweight or obesity (Silverwood et al., 2015). These findings, combined with the knowledge that obesity is growing in prevalence and that older adults (who tend to be more affected by osteoarthritis) continue to make up a larger portion of the population, are sobering facts that indicate that exercise professionals are more likely than not to work with individuals who suffer from knee pain brought on by joint deterioration.

Rheumatoid Arthritis

While osteoarthritis is the most common affliction of the joints, rheumatoid arthritis is another condition that may be present among older clientele. Rheumatoid arthritis is a chronic autoimmune disease that results in inflammation of the **synovium,** leading to long-term joint damage, chronic pain, and loss of function or disability (Arthritis Foundation, 2019). In comparison to osteoarthritis, rheumatoid arthritis, which is an autoimmune disease and has a more systemic effect, may manifest itself in the development of heart and lung disease and diabetes. As with osteoarthritis, the quality of life for individuals with rheumatoid arthritis can be improved with exercises that are designed to maintain muscle strength, joint range of motion (ROM), and cardiovascular function.

Symptoms

Many of the symptoms and treatment strategies for osteoarthritis and rheumatoid arthritis are similar and include the following:

▸ *Pain:* Many people equate the pain of arthritis to a nagging, dull toothache. The pain of osteoarthritis is often asymmetrical (e.g., only one knee), although it is not uncommon to feel pain in both joints. Clients who have a high tolerance for pain are able to participate in more activity.

▶ *Decreased ROM:* Another common symptom of arthritis is decreased ROM. Sometimes, this occurs because of a shortening of muscle fibers associated with inactivity; other times it is due to joint destruction. A client may try to protect the joint by becoming inactive, causing further shortening of the muscle fibers.

▶ *Joint instability:* The affected joint often becomes unstable as a result of overstretching the supportive ligaments that protect it. This occurs more often with rheumatoid arthritis than osteoarthritis.

▶ *Muscle weakness:* Muscle weakness is common in older adults with arthritis because they often think that they protect the joint by not exercising. On the contrary, a lack of physical activity leads to other physical problems and can worsen the symptoms of arthritis.

▶ *Diminished endurance:* Just as muscle weakness occurs as a result of inactivity, cardiorespiratory endurance is lower in sedentary persons with arthritis. Many individuals with arthritis do not understand the value of maintaining good cardiorespiratory endurance and think that exercise will do more harm than good.

While this chapter introduces two forms of arthritis, the main focus from this point on will be on osteoarthritis, as it is the type of arthritis most likely to affect the broadest range of older adults.

Exercise Guidelines for Clients with Arthritis

A meta-analysis of the literature strongly supports that exercise is a cornerstone of therapy for persons with arthritis for improving pain and physical function (Goh et al., 2019). No matter how severe the condition, it is extremely important for older clients with osteoarthritis to participate in physical-activity programs, as a deterioration in fitness will clearly worsen their condition. People with arthritis who are deconditioned lose strength, flexibility, and endurance, all of which are needed to overcome the pain and physical limitations associated with this disease.

In addition to the guidelines summarized in Table 9-12, exercise professionals should adhere to the following.

Flexibility

People reluctant to move a painful joint may experience extreme tightness in the muscles, ligaments, and tendons that surround it. Although protecting the joint from further injury is important, immobilizing the joint may do more harm than good by increasing the tightness/stiffness in and around it. Therefore, flexibility exercises are an essential component of the exercise program for an older adult with arthritis.

Follow these general guidelines when developing a flexibility program:

▶ *Avoid exercises that provoke pain:* Discontinue flexibility exercises that cause immediate pain, or pain that develops within 24 to 48 hours after exercise.

▶ *Teach clients to distinguish between soreness and pain:* Soreness, which often occurs when sedentary people begin an exercise program, is usually located in the muscle. Pain originates in the joint and indicates that the client may have exercised that joint too strenuously. Soreness will ease after the first few weeks of the program, but pain will last longer than a few weeks and may result in further joint damage.

▸ *Respect the client's tolerance for static stretching*: Each client has an individual threshold for holding a static stretch. Some will be able to hold a stretch for six to eight seconds, others longer.

▸ *Pay attention to the client's overall posture and joint mechanics*: Make sure flexibility exercises are executed correctly with proper form, and do not allow the client to bounce during the stretch.

Strength Exercises

It is a misconception that strength exercises will do more harm than good for clients with arthritis. The American College of Rheumatology and the Arthritis Foundation recommend muscular training, among other forms of physical exercise, in the non-pharmacologic treatment of arthritis (Kolasinski et al., 2020). Strength exercises help people to better cope with their arthritis by improving muscle function and reducing the load on the joint. Furthermore, performing strength training with arthritic joints can improve functional mobility.

Follow these general strength-training guidelines for older adults with arthritis:

▸ *Avoid pain and painful ROM*: Excessive weight training can cause an inflammatory response that results in pain and reduced mobility. Therefore, make sure the client experiences no pain during the activity (i.e., discomfort or soreness is acceptable, but there should be no pain).

▸ *Consider using isometric exercises to build strength in affected joints, particularly during the initial phase of training*: If the joints are severely damaged, isometric exercise may be the preferred method of muscular conditioning. Isometric muscle actions should last approximately six to eight seconds and be performed two to three times for each muscle group. Isometric exercises can be done with or without weights, depending on the client's initial levels of strength.

▸ *Progress to moderate-intensity resistance training*: Once clients adapt to isometric resistance training, they should begin participating in moderate-intensity progressive resistance training of all the major muscle groups. All exercises should be performed within a pain-free ROM.

Cardiorespiratory Endurance

Clearly, the best cardiorespiratory exercise for a client with arthritis is one that does not cause pain. People who have arthritis have successfully performed water exercise for years. Some fitness facilities even have swim programs designed specifically for people with arthritis. The pool temperature is elevated and participants perform different exercises in the water. (Note: The pool also can be used to develop flexibility and strength.)

Cardiorespiratory exercise equipment that can be used by most clients with arthritis without causing high levels of pain includes the arm ergometer (particularly for clients who have knee or hip arthritis), recumbent bike, and recumbent stepper. These machines do not excessively overload the joints and can usually be used for several minutes without pain. A combination arm-leg device such as a cycle ergometer or recumbent stepper with arm action may be a popular choice because clients can use their arms and legs to propel them.

These devices more evenly distribute the load between the upper and lower body, reducing the stress on the hip and knee joints.

Follow these general guidelines for improving the cardiorespiratory endurance of older clients with arthritis:

▸ *Choose activities with smooth, repetitive motions:* Swimming, cycling, and walking are good options.

▸ *Avoid high-impact activities during acute flare-ups:* Jogging or other jarring activities, such as high-impact aerobics or jumping rope, are contraindicated during periods of acute flare-ups for this clientele. There is no strong evidence that suggests that individuals with arthritis cannot participate in high-intensity activities. However, since the majority of individuals with arthritis have low cardiorespiratory fitness, they should start at intensities that avoid aggravating joint symptoms.

▸ *If necessary, start with intervals of exercise and progress to longer durations:* Use interval-training or circuit-training routines with clients who are unable to tolerate continuous activity. For example, a client might spend one minute on the recumbent cycle, followed by a 30-second rest, and then complete another minute on the recumbent cycle. The client may do this for five or 10 minutes and then move to a new machine that uses different joints, such as the arm ergometer.

▸ *Keep the intensity level within the client's comfort zone:* The duration and frequency of exercise is more important than the intensity. Encourage 60-minute exercise sessions that allow the client to take periodic breaks. The client may be actually exercising for only 30 minutes, but still need a full 60 minutes to incorporate rest periods.

▸ *Avoid strenuous exercise during a flare-up:* A client with rheumatoid arthritis may occasionally have an acute flare-up. This is called an exacerbation, which means that the arthritis has worsened. This has nothing to do with the exercise program but is instead part of the disease's progression. Gentle full-ROM exercises are appropriate during these periods (ACSM, 2018).

▸ *Ask the client about fatigue levels and proceed accordingly:* Clients with arthritis will often fatigue easily. This may be due to a number of problems, including a low fitness level, side effects from certain medications, and not sleeping well at night. Be sure not to cause excessive fatigue during the early stages of the program when the client is at high risk for dropping out.

TABLE 9-12

Exercise Guidelines Summary for Clients with Arthritis

Cardiorespiratory Training	
Frequency	▸ 3–5 days per week
Intensity	▸ Below VT1 HR; can talk comfortably; RPE 0.5–4 (0–10 scale)
	▸ Moderate (40–59% HRR or $\dot{V}O_2R$) to vigorous (≥60% HRR or $\dot{V}O_2R$) intensity*
	▸ Light intensity (e.g., 30–39% HRR or $\dot{V}O_2R$) may be necessary for deconditioned clients with arthritis.

Continued on the next page

TABLE 9-12 *(continued)*

Cardiorespiratory Training	
Time	▸ Minutes per session will be dictated by the client's tolerance to exercise. ▸ At least 150 minutes per week of light or moderate intensity, 75 minutes of vigorous intensity, or a combination of the two

Type	▸ A variety of low-impact rhythmic large-muscle-group exercise:
	  ▪ Walking
	  ▪ Cycling
	  ▪ Swimming
	▸ High-impact activities such as running are not recommended for those with lower-extremity arthritis.

Progression	▸ Progress following the ACE Integrated Fitness Training Model based on client goals and availability.

Muscular Training	
Frequency	▸ 2–3 days per week
Intensity	▸ 50–80% 1-RM, with lower initial intensities
Time	▸ 2–4 sets of 8–12 repetitions
Type	▸ All major muscle groups ▸ Include machines, free weights, and body weight ▸ Perform all exercises within a pain-free range of motion.
Progression	▸ Progress following the ACE Integrated Fitness Training Model based on client goals and availability.

*Moderate intensity = Heart rates <VT1 where speech remains comfortable and is not affected by breathing; Vigorous intensity = Heart rates from ≥VT1 to <VT2 where clients feel unsure if speech is comfortable.

Note: HR = Heart rate; RPE = Rating of perceived exertion; HRR = Heart-rate reserve; $\dot{V}O_2R$ = Oxygen uptake reserve; 1-RM = One-repetition maximum; VT1 = First ventilatory threshold; VT2 = Second ventilatory threshold

Source: American College of Sports Medicine (2018). *ACSM's Guidelines for Exercise Testing and Prescription* (10th ed.). Philadelphia: Wolters Kluwer.

LOW-BACK PAIN

Low-back pain (LBP) is a common complaint among individuals of all ages but may become a chronic problem for older persons who also have arthritis. Previously, LBP was considered a generally short-lasting condition with spontaneous recovery as the most likely outcome. Because of the complexity of providing specific diagnoses for LBP, it became common to classify it according to the duration of the pain [i.e., acute (lasting fewer than three months in duration) or chronic (lasting longer than three months)], with chronicity being considered relatively uncommon. More recently, however, LBP is considered to be a recurring or persistent condition with a fluctuating course over time (Lemeunier, Leboeuf-Yde, & Gagey, 2012). LBP has been shown to be a major problem globally, with the highest prevalence among males (Fatoye, Gabrye, & Odeyemi, 2019).

Exercise Guidelines for Clients with Low-back Pain

Exercises for clients experiencing an exacerbation of LBP should be developed by the client's physician and/or physical therapist. However, once the client is cleared to return to full physical activity, exercise professionals can play an important role in preventing another occurrence of LBP.

▶ *Prevent deconditioning of the muscles surrounding the spine:* A major goal of an exercise program for persons with chronic LBP is to prevent deconditioning. The person may avoid movement for fear of re-injuring the back; in the interim, the muscles weaken and the low back loses some of its extensibility.

▶ *Avoid painful ROM:* The exercise program must remain within the client's pain threshold and should not exacerbate any underlying conditions. Sharp pain may be an indication that the exercise is harmful to the condition.

▶ *Choose low- or nonimpact activities:* Cardiorespiratory exercise that puts minimal stress on the back may help to maintain cardiorespiratory endurance. Walking or recumbent cycling while maintaining good posture may be good modalities for mitigating LBP in some clients. Also, consider adding pole walking (e.g., Nordic walking) as an effective way to participate in an aerobic activity that helps to unload the spine. Check with each client to determine which type of exercise produces the least amount of pain or discomfort.

▶ *Focus on core function and fundamental movements:* Strength and flexibility exercises may be helpful for some clients with LBP (see pages 270–271). Be sure to check with the client's physician or physical therapist regarding any contraindications and exercise limitations for an older client with LBP. Exercises that focus on core function and functional movement patterns are ideal for working with clients who have chronic LBP.

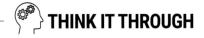 **THINK IT THROUGH**

Mobility Limitations

Many older clients have mobility limitations, whether due to arthritis, LBP, obesity, balance problems, or a number of other issues. How will you address these limitations in your training sessions? Spend some time developing a plan for helping clients with mobility problems achieve success in their workouts. For example, how will you modify floor exercises for clients who cannot make it down to the floor? What will you do to accommodate individuals who use mobility-assistance devices such as canes or walkers?

Metabolic Disorders

The three most common metabolic disorders seen in older adults are diabetes, obesity, and osteoporosis. The following statistics shed light on this sobering trend:

▶ The overall prevalence of diabetes has risen sharply in the U.S. since 1999 (i.e., from 1999 to 2016, the prevalence of diagnosed diabetes rose from 9.5% to 12%) [Centers for Disease Control and Prevention (CDC), 2020]. Diabetes is prevalent in 26.8% of the population who are 65 years or older (CDC, 2020).

▶ The number of older adults (>60 years) categorized as having obesity [body mass index (BMI) ≥30 kg/m²] is 42.8%, with almost 6% categorized as having extreme obesity (BMI ≥40 kg/m²) (Hales et al., 2020).

▶ Approximately 10 million Americans over the age of 50 have osteoporosis, with an additional 43 million diagnosed with **osteopenia** or low bone mass (Wright et al., 2014).

DIABETES

Diabetes is characterized by reduced **insulin** secretion by the pancreatic beta cells and/or reduced sensitivity to insulin. Diabetes causes abnormalities in the metabolism of carbohydrate, protein, and fat and, if left untreated, can be deadly. This is of particular concern since the symptoms of diabetes are not always evident in the early stages. Overall, the risk for death among people with diabetes is about twice that of people of similar age but without diabetes (Röckl et al., 2017). However, there is a significant decline in the incidence of deaths caused by diabetes, which means those with diabetes will be living longer, many with significant chronic comorbidities (Gregg et al., 2014).

People with diabetes are at greater risk for numerous health problems, including kidney failure, nerve disorders, and eye problems, and are two to four times more likely to develop CVD. Prolonged and frequent elevation of blood sugar can damage the capillaries, a condition called microangiopathy that leads to poor circulation. In addition, people with diabetes are at greater risk for permanent nerve damage, which can lead to **peripheral neuropathy** and retinopathy.

There are two main types of diabetes. **Type 1 diabetes** is caused by the destruction of the insulin-producing beta cells in the pancreas, which leads to little or no insulin secretion. Type 1 diabetes generally occurs in childhood and regular insulin injections are required to regulate blood glucose levels.

The typical symptoms of type 1 diabetes are excessive thirst and hunger, frequent urination, weight loss, blurred vision, recurrent infections, and fatigue. During periods of insulin deficiency, a higher-than-normal level of glucose remains in the blood because of reduced uptake and storage. A portion of the excess glucose is excreted in the urine, which leads to increased thirst and appetite and weight loss. Elevated blood glucose is a condition known as hyperglycemia.

Type 2 diabetes is the most common form of diabetes, affecting 90 to 95% of all patients with diabetes (CDC, 2020). It typically occurs in adults who have overweight and is characterized by **insulin resistance,** a reduced sensitivity of insulin target cells to available insulin. Consequently, as the need for insulin rises, the pancreas gradually loses its ability to produce sufficient amounts of it, leading to type 2 diabetes. Unfortunately, increasing numbers of children are being diagnosed with type 2 diabetes, making the once-common term "adult-onset diabetes" obsolete. Some people with type 2 diabetes never exhibit any of the classic symptoms of diabetes. Treatment usually includes diet modification, exercise, and medication.

Type 2 diabetes also is characterized by frequent states of hyperglycemia, but without the increased **catabolism** of fats and proteins. Because a majority of individuals with type 2 diabetes have obesity or a history of obesity, it is important to note that this condition is often reversible with permanent weight loss.

Effective Diabetes Control

Long-term regulation of blood glucose levels is necessary to effectively control diabetes. In type 1 diabetes, glucose regulation is achieved through regular glucose assessment, proper diet, exercise, and appropriate insulin medication. For type 2 diabetes, it is achieved through lifestyle changes centered around proper diet, weight management, exercise, and oral hyperglycemic agents or insulin if needed. A well-designed diet and exercise regimen can result in weight loss and weight control, improved circulation and cardiorespiratory fitness, a reduced need for medication, improved self-image, and a better ability to deal with stress.

Exercise Guidelines for Clients with Diabetes

In addition to the guidelines summarized in Table 9-13, exercise professionals should adhere to the following:

▸ *Emphasize frequency and duration:* The intensity, frequency, and duration of exercise will depend to a large extent on the severity of the diabetes and the client's initial fitness level. In general, emphasize frequency and duration over intensity.

▸ *Clients with obesity should follow guidelines for obesity:* If a client has type 2 diabetes as well as overweight or obesity, follow the guidelines presented here along with the guidelines recommended for obesity on pages 368–370.

▸ *Encourage self-care for the feet:* A common side effect of type 1 diabetes is foot ulcers. Diabetes causes deterioration of the small blood vessels in the feet, diminishing blood flow to these tissues and resulting in foot ulcers. Foot ulcers can last several months or longer and are exacerbated by high-impact exercise, such as jogging. Discourage clients with foot problems from participating in weight-bearing, jarring exercises such as jogging or racquet sports.

▸ *Ensure that clients understand their own glucose medication–management as it relates to exercise:* Be aware that clients with type 1 diabetes must coordinate insulin shots and food intake with their exercise program. Too much exercise, too much insulin, or too little food can cause glucose levels to drop to a dangerously low level. Low blood sugar levels (<70 mg/dL) prior to initiating an exercise session is a relative contraindication and most diabetic clients who use insulin will need to ingest up to 15 grams of carbohydrate before an acute bout of exercise if blood glucose levels are ≤100 mg/dL.

▸ *Know the signs and symptoms of hypoglycemia:* An exercise professional's major concern when working with older clients with type 1 diabetes should be a condition known as **hypoglycemia,** or what some experts call an insulin reaction. This is defined as a blood glucose level less than 70 mg/dL. An extremely dangerous situation could develop when blood glucose levels drop below this value. Table 9-14 describes the signs and symptoms of an insulin reaction. Exercising under these conditions is a serious hazard and should be avoided until food is consumed and glucose levels rise above 100 mg/dL. Refer to Table 9-15 for guidelines on what to do if a client is having an insulin reaction.

▸ *Provide time for clients to monitor their blood glucose levels before, during, and after exercise:* In older individuals with type 2 diabetes, the occurrence of hypoglycemic unawareness and declining cognitive function is a critical factor in exercise blood glucose management (ACSM, 2018). Become familiar with a small, pocket-size device called a glucometer that measures blood glucose levels with a single drop of blood. Clients who have trouble regulating their glucose levels should bring a glucometer to the exercise session so that blood glucose levels can be checked before, during, and after the activity. If blood glucose levels drop below 100 mg/dL, a small snack (e.g., orange juice or snack bar) should be consumed before the exercise session continues. Clients who present with hyperglycemia (≥300 mg/dL) but feel good and have no ketones present (blood or urine) may continue to exercise up to a moderate intensity (ACSM, 2018). Exercise should be postponed if both hyperglycemia and ketones are present. It is also suggested that individuals with type 1 diabetes test for urine ketones when blood glucose levels are ≥250 mg/dL prior to beginning an exercise session.

▸ *Be aware of the client's medications and their potential effects on exercise:* Clients who have type 1 diabetes and are taking beta blockers for a heart condition have a higher risk for developing hypoglycemia because the drugs mask the symptoms of an insulin reaction.

TABLE 9-13

Exercise Guidelines Summary for Clients with Diabetes

Cardiorespiratory Training	
Frequency	▸ 3–7 days per week ▸ 3 days of vigorous or 5 days of moderate intensity (greater regularity may facilitate diabetes management)

Intensity	▸ Moderate intensity
	  ▪ Below VT1 HR; can talk comfortably
	  ▪ 40–59% HRR or $\dot{V}O_2R$
	  ▪ RPE 3–4 (0–10 scale)
	▸ Vigorous intensity
	  ▪ HR from VT1 to just below VT2
	  ▪ 60–89% HRR or $\dot{V}O_2R$
	  ▪ RPE 5–6 (0–10 scale)

Time	▸ Type 1 diabetes
	  ▪ 150 minutes/week at moderate intensity; 75 minutes at vigorous intensity, or combination of both
	▸ Type 2 diabetes
	  ▪ 150 minutes/week at moderate intensity

Type	▸ A variety of rhythmic large-muscle-group exercises
Progression	▸ Progress following the ACE Integrated Fitness Training Model based on client goals and availability.
Muscular Training	
Frequency	▸ A minimum of 2 nonconsecutive days per week, preferably 3
Intensity	▸ 50–85% 1-RM (lower intensity to start)

TABLE 9-13 *(continued)*

Muscular Training	
Time	▶ 1–3 sets of 8–10 repetitions (10–15 repetitions to start)
Type	▶ All major muscle groups ▶ At least 8–10 exercises to near fatigue ▶ Resistance machines and free weights
Progression	▶ Progress following the ACE Integrated Fitness Training Model based on client goals and availability.

Note: VT1 = First ventilatory threshold; HR = Heart rate; HRR = Heart-rate reserve; $\dot{V}O_2R$ = Oxygen uptake reserve; RPE = Rating of perceived exertion; VT2 = Second ventilatory threshold; 1-RM = One-repetition maximum

Source: American College of Sports Medicine (2018). *ACSM's Guidelines for Exercise Testing and Prescription* (10th ed.). Philadelphia: Wolters Kluwer.

TABLE 9-14

Symptoms of an Insulin Reaction (Hypoglycemia)

▶ Anxiety, uneasiness
▶ Insomnia
▶ Irritability
▶ Nausea
▶ Extreme hunger
▶ Confusion
▶ Double vision
▶ Sweating, palpitations
▶ Headache
▶ Loss of motor coordination
▶ Pale, moist skin
▶ Strong, rapid pulse

TABLE 9-15

What to Do If a Client Is Having an Insulin Reaction

▶ Stop the activity immediately.
▶ Have the client consume a quickly absorbing carbohydrate, such as fruit juice, jelly beans, or soda (not diet soda).
▶ Have the person sit down and check their blood glucose level with a glucometer.
▶ Allow the client to rest and return to normal function.
▶ When the client feels better, have them recheck the blood glucose level.
▶ If the blood glucose level is above 100 mg/dL, and the client feels better, resume activity.

OBESITY

The pervasiveness of obesity in the older adult population has been under-studied, even though one-third or more of U.S. adults aged 60 years and older have body weights in the obese range [body mass index (BMI) >30 kg/m^2] (Porter Starr et al., 2016). Often, overweight and obesity are described simplistically as the result of an imbalance between calories consumed (energy intake) and calories expended (energy expenditure). An increased energy intake, without an equal increase in energy expenditure, leads to an increase in weight.

Similarly, decreased energy expenditure with no change in energy intake will also result in an energy imbalance and lead to weight gain. While these are contributing variables, obesity is a multifactorial disease involving a complex interplay among environmental, behavioral, genetic, and hormonal factors. With a multidimensional view of health and wellness, exercise professionals are in a unique position to offer much-needed support as key allies in the fight against obesity.

Once associated with high-income countries, obesity is now also prevalent in low- and middle-income countries. Worldwide projections by the WHO (2020) indicate that 1.9 billion people age 18 years or older have overweight, with approximately 650 million of them having obesity. Some contributing factors to this epidemic can be attributed largely to the progression from a rural lifestyle to a highly technological urban existence, and the tempting capacity of the modern environment to encourage individuals to eat more and move less. Almost all countries are experiencing this dramatic increase in overweight and obesity.

Excess body weight is associated with an increased likelihood to develop heart disease, hypertension, type 2 diabetes, sleep disorders, gallstones, breathing problems, musculoskeletal disabilities, and certain forms of cancer (endometrial, breast, and colon) (National Institutes of Health, 2012). It is also associated with reduced life expectancy and early mortality (ACSM, 2018). In addition, obesity has a deleterious effect on the economy of all countries, as it increases the associated costs for treating the related diseases.

Exercise Guidelines for Clients with Obesity

In addition to the guidelines summarized in Table 9-16, exercise professionals should adhere to the following:

▸ *Progress to a frequency of at least five days per week:* Exercising three days per week is a good start for clients with obesity who are over the age of 65. As the client adapts to the program, progressively work up to five days per week, varying the program on alternating days can help to prevent boredom.

▸ *Start with shorter bouts of exercise:* The higher the level of obesity, the more difficult it will be to exercise. For this reason, it is important to encourage clients to move more, sit less, and successfully complete bouts of exercise of any duration. Start with an amount of exercise that can be comfortably completed using multiple components of fitness and gradually increase the frequency and duration. For example, a client may begin with three, 10-minute bouts of exercise: 10 minutes of cardiorespiratory activity (e.g., stationary cycling), 10 minutes of muscular training (e.g., fundamental movements such as squats, presses, and pulls), and 10 minutes of flexibility exercises. Add minutes to each area of fitness as the client becomes more capable and comfortable with the program. Provide as much rest as is necessary to prevent premature fatigue. The major objective of exercise for clients with obesity is to keep them moving, so intensity should not be a primary focus of the program, especially during the early stages. Use RPE to gauge exercise intensity.

▸ *Focus on muscular training:* Muscular training to improve strength and muscular function should be a cornerstone of programming. Due to possible frailty, start with higher repetitions (10 to 15) for one set.

▸ *Introduce weight-bearing exercise slowly:* Weight-bearing activities may be difficult for the novice exerciser who has obesity. Try to incorporate non-weight-bearing activities, such as water exercise, arm and leg cycling, and machine-assisted muscular training.

▸ *Start off with low-intensity exercise:* Clients with obesity will be more susceptible to injury, fatigue, and dehydration because of their excess weight. Because these conditions make people more likely to drop out of the program, do not ask this clientele to exercise too strenuously.

▸ *Be respectful of the client's physical challenges and emotional struggles:* People with obesity generally have very low self-esteem, so be generous with meaningful praise and encouragement, and avoid placing the client in an uncomfortable situation.

▸ *Incorporate strategies to encourage healthy eating:* Develop educational talking points on dietary guidelines for this clientele.

TABLE 9-16

Exercise Guidelines Summary for Clients with Overweight and Obesity

Cardiorespiratory Training	
Frequency	▸ At least 5 days per week

Intensity	▸ Initially moderate intensity
	  ▪ Below VT1 HR; can talk comfortably
	  ▪ 40–59% HRR or $\dot{V}O_2R$
	  ▪ RPE 3–4 (0–10 scale)
	▸ Progress to vigorous intensity
	  ▪ HR from VT1 to just below VT2; cannot say more than a few words without pausing for a breath
	  ▪ RPE 5–6 (0–10 scale)

Time	▸ Initially progress to at least 30 minutes per day ▸ Increase to 60 minutes or more per day ▸ For weight-loss maintenance, achieve a weekly goal of at least 250 minutes ▸ Multiple daily bouts of activity can be used to achieve target

Type	▸ Rhythmic large-muscle-group exercise, such as:
	  ▪ Walking
	  ▪ Cycling
	  ▪ Swimming

Progression	Progress following the ACE Integrated Fitness Training Model based on client goals and availability.
Muscular Training	
Frequency	▸ 2–3 nonconsecutive days per week
Intensity	▸ 60–70% 1-RM (gradually increase to enhance muscle mass and strength)
Time	▸ 2–4 sets of 8–12 repetitions
Type	▸ All major muscle groups ▸ Resistance machines and free weights

Continued on the next page

TABLE 9-16 *(continued)*

Muscular Training	
Progression	▸ Progress following the ACE Integrated Fitness Training Model based on client goals and availability.

Note: VT1 = First ventilatory threshold; HR = Heart rate; HRR = Heart-rate reserve; V̇O₂R = Oxygen uptake reserve; RPE = Rating of perceived exertion; VT2 = Second ventilatory threshold; 1-RM = One-repetition maximum

Source: American College of Sports Medicine (2018). ACSM's Guidelines for Exercise Testing and Prescription (10th ed.). Philadelphia: Wolters Kluwer.

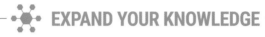 **EXPAND YOUR KNOWLEDGE**

Sarcopenic Obesity

In the older adult, obesity may be compounded by the loss of muscle mass and function. **Sarcopenic obesity** is defined as having both **sarcopenia** (the age-related loss of muscle mass and either low muscular strength or low physical performance) and obesity. With age, there is a decline of **fat-free mass** and **resting energy expenditure** (Amdanee et al., 2018), as well as a decline of 30 to 50% in skeletal muscle mass and function by the time individuals reach approximately 80 years of age (Akima et al., 2001). As there is a lack of a consistent definition for either sarcopenia or obesity, an accurate prevalence rate is challenging to determine.

Individuals with sarcopenic obesity are at higher risk for developing frailty and disability (Tyrovolas et al., 2016). The risk of falls, fractures, depression, and decreased mobility increase with the presence of sarcopenic obesity (Benjumea et al., 2018; Chang et al., 2017; Steihaug et al., 2017; Tanimoto et al., 2014). It has also been found that low or declining muscle mass is emerging as a negative predictive factor associated with higher morbidity and mortality in older individuals with obesity (Zhang et al., 2019). Working to improve muscular function while preventing further weight gain is paramount to improving sarcopenic obesity.

OSTEOPOROSIS

Osteoporosis is a metabolic bone disease that affects about 10 million older adults (Wright et al., 2014). It is characterized by a gradual reduction in bone mass, which can eventually lead to bone fractures and pain, especially in the back and in weight-bearing bones. Osteopenia is a less severe condition associated with osteoporosis and occurs when bone mineral density is lower than normal but has not yet reached osteoporotic levels. People with osteopenia are at an elevated risk for developing osteoporosis. Like hypertension, osteoporosis has been referred to as a silent disease because there are frequently no clinical symptoms until a fracture occurs.

Osteoporosis and osteopenia greatly increase the risk of fractures, especially in elderly women. Fractures associated with osteoporosis are often seen in the thoracic vertebrae (i.e., compression fractures that lead to excessive **kyphosis**), the neck of the femur (hip), and the wrist. Fractures of the hip, typically due to a fall, are devastating, as they reduce individuals' quality of life and are associated with a 30% one-year mortality rate in women and a 43% one-year mortality rate in men (Guzon-Illescas et al., 2019). Osteoporotic fractures can also occur through routine bending, lifting, and even coughing. Fortunately, there is compelling evidence that bone mineral density increases, and the risk of falls and fractures decreases, with regular participation in physical activity (Watson et al., 2018).

Exercise Guidelines for Clients with Osteoporosis

In addition to the guidelines summarized in Table 9-17, exercise professionals should adhere to the following:

▸ *Avoid excessive twisting, bending, and compression of the spine:* Clients with osteoporosis at high risk of fracture should not perform exercises involving twisting, bending, and compression of the spine, which increase the risk of spine fracture. Trunk extension exercises and abdominal stabilization exercises can be done safely.

▸ *Encourage weight-bearing activity:* Clients with osteoporosis can safely perform a variety of cardiorespiratory physical activities and muscular training. Intensity of the exercise sessions should initially be light to moderate and progressively increase based on the individual's capability.

▸ *Avoid movements or environments that could lead to a fall:* Quick, jarring movements or exercise on slick surfaces or around tripping hazards should be avoided to minimize the risk of a fall or fracture.

▸ *Take extra precaution with back exercises:* If excessive kyphosis is present, avoid excessive overloading of the back. Unsupported flexion at the spine could cause excessive loading of the lower vertebrae. Be careful when performing any back exercises, and if the client complains of pain, stop the activity.

TABLE 9-17

Exercise Guidelines Summary for Clients with Osteoporosis

Cardiorespiratory Training	
Frequency	▸ 4–5 days per week
Intensity	▸ Moderate (40–59% HRR or $\dot{V}O_2R$) intensity,* although some clients may be able to tolerate more intense exercise ▸ Below VT1 HR; can talk comfortably; RPE 3–4 (0–10 scale)
Time	▸ Begin with 20 minutes and gradually progress to a minimum of 30 minutes and a maximum of 45–60 minutes
Type	▸ Emphasize weight-bearing, large-muscle-group activities, such as: ▪ Walking ▪ Stair climbing/descending
Progression	▸ Progress following the ACE Integrated Fitness Training Model based on client goals and availability.
Muscular Training	
Frequency	▸ Start with 1–2 nonconsecutive days and possibly progress to 2–3 days per week.
Intensity	▸ Adjust resistance so that the last 2 repetitions are challenging to perform. ▸ High-intensity training is beneficial for those who can tolerate it.

Continued on the next page

TABLE 9-17 *(continued)*

Muscular Training	
Time	▸ Begin with 1 set of 8–12 repetitions and increase to 2 sets after approximately 2 weeks; no more than 8–10 exercises per session
Type	▸ Exercises involving each major muscle group with an emphasis on bone-loading forces ▸ Exercises while standing that emphasize balance, gait, and functional movements
Progression	▸ Progress following the ACE Integrated Fitness Training Model based on client goals and availability.

*Moderate intensity = Heart rates <VT1 where speech remains comfortable and is not affected by breathing; Vigorous intensity = Heart rates from ≥VT1 to <VT2 where clients feel unsure if speech is comfortable.

Note: HRR = Heart-rate reserve; $\dot{V}O_2R$ = Oxygen uptake reserve; VT1 = First ventilatory threshold; HR = Heart rate; RPE = Rating of perceived exertion; VT2 = Second ventilatory threshold

Source: American College of Sports Medicine (2018). *ACSM's Guidelines for Exercise Testing and Prescription* (10th ed.). Philadelphia: Wolters Kluwer.

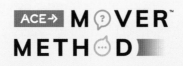

The Initial Consultation

Joan is a 75-year-old retired schoolteacher who provides care for her two youngest grandchildren three days per week for eight hours each day. Joan loves having this time with her grandchildren and has noticed that it has been getting more challenging for her to move around while caring for them. Joan has had pain in her hip and knee joints for the past five years and was recently diagnosed as having both osteoporosis and osteoarthritis. Joan has filled out health and exercise history forms and has received medical clearance from her doctor to begin a moderate-intensity exercise program. You have had the chance to review Joan's paperwork and are meeting in person for the first time to discuss exercise program goals and concerns, as she is apprehensive about beginning an exercise program.

The following is an example of how to use the principles of the ACE Mover Method™ and the ACE ABC Approach™ during an initial consultation. The purpose of this meeting is to use a collaborative, client-centered approach to identify the client's needs, build rapport, and begin working toward the desired behavior change.

ACE→ ABC APPROACH

Ask: The initial consultation begins with asking powerful open-ended questions. The use of open questioning unlocks the door to a collaborative discussion involving the exploration of the client's expectations.

Exercise Professional: Hi, Joan! It is great to meet you. Thank you for taking the time to complete all of the paperwork I sent you and for following through with contacting your doctor to find out if she has any specific exercise guidelines to follow. I appreciate your effort!

Client: You're welcome and it is nice to meet you also! There was quite a bit of paperwork to fill out and it took me a few days to get in touch with my doctor, but I was able to get it all done. I was surprised by how much information I needed to get started with exercise and am glad to know that my safety is a priority.

Exercise Professional: Your safety and your goals, along with enjoyment of this exercise program, will be the top priorities as we move forward. I have had the chance to review the information you sent me and am curious to know what you would like to achieve by working together.

Client: I have been wanting to begin an exercise program for quite some time but until recently never felt much of a reason to be more active. I always thought I was active when I was teaching because I was moving around a lot, but since retiring I have not been regularly active at all. The main reason for me contacting you is that recently, due to some life changes, I have been taking care of my grandchildren multiple days per week for at least eight hours a day and it has been exhausting. That said, it's the best part of my week and I am so lucky to have this time with my family! However, I have noticed that it is hard for me to keep up with all that my grandkids want to do, including playing, holding them, and going on walks while sometimes pulling them in a wagon. Having the strength and endurance to do things with my family is important to me and I don't want to have to tell my grandchildren "no" simply because I can't keep up with them.

Exercise Professional: Getting the most out of this time with your grandchildren is important to you and working together with an exercise professional will help give you the tools you need to develop the strength and endurance you require to keep up with all the fun they want to have. What else would you like to achieve?

Client: You summed it up nicely. Success for me would be moving more easily without pain and for longer periods. I have been extra hesitant with my activity since my diagnosis of osteoarthritis and osteoporosis because I cannot afford to get hurt, as my family is depending on me.

Break down barriers: The client has shared a great deal of information about what she would like to achieve in working together and about her concerns. Now is the time to ask more questions to better understand the client's barriers to being more active.

Exercise Professional: Being more active with your grandchildren is important to you and you want to be able to keep up with them. Beginning an exercise program will help you with this goal. What will be the most challenging part of this process for you?

Client: I think the most challenging thing for me will be overcoming my fear that being more active and adding exercise to my weekly routine will create more pain in my life. Like I said, my family depends on me and I don't want to let them down. Currently, the more I move the more pain I seem to have. I know it is safe for me to exercise because my doctor told me it is and I trust her, but it seems like doing more of what hurts is not a good idea.

Exercise Professional: Thank you for sharing your concerns with me and I appreciate your honesty. What do you already know about the connection between exercise and joint health?

Client: I don't know much at this point, but I do know that being more active is good for my bones and will make them stronger. About the arthritis, I have been reading up on the condition itself and know that this is where my joint pain is coming from. The resources I have been reading also recommend exercise, but I am still hesitant. What else do you think is important for me to know?

Exercise Professional: It sounds like you are actively seeking more information about your conditions and still have some open questions. Arthritis is a common cause of joint pain and the type you have is related to the condition of the joint. Osteoporosis, on the other hand, is a metabolic bone disease related to your bones becoming less dense. The reason you will see exercise mentioned along with treatments for both conditions is because an appropriately designed and personalized exercise program can be safe and effective for supporting your bones and joints. We will work together to take a step-by-step approach to build muscular strength and endurance to support proper alignment and function of your joints and help you to move more easily, and we will do this without creating more pain. Does that make sense?

Client: That does make sense. It sounds like the key is to have a personalized program. The thought of following a program that is just for me and built around my needs sounds like a good idea.

Collaborate: Now that the client's program expectations have been identified and potential barriers have been addressed, the client and exercise professional can collaborate to discuss the next steps.

Exercise Professional: Exactly! The key for us will be to maintain open communication about your progress, energy and pain levels, and enjoyment while implementing evidence-based programming into your weekly routine. What would you like your next steps to be regarding your exercise program?

Client: My initial thought was that I could meet with you in the mornings on the days when I am not caring for my grandkids. I thought two days per week to start would be realistic and I really want to make sure the exercises we do don't hurt. If things go well, I could potentially do three times per week.

Exercise Professional: Two exercise sessions per week is a good start and if you adapt as I believe you will, I will make myself available for the third day if and when you are ready. We will communicate about your pain levels continuously during and after exercise to make sure your intensity level is appropriate. It is also important for you to distinguish the difference between joint pain and muscle soreness.

In this scenario, the exercise professional and client work together to explore client expectations, identify barriers to becoming more physically active, and collaborate on next steps. Also, the exercise professional uses **elicit-provide-elicit** to find out what the client already knows about bone and joint health and exercise, provide additional information, and ensure the information provided makes sense to the client all within a client-centered initial interaction that builds and strengthens rapport.

MENOPAUSE

While **menopause** is not a health condition or a disease, it marks a time in a woman's life when associated physiological changes make her more susceptible to certain health problems such as osteoporosis and heart disease. Menopause literally means the "permanent pause of menses." It is the point in a woman's life that signifies the end of her reproductive capabilities. Biologically speaking, menopause is the last stage of a gradual process in which the ovaries reduce their production of the female sex hormones **estrogen** and **progesterone.**

The average age of women at menopause is 51 years, although it can occur as early as age 40 and as late as the early 60s. Unless it is surgically induced [hysterectomy with bilateral oophorectomy (removal of both ovaries)] or chemically hastened [with prescription drugs that shut down hormone production (e.g., some cancer medications or hormone therapies that treat other disorders)], menopause does not occur suddenly. A period called **perimenopause** usually begins three to five years before the final menstrual cycle. Menopause is considered complete when a woman has been without periods for one year. Women now have a life expectancy of approximately 80 years. As such, women can expect to live some 30 to 40 years in the postmenopausal state.

Hormones and Menopause

Declining levels of the female sex hormone, estrogen, is a predominant factor in the symptoms associated with menopause, as it affects about 300 different tissues throughout the body. Estrogen's many functions include the development of the uterus and breasts and distribution of body fat on the hips and thighs. It is also involved in the tissues of the central nervous system (including the brain), bones, liver, and urinary tract. Estrogen has different forms—the most potent form is estradiol, followed by estrone and estriol. The other major female sex hormone, progesterone, is necessary for thickening and preparing the uterine lining for the fertilized egg.

During her mid-30s, a woman's ovaries begin to decline their hormone production. In the late 40s, the process accelerates and her hormones fluctuate more, causing irregular menstrual cycles and unpredictable episodes of heavy bleeding (perimenopause). Typically, by the early to mid-50s, periods finally end altogether.

Estrogen production does not completely stop after menopause. When ovaries are no longer functional, the source of estrogens in postmenopausal women comes from the conversion of androgens (male sex hormones, such as **testosterone**) by the **enzyme** aromatase. This enzyme is present in multiple structures including adipose tissue, muscle, brain, blood vessels, skin, bone, and uterus and breast tissue.

Symptoms

The symptoms associated with perimenopause and menopause are not caused as much by low estrogen levels, but by fluctuations of high and low estrogen. At menopause, hormone levels do not always decline uniformly. Instead, they alternately rise and fall. These changing ovarian hormone levels affect other glands and tissues in the body, including the breasts, vagina, bones, blood vessels, gastrointestinal tract, urinary tract, and skin. Accordingly, the process of menopause affects a woman as a whole, not just her reproductive organs.

Menopause is an individualized experience that each woman experiences in her own way. Some women notice little difference in their bodies or moods, while others find the change extremely disruptive. As the ovaries become less functional, they produce less estrogen and progesterone, which affect virtually all tissues in the body. For some women, a gradual decrease of estrogen allows the body to slowly adjust to the hormonal change. For others, a sudden decrease in estrogen levels occurs, causing severe symptoms. The following sections include some of the most frequently reported symptoms experienced as women progress through menopause.

VASOMOTOR SYMPTOMS

Vasomotor symptoms (VMS) (i.e., hot flashes and night sweats) are reported by an estimated 70 to 80% of women at some point during the menopausal transition (Gibson et al., 2011). They occur sporadically and often start a year or two before menopause and last, on average, for a total duration of four years (Freeman, Sammel, & Sanders, 2014). A hot flash is a sudden sensation of intense heat in the upper part or all of the body. There may also be heart palpitations, anxiety, irritability, and even feelings of panic associated with a hot flash. The sensation of heat is often followed by profuse sweating and then cold shivering as the body temperature readjusts. Hot flashes can be as mild as a light blush or severe enough to require a change of clothes from profuse sweating.

CHANGES IN MOOD

There appears to be an association between VMS and mood. Women often report distress and embarrassment due to VMS, particularly when they occur in public. VMS may precede a negative mood by triggering feelings of lack of control, embarrassment, and shame, or by disturbed sleep, leading to functional impairment (Gibson et al., 2011). It has been found that there is a bidirectional association between vasomotor and depressive symptoms during perimenopause, meaning women with depressive symptoms are more likely to develop VMS, and women with VMS are more likely to develop depressive symptoms (Worsley et al., 2014).

Thus, exercise professionals should take note that women with VMS may be at increased risk for subsequent negative mood symptoms, as well as for sleep difficulty that may have a broad impact on mood, health, and daily functioning.

VAGINAL AND URINARY TRACT CHANGES

Within five years after menopause, tissues in the vaginal and urinary tract may change. Lower levels of estrogen may cause the vagina to lose elasticity, causing it to become smaller, thinner, and more fragile. Lower levels of estrogen may also cause a change in the acidity of the vagina, resulting in an increased risk of infection. Collectively, these symptoms affect up to 80% of menopausal women and significantly impact their quality of life (Palma et al., 2016).

Exercise, coughing, laughing, or lifting heavy objects can put pressure on the bladder and cause small amounts of urine to leak—a condition called **stress urinary incontinence (SUI).** The incidence of SUI in middle-aged and older women is about 3.5% (Alperin et al., 2019). Having overweight or obesity and a lack of regular exercise may contribute to this condition. It is important to note, however, that SUI is not a normal part of aging. Rather, it is usually a treatable condition that warrants medical evaluation. Pelvic floor training through **Kegel exercises** can help reduce the severity of SUI.

📖 APPLY WHAT YOU KNOW

Kegel Exercise

A Kegel exercise is performed simply by contracting the pelvic muscles, as if trying to stop urine flow in midstream. It is recommended to attempt 60 to 80 Kegel contractions per day, alternating quick squeezes and longer isometric contractions. Kegel exercises may be performed in the following manner:

▶ *Long holds:* Hold for 5 seconds, relax for 5 seconds, working up to a 10-second hold with a 1-second rest period; increase to 30 repetitions

▶ *Short holds:* Hold 1 to 2 seconds, building up to 30 repetitions

WEIGHT GAIN

Many women will experience visible changes with menopause that may include a thickening of the waist, loss of muscle mass, and an increase in fat tissue. Clients who have never had a weight problem before or who typically gain weight in other areas, may experience a focused increase of body fat at the waistline. Weight gain is not a direct result of menopause but is instead related to aging and lifestyle changes. A lack of physical activity and an increase in the number of daily calories consumed are more likely causes. Additionally, the "sudden" weight gain many women report may be due to the new deposition of body fat around the torso. This redistribution of body fat causes an "apple" (male-type pattern) versus a "pear" (female-type pattern) shape, which elevates a postmenopausal woman's risk for heart disease. A decline in estrogen allows the influence of a woman's circulating testosterone to surface. This scenario allows for a more male-type body-fat storage pattern. In other

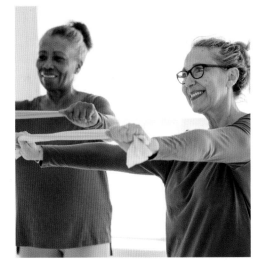

words, there is a shift in fat accumulation to the abdomen (as opposed to the hips and thighs), and an increase in blood triglyceride and cholesterol levels (Anagnostis et al., 2015). All of these changes increase the risk of heart disease for postmenopausal women compared to women who have yet to make the transition.

Postmenopause Health Concerns

Although menopause itself is not considered an unhealthful event, there are two conditions that are more common in postmenopausal women due to the long-term effects of estrogen deficiency—osteoporosis and heart disease. See the related sections in this chapter for more details on these conditions.

Management of Menopause

Menopause is a natural process. It does not necessarily require treatment unless menopausal symptoms are bothersome to the point of affecting a woman's quality of life. The most effective treatment for VMS is menopausal hormone therapy (MHT). The risks and benefits of MHT depend on duration of exposure to the treatment. Some risks (e.g., stroke) are only apparent after one to two years of treatment. Some risks (e.g., breast cancer) increase with longer duration of treatment, while others (e.g., CAD) appear to decrease over time. The standard recommendation for duration of MHT use has been five years or less (and not beyond age 60 years) (Baber et al., 2016).

Exercise Guidelines for Clients in Menopause

Barring no other health conditions, clients going through menopause, as well as postmenopausal women, can follow the guidelines established for healthy adults (see Chapter 8). The hormonal fluctuations of menopause cause a number of side effects, including an increased appetite and, when paired with a lack of physical activity, a loss of lean tissue, which in turn lowers metabolic rate. A lower metabolic rate can lead to increased body fat. Thus, weight gain after menopause is more likely in sedentary women. A regular exercise program can help with weight management and help to decrease a postmenopausal woman's risk of CVD and osteoporosis.

▸ *Ask clients how they are feeling at the beginning of each session:* A woman suffering with menopause symptoms may be experiencing fatigue due to sleep disturbances and hot flashes (night sweats). Thus, the workout might need to be modified for a client who finds it difficult to summon the energy for an intense workout.

▸ *Focus on land-based, weight-bearing exercise:* In general, cardiorespiratory activity should focus on a variety of weight-bearing exercises (e.g., walking, running, and stepping). However, exercise professionals should be mindful of the potential for SUI in postmenopausal clients and provide options for non-impact exercise to reduce the risk of leakage that can accompany the jarring of impact.

▸ *Incorporate muscular training to promote increased muscle strength and bone mass:* Focus on exercises that load the spine and enhance posture (e.g., lat pull-downs, seated rows, and abdominal and low-back exercises). In addition, exercises to protect and strengthen the hips are important (e.g., squats and hip abductor exercises). Balance training should also be a focus of programming for postmenopausal women.

▸ *Enhance daily function through exercise:* Overall fitness goals for clients who are going through or who have gone through menopause include:

- Protecting bone mass and reversing bone loss
- Enhancing cardiovascular function
- Striving for a healthy body composition
- Sustaining exercise as a means of boosting quality of life
- Fall prevention and balance training

Neurological Disorders

DEMENTIA AND ALZHEIMER'S DISEASE

Exercise professionals who specialize in working with senior clients will undoubtedly be exposed to a number of older adults who have memory loss and several different types of cognitive impairments. When a person loses memory and other intellectual capacities (e.g., orientation, attention, calculation, language, and motor skills), it is called **dementia. Alzheimer's disease (AD)** is the most common cause of dementia in older adults. Numerous risk factors for AD have been identified by epidemiologic studies. The most common risk factors for the development of AD are older age, genetics and family history. Age is a major risk factor (32% of individuals have AD over age 85), but some persons are more at risk than others because of their family history (family history in first-degree relatives being the main factor) (Wolters et al., 2017; Hebert et al., 2013). Brain scans of people with AD exhibit structural changes, including neurofibrillary tangles (twisted fragments of protein within nerve cells that clog up the cell), neuritic plaques (abnormal clusters of dead and dying nerve cells, other brain cells, and protein), and senile plaques (areas where products of dying nerve cells have accumulated around protein).

Exercise professionals interested in working with older adults can play a vital role in helping to prevent or mitigate advancing stages of dementia through helping clients with healthy lifestyle behaviors. There is an increasing research interest in possible non-pharmacological interventions, such as lifestyle changes, that can modify vascular risk factors and enhance protective factors through predominantly physical exercise, cognitive stimulation, and healthy diet. A meta-analysis of 19 research studies in humans found that cardiorespiratory exercise

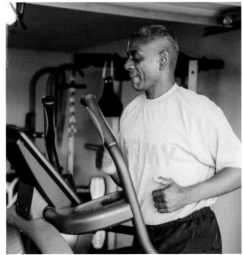

training may delay the deterioration in cognitive function that individuals who are at risk for or have Alzheimer's disease exhibit (Panza et al., 2018). Other forms of exercise, such as muscular training, have very limited amounts of data to support the promotion of brain health. Liu-Ambrose et al. (2010) found that muscular training aided the executive cognitive function of selective attention and conflict resolution among senior women. Nagamatsu et al. (2012) demonstrated that muscular training is associated with modest cognitive benefits in those with cognitive deficiency.

Exercise Guidelines for Clients in the Early Stages of Dementia

▸ *Be understanding of memory loss:* During the early stages of dementia, the client may forget to come to an exercise session or how to do certain exercises. Be patient, understanding, and sensitive to the mental anguish that the person is experiencing. Memory loss is one of the most devastating conditions that older adults may experience during their lifetime. Provide moral support and make regular phone calls to remind them of their exercise class or session.

▸ *Reach out to clients regularly to maintain contact:* Depression is common in this clientele and may lead to a higher dropout rate. To reduce the likelihood of clients dropping out of the program, contact them regularly and make sure their caregivers understand the importance of the exercise program.

▸ *Keep exercise programs simple:* Replace complex exercise routines with simpler activities, such as walking, stationary cycling, and basic stretches. Free weights, treadmills, and other pieces of equipment that require steady control of the body could be dangerous to clients with cognitive impairments or disorders.

▸ *Reward clients often:* Part of the focus of an exercise program for clients with dementia is keeping them interested. Provide lots of meaningful verbal praise and positive reinforcement (e.g., birthday card, phone calls, short letters, and client-of-the-week awards) to encourage adherence.

▸ *Focus on time of day and frequency and duration of exercise:* The intensity of the exercise program is not as important as the frequency and duration. The frequency of exercise should be five days per week, preferably at the same time each day, so that the client develops a structured exercise routine. Mornings are typically better than afternoons since the client will be rested in the morning and may experience more agitation and fatigue as the day progresses.

Exercise Guidelines for Clients in the Later Stages of Dementia

▸ *Plan for emotional outbursts:* Clients with Alzheimer's disease may sometimes exhibit extreme outbursts of anger and physical aggression. Be aware that this behavior has nothing to do with the exercise program. These acts of aggression occur randomly and often will last only a few minutes. If the client disrupts a class, remove them from the group until they have calmed down. Understand that these outbursts are a symptom of the disease and the client often does not understand what they are saying.

▸ *Know when to change settings:* Memory loss will become more pronounced during the later stages of a progressive cognitive disorder. When this occurs, the client may have to switch from a group exercise class to individual training sessions.

▸ *Allow the caregiver to be present during the exercise program:* A person with severe dementia often will not want to be left alone with anyone but the caregiver with whom they are most familiar.

▸ *Stick with the same routine:* It is important to provide a structured exercise routine with little variation for a client in the later stages of a cognitive disorder. An introduction to new activities may confuse them.

▸ *Never leave a client with Alzheimer's disease alone:* They will often wander to other parts of the facility.

▸ *Consider playing relevant music:* Playing music from the client's generation during the exercise session will occasionally bring back memories and may be a good way to keep them interested in the program.

PARKINSON'S DISEASE

Although **Parkinson's disease (PD)** can occur in younger populations, it is most often seen in individuals older than 50. PD is the second most prevalent neurodegenerative disease and is estimated to affect more than 1.2 million people in the U.S. by 2030 (Marras et al., 2018). A chronic, progressive disease that causes movement and postural problems, the condition is caused by a shortage of a chemical produced by the brain called **dopamine,** which is responsible for transmitting messages across nerve pathways in the brain. When there is not enough dopamine available for the brain to send these messages, voluntary muscle movement and coordination are affected. Gait disorders are a hallmark of PD. A slow, short-stepped, shuffling, forward-stooped gait with asymmetrical arm swing is quickly recognizable to clinicians and varies according to the progression of the disease (Ospina et al., 2019). Tremor (shaking), muscle rigidity, and the loss of postural reflexes also characterize the condition. During the early stages of PD, shaking is isolated to the hands. Other symptoms include slowness in ambulation and dressing, difficulty getting out of a chair, and difficulty in starting movements.

Epidemiologic evidence suggests that regular participation in moderate- to vigorous-intensity exercise may protect against PD (Fang et al., 2018).

Exercise Guidelines for Clients with Parkinson's Disease

In addition to the guidelines summarized in Table 9-18, exercise professionals should adhere to the following:

▸ *Incorporate relaxation and flexibility:* Relaxation techniques appear to be very helpful in reducing tremors. Begin relaxation in the supine position and gradually progress to sitting and standing. Flexibility exercises also are an important part of the exercise program. Clients with PD will exhibit a great deal of muscle tightness and may need some assistance with flexibility routines.

▶ *Take precautions to deal with lack of balance:* Since balance is a major problem for people with PD, take every precaution to assure that the exercise environment is safe and that there is a minimal risk of the client falling. Always be in close contact with the client in case they lose balance. If the client is participating in group exercise classes, recommend that they hold onto a railing or chair or sit down during the exercise routine. Balance exercises must be an integral part of the exercise program. Both static and dynamic balance exercises should be incorporated into the routine while sitting and standing.

▶ *Allow extra time:* Clients with PD usually have a delay when starting a movement, so allow more time to initiate movements.

▶ *Focus on breathing:* Breathing exercises also are important for persons with PD. Teach the client to use diaphragmatic and pursed-lip breathing, and have them practice expiring air (e.g., blowing out candles) to strengthen respiratory muscles.

▶ *Incorporate multiple activities:* Encourage participation in cardiorespiratory and strength exercises to prevent secondary conditions, such as osteoporosis and muscle atrophy. Be sure that the machines and equipment selected are safe for a clientele with a high risk of falling. Water exercise is extremely beneficial to this clientele and helps eliminate the risk of a serious fall while performing strength and balance exercises. However, keep in mind that clients with PD may have difficulty dressing and undressing, and may not want to go through this burden in order to swim. Be sure the pool temperature is at least 86° F (30° C).

TABLE 9-18

Exercise Guidelines Summary for Clients with Parkinson Disease

Cardiorespiratory Training	
Frequency	3 days per week
Intensity	▶ Moderate intensity ▶ 40–59% HRR or $\dot{V}O_2R$ ▶ Below VT1 HR, can talk comfortably; RPE 3–4 (0–10 scale)
Time	30 minutes of accumulated or continuous exercise
Type	Rhythmic large-muscle-group activities, such as: ▶ Walking ▶ Cycling ▶ Swimming ▶ Dancing
Progression	Progress following the ACE Integrated Fitness Training Model based on client goals, availability, and disease progression.

TABLE 9-18 *(continued)*

Muscular Training	
Frequency	2 to 3 days per week
Intensity	▸ Lower intensity for beginners to improve strength (40–50% 1-RM) ▸ 60–70% 1-RM for more advanced exercisers
Time	At least 1 set of 8–12 repetitions (10–15 repetitions to start)
Type	All major muscle groups ▸ Avoid free weights and focus on machines, body weight and other resistance equipment ▸ Emphasize the extensor muscles of hip and trunk for maintaining posture ▸ Focus on mobility and fall prevention
Progression	Progress following the ACE Integrated Fitness Training Model based on client goals, availability, and disease progression.

*Moderate intensity = Heart rates <VT1 where speech remains comfortable and is not affected by breathing; Vigorous intensity = Heart rates from ≥VT1 to <VT2 where clients feel unsure if speech is comfortable.

Note: HRR = Heart-rate reserve; $\dot{V}O_2R$ = Oxygen uptake reserve; HR = Heart rate; RPE = Rating of perceived exertion; 1-RM = One-repetition maximum; VT1 = First ventilatory threshold; VT2 = Second ventilatory threshold

Source: American College of Sports Medicine (2018). *ACSM's Guidelines for Exercise Testing and Prescription* (10th ed.). Philadelphia: Wolters Kluwer.

THINK IT THROUGH

Responding to Injuries

Despite careful risk-prevention measures, clients sometimes fall during exercise. Review important safety and first-aid procedures for treating musculoskeletal injuries and develop a plan of action to deal with the unfortunate possibility that a client may fall while completing a workout with you. This should include checking to make sure you have access to a first-aid kit and an emergency procedure policy for contacting emergency medical services, if required.

APPLY WHAT YOU KNOW

Instructional Strategies for Working with Clients Who Have a Neurological Cognitive Disorder

The following instructional strategies will help you design a program that will lower the frustration level of clients with neurological disorders, as well as your own.

▸ *Explain each movement clearly and frequently:* Many clients with neurological impairments will need a frequent explanation of the activity. They will often forget how to perform certain movements and will need to be reminded regularly. Repetition is very important with this group. It may seem boring to the exercise professional but will make the client more successful.

▸ *Keep the exercise routine structured:* For some clients with dementia, a structured exercise routine (e.g., the same room, same equipment, same music, and same professional) may need to be established. New activities or surroundings can be frightening for some clients and will agitate others. Do not change the exercise routines on a regular basis, as doing so may frustrate a client with memory loss.

▸ *Slow down all activities:* Everything will have to be slowed down (e.g., speech, tempo, and activity) for some clients with dementia. This is especially true for clients with PD.

▸ *Touching is a double-edged sword:* Some clients will like to be touched; others will become agitated. The exercise professional may try to show a client a correct movement and the client may become offended. Keep track of which clients are and are not comfortable being touched. As a client gets to know the exercise professional, they may become more willing to be touched during a workout.

▸ *Avoid talking down to the client:* Many exercise professionals talk to older clients with neurological disorders as if they are children, since some of the behaviors are similar to what may be observed in children. This may offend the client or their caregiver. Always treat adult clients like adults.

▸ *Always listen and be responsive:* Occasionally, clients with dementia will say something that does not make sense. Instead of laughing or becoming distracted, understand that this is part of the disease process and respond to the client in an appropriate manner.

▸ *Do not tolerate verbal or physical abuse:* If a client is verbally or physically abusive to you or other members of a fitness facility or class, understand that although this is part of the disorder, it should not be permitted. Respond to such situations appropriately and remove the client from the setting until they calm down.

Visual and Auditory Disorders

Sensory impairment is one of the most common chronic conditions of later life, and both vision and hearing impairment increase with age, as does the prevalence of dual sensory loss (vision and hearing deficits presenting in the same individual). As such, a significant portion of the older U.S. population suffers from vision impairment, hearing impairment, or both. The National Institute on Deafness and Other Communication Disorders (NIDCD, 2020) reports that approximately one in three people in the U.S. between the ages of 65 and 74 has hearing loss, nearly half of those older than 75 have difficulty hearing, and diseases of the eyes, such as **presbyopia,** cataracts, glaucoma, and age-related macular degeneration increase with age. Visual and auditory problems increase the likelihood of falls in the older adult (Gopinath et al., 2016). Therefore, when working with clients who have visual and auditory problems, ensuring that the environment is safe and that communication is as clear as possible are priorities.

Suggestions for Working with Older Adults with Visual Problems

- Use brightly colored tape (e.g., hot pink or yellow, depending on the background color) to mark objects above and below eye level:
  - Because many older clients will not have a good vertical range of vision, machines that contain parts higher than the client's eye level or lower than their knees may be bumped into. Objects left in the middle of the floor have the potential to cause a fall.
  - The display panel on some pieces of exercise equipment may be difficult to see for clients with visual problems. Use brightly colored tape to mark the dials or make arrows that show the client which button to press to increase or decrease time or intensity.
- *Avoid potential trips and falls by choosing the right machines:* Certain types of exercise machines, such as a treadmill, may be hazardous for clients with poor eyesight. To increase safety, use equipment that requires a sitting position, such as a stationary cycle or a recumbent stepper.
- *Use both verbal and physical-guidance instruction techniques:* Because clients with visual impairments may not be able to clearly see movements, verbal instructions must be precise. Physically guide the client through the correct movement to make the verbal instructions clearer.
- *Avoid rearranging equipment:* Clients with visual impairments often use certain pieces of equipment as markers for where they are located in a room. Inform them if any equipment is moved or rearranged.

Suggestions for Working with Older Adults with Auditory Problems

- *Always face the client when speaking:* Some older adults may be able to read lips, and, when this is combined with the little hearing they have, they will be better able to follow instructions.
- *Never eat or chew gum while working with the client:* This will make it difficult for the client to understand the exercise professional's speech.
- *Provide a distraction-free environment:* Reduce background noise or move to a quiet area while talking to the client.
- *Keep hands away from the face when speaking:* If the exercise professional blocks their mouth, a client who can read lips will be unable to understand.
- *Speak in a normal tone and volume:* Do not shout at the client, but speak with a normal, clear tone. Shouting will distort the sound of a voice.
- *Use a combination of visual cues and verbal instructions:* Clients with hearing impairments respond well to visual cues (e.g., pictures of the exercises and demonstrations).

📖 APPLY WHAT YOU KNOW

Networking with Healthcare Professionals

Creating a dynamic, professional network with local healthcare providers such as geriatric physicians, internists, physical therapists, orthopedic specialists, nutritionists, and mental health specialists will provide exercise professionals with important resources for their senior clients and their own practices. Exercise professionals can call upon the healthcare providers' expertise and request their input on program components. Advice can be sought on such things as the level of cardiorespiratory conditioning appropriate for seniors with heart- and lung-related restrictions, and on the safety of specific exercises for muscle and joint conditions. Take the time to establish a relationship of trust and reliability within this network. This is an ongoing process that takes time and careful attention to detail but offers a great deal in return. Adequately involving area health professionals increases a program's safety and credibility. It can also increase participation through direct referrals from these healthcare professionals. Literature from numerous health-related disciplines strongly supports the belief that the right kind of exercise can improve many aspects of health. Therefore, if area healthcare professionals are aware of an exercise professional who offers safe and effective exercise programming for seniors, they will be motivated to refer patients to that program.

Living in an area with close access to a college or university is an added benefit for an exercise professional. It is a good practice to include health and exercise professionals from surrounding academic institutions in the senior services network. This relationship can be mutually beneficial, offering the exercise professional access to current information in the field of exercise and aging, and providing research faculty an opportunity to involve your group in appropriate research projects. For more information on business networking with healthcare providers and other exercise professionals, refer to *The Professional's Guide to Health and Wellness Coaching* (ACE, 2019) and the *ACE Medical Exercise Specialist Manual* (ACE, 2015).

SUMMARY

Older adults constitute the fastest growing segment of the population. More and more older persons with chronic conditions are electing to remain physically active. Despite potential physical limitations, older adults are interested in quality exercise programs delivered by competent exercise professionals. As a result of these demographic shifts, health coaches and exercise professionals will emerge as major players in health promotion among older adults in the coming years. For more information on fitness programming for older adults with chronic conditions, contact your local heart association, lung association, diabetes association, and arthritis association, or log onto the National Center on Physical Activity and Disability website at www.ncpad.org.

REFERENCES

Akima, H. et al. (2001). Muscle function in 164 men and women aged 20–84 yr. *Medicine Science Sports & Exercise,* 33, 220–226.

Aladin, A. et al. (2019). Alcohol consumption and risk of hypertension. *Journal of the American College of Cardiology,* 73, 9.

Alperin, M. et al. (2019). The mysteries of menopause and urogynecologic health: Clinical and scientific gaps. *Menopause,* 26, 1, 103–111.

Amdanee, N. et al. (2018). Age-associated changes of resting energy expenditure, body composition and fat distribution in Chinese Han males. *Physiological Reports,* 6, 23, e13940.

American College of Sports Medicine (2018). *ACSM's Guidelines for Exercise Testing and Prescription* (10th ed.). Philadelphia: Wolters Kluwer.

American Council on Exercise (2019). *The Professional's Guide to Health and Wellness Coaching.* San Diego: American Council on Exercise.

American Council on Exercise (2015). *ACE Medical Exercise Specialist Manual.* San Diego: American Council on Exercise.

Anagnostis, P. et al. (2015). The effect of menopause and gender on lipids and HDL cholesterol subfractions in apparently healthy pre- and postmenopausal women and men. *Maturitas,* 81, 1, 214.

Aronow, W.S. et al. (2011). ACCF/AHA 2011 Expert consensus document on hypertension in the elderly: A report of the American College of Cardiology Foundation Task Force on Clinical Expert Consensus Documents. *Circulation,* 123, 2434–2506.

Arthritis Foundation (2019). *Arthritis by the Numbers: Book of Trusted Facts and Figures.* Atlanta: Arthritis Foundation.

Baber, R.J. et al. (2016). 2016 IMS Recommendations on women's midlife health and menopause hormone therapy, *Climacteric,* 19, 2, 109–150.

Barbour, K.E. et al. (2017). Vital signs: Prevalence of doctor-diagnosed arthritis and arthritis-attributable activity limitation—United States, 2013–2015. *Morbidity and Mortality Weekly Report,* 66, 246–253.

Beauchamp, M.K. et al. (2017). Pulmonary rehabilitation with balance training for fall reduction in chronic obstructive pulmonary disease: Protocol for a randomized controlled trial. *JMIR Research Protocols,* 6, 11, e228.

Benjamin, E.J. et al. (2019). Heart disease and stroke statistics—2019 update: A report from the American Heart Association. *Circulation,* 139, 10, e56–528.

Benjumea, A.M. et al. (2018). Dynapenia and sarcopenia as a risk factor for disability in a falls and fractures clinic in older persons. *Open Access Macedonia Journal of Medical Sciences,* 6, 2, 344–349.

Bronas, U.G. et al. (2009). Design of the multicenter standardized supervised exercise training intervention for the claudication: Exercise vs endoluminal revascularization (CLEVER) study. *Vascular Medicine,* 14, 313–321.

Carpio-Rivera, E. et al. (2016). Acute effects of exercise on blood pressure: A meta-analytic investigation. *Arquivos Brasileiros de Cardiologia,* 106, 5, 422–433.

Centers for Disease Control and Prevention (2020). *National Diabetes Statistics Report 2020: Estimates of Diabetes and its Burden in the United States.* Washington, D.C.: Centers for Disease Control and Prevention.

Chang, K.V. et al. (2017). Is sarcopenia associated with depression? A systematic review and meta-analysis of observational studies. *Age and Ageing,* 46, 5, 738–746.

Ciolac, E.G. (2012). High-intensity interval training and hypertension: Maximizing the benefits of exercise? *American Journal of Cardiovascular Disease,* 2, 102–110.

Dean, C. (2012). Group task-specific circuit training for patients discharged home after stroke may be as effective as individualized physiotherapy in improving mobility. *Journal of Physiotherapy,* 58, 269.

Dogra, S., Meisner, B.A., & Baker, J. (2008). Psychosocial predictors of physical activity in older aged asthmatics. *Age and Ageing,* 37, 449–454.

Fang, X. et al. (2018). Association of levels of physical activity with risk of Parkinson disease: A systematic review and meta-analysis. *Journal of America Medical Association Network Open,* 1, 5, 1–25.

Fatoye, F., Gebrye, T. & Odeyemi, I. (2019). Real-world incidence and prevalence of low back pain using routinely collected data. *Rheumatology International,* 39, 619–626.

Fejer, R. & Ruhe, A. (2012). What is the prevalence of musculoskeletal problems in the elderly population in developed countries? A systematic critical literature review. *Chiropractic & Manual Therapies,* 20, 31.

Fernandez-Gonzalo, R. et al. (2016). Muscle, functional and cognitive adaptations after flywheel resistance training in stroke patients: A pilot randomized controlled trial. *Journal of NeuroEngineering and Rehabilitation*, 13, 1, 1–11.

Freeman, E.W., Sammel, M.D., & Sanders, R.J. (2014). Risk of long-term hot flashes after natural menopause: Evidence from the Penn Ovarian Aging Study cohort. *Menopause*, 21, 924–932.

Fuchs, F.D. et al. (2012). Proof of concept in cardiovascular risk: The paradoxical findings in blood pressure and lipid abnormalities. *Vascular Health & Risk Management*, 8, 437–442.

Gibson, C.J. et al. (2011). Negative affect and vasomotor symptoms in the study of women's health across the nation (SWAN) daily hormone study. *Menopause*, 18, 1270–1277.

Global Initiative for Asthma (GINA) (2020). *Global Strategy for Asthma Management and Prevention.* http://www.ginasthma.org.

Goh, S. et al. (2019). Relative efficacy of different exercises for pain, function, performance and quality of life in knee and hip osteoarthritis: Systematic review and network meta-analysis. *Sports Medicine*, 49, 743–761.

Gopinath, B. et al. (2016). Hearing and vision impairment and the 5-year incidence of falls in older adults. *Age and Ageing*, 45, 3, 409–414.

Gregg, E.W. et al. (2104). Changes in diabetes-related complications in the United States, 1990–2010. *New England Journal of Medicine*, 370, 1514–1523.

Guzon-Illescas, O. et al. (2019). Mortality after osteoporotic hip fracture: Incidence, trends, and associated factors. *Journal of Orthopaedic Surgery and Research*, 14, 203, 1–9.

Hales, C.M. et al. (2020). Prevalence of obesity and severe obesity among adults: United States, 2017–2018. *National Center for Health Statistics Data Brief*, 360, 1–8.

Hamburg, N.M. & Balady, G.J. (2011). Exercise rehabilitation in peripheral artery disease: Functional impact and mechanisms of benefits. *Circulation*, 123, 87–97.

Hebert, L.E. et al. (2013). Alzheimer disease in the United States (2010-2050) estimated using the 2010 Census. *Neurology*, 80, 19, 1778–1783.

Heron, M. (2019). Deaths: Leading causes for 2017. *National Vital Statistics Reports*, 68, 6, 1–76.

Jafarzadeh, S.R. & Felson, D.T. (2018). Updated estimates suggest a much higher prevalence of arthritis in United States adults than previous ones. *Arthritis & Rheumatology*, 70, 2, 185–192.

Kolasinski, S.L. et al. (2020). American College of Rheumatology/Arthritis Foundation guideline for the management of osteoarthritis of the hand, hip, and knee. *Arthritis and Rheumatology*, 72, 2, 149–162.

Kraus, W.E. et al. (2019). Physical activity, all-cause and cardiovascular mortality, and cardiovascular disease. *Medicine & Science in Sports & Exercise*, 51, 6, 1270–1281.

Lemeunier, N., Leboeuf-Yde, C., & Gagey, O. (2012). The natural course of low back pain: A systematic critical literature review. *Chiropractic & Manual Therapies*, 20, 33.

Liu-Ambrose, T. et al. (2010). Resistance training and executive functions: A 12-month randomized controlled trial. *Archives of Internal Medicine*, 170, 2, 170–178.

Marras, C. et al. (2018). Prevalence of Parkinson's disease across North America. *npj Parkinson's Disease*, 4, 21, 1–7.

Nagamatsu, L.S. et al. (2012). Resistance training promotes cognitive and functional brain plasticity in seniors with probable mild cognitive impairment. *Archives of Internal Medicine*, 172, 8, 666–668.

National Asthma Education and Prevention Program (2007). Expert Panel Report 3 (EPR-3): Guidelines for the diagnosis and management of asthma: Summary report. *Journal of Allergy & Clinical Immunology*, 120, S94–138.

National Institute on Deafness and Other Communication Disorders (2020). *Age-related Hearing Loss.* https://www.nidcd.nih.gov/health/age-related-hearing-loss

National Institutes of Health (2012). *What Are Overweight and Obesity?* www.nhlbi.nih.gov/health/dci/Diseases/obe/obe_whatare.html

Norgren, L. et al. (2007). Inter-society consensus for the management of peripheral arterial disease (TASC II). *European Journal of Vascular & Endovascular Surgery*, 33, S1–S75.

O'Donnell, M.E. et al. (2011). Optimal management of peripheral arterial disease for the non-specialist. *Ulster Medical Journal*, 80, 33–41.

O'Keefe, J.H., Carter, M.D., & Lavie, C.J. (2009). Primary and secondary prevention of cardiovascular diseases: A practical evidence-based approach. *Mayo Clinic Proceedings*, 84, 741–757.

Oliveira, C.C. et al. (2015). Falls by individuals with chronic obstructive pulmonary disease: A preliminary 12-month prospective cohort study. *Respirology, 20,* 7, 1096–1101.

Ospina, B.M. et al. (2019). Age matters: Objective gait assessment in early Parkinson's disease using an RGB-D camera. *Parkinson's Disease, 2019,* 1–9.

Palma, F. et al. (2016). Vaginal atrophy of women in postmenopause: Results from a multicentric observational study: The AGATA study. *Maturitas, 83,* 40–44.

Panza, G.A., et al. (2018). Can exercise improve cognitive symptoms of Alzheimer's disease? *Journal of American Geriatrics Society, 66,* 3, 487–495.

Parsons, J.P. et al. (2013). An official American Thoracic Society clinical practice guideline: Exercise-induced bronchoconstriction. *American Journal of Respiratory and Critical Care Medicine, 187,* 1016–1027.

Porter Starr, K.N. et al. (2016). Challenges in the management of geriatric obesity in high risk populations. *Nutrients, 8,* 5, 262.

Reed, C.E. (2010). Asthma in the elderly: Diagnosis and management. *Journal of Allergy and Clinical Immunology, 126,* 681–687.

Reid, W.D. et al. (2012). Exercise prescription for hospitalized people with chronic obstructive pulmonary disease and comorbidities: A synthesis of systematic reviews. *International Journal of Chronic Obstructive Pulmonary Disease, 7,* 297–320.

Roberts, A.W. et al. (2018). The population 65 years and older in the United States. *American Community Survey Reports,* 1–25.

Röckl, S. et al. (2017). All-cause mortality in adults with and without type 2 diabetes: Findings from the national health monitoring in Germany. *BMJ Open Diabetes Research & Care, 5,* 1, e000451.

Silverwood, V. et al. (2015). Current evidence on risk factors for knee osteoarthritis in older adults: A systematic review and meta-analysis. *Osteoarthritis and Cartilage, 23,* 507–515.

Song, P. et al. (2019). Global, regional, and national prevalence and risk factors for peripheral artery disease in 2015: An updated systematic review and analysis. *Lancet: Global Health, 7,* 8, e1020–e1030.

Steihaug, O.M. et al. (2017). Sarcopenia in patients with hip fracture: A multicenter cross-sectional study. *PLoS One, 12,* 9, e0184780.

Sveaas, S.H. et al. (2017). Effect of cardiorespiratory and strength exercises on disease activity in patients with inflammatory rheumatic diseases: A systematic review and meta-analysis. *British Journal of Sports Medicine, 51,* 1065–1072.

Tanimoto, Y. et al. (2014). Sarcopenia and falls in community-dwelling elderly subjects in Japan: Defining sarcopenia according to criteria of the European working group on sarcopenia in older people. *Archives of Gerontology and Geriatrics, 59,* 2, 295–299.

Treat-Jacobson, D. et al. (2019). Optimal exercise programs for patients with peripheral artery disease: A scientific statement from the American Heart Association. *Circulation, 139,* 4, e10–33.

Tyrovolas, S. et al. (2016). Factors associated with skeletal muscle mass, sarcopenia, and sarcopenic obesity in older adults: A multi-continent study. *Journal of Cachexia, Sarcopenia and Muscle, 7,* 312–321.

Wang, Q. et al. (2018). Physical activity patterns and risk of type 2 diabetes and metabolic syndrome in middle-aged and elderly Northern Chinese adults. *Journal of Diabetes Research, 7198274.*

Watson, S. et al. (2018). High-intensity resistance and impact training improves bone mineral density and physical function in postmenopausal women with osteopenia and osteoporosis: The LIFTMOR randomized controlled trial. *Journal of Bone and Mineral Research, 33,* 2, 211–220.

Whelton, P.K. et al. (2017). 2017 ACC/AHA/AAPA/ABC/ACPM/AGS/APhA/ASH/ASPC/NMA/PCNA guideline for the prevention, detection, evaluation, and management of high blood pressure in adults: A report of the American College of Cardiology/American Heart Association Task Force on Clinical Practice Guidelines. *Journal of the American College of Cardiology,* Nov 7. pii: S0735-1097 (17) 41519-1.

Whitehurst, M. (2012). High-intensity interval training: An alternative for older adults. *American Journal of Lifestyle Medicine, 6,* 382–386.

Whiteneck, G. (2006). Conceptual models of disability: Past, present, and future. In: Field, M., Jette, A., & Martin L. (Eds.) *Workshop on Disability in America: A New Look—Summary and Background Papers.* Washington, D.C.: National Academies Press; pp. 50–66.

Wolters, F.J. et al. (2017). Parental family history of dementia in relation to sub-clinical brain disease and dementia risk. *Neurology, 88,* 1642–1649.

World Health Organization (2020). *Obesity and Overweight*. www.who.int/news-room/fact-sheets/detail/obesity-and-overweight

World Health Organization (2001). *International Classification of Functioning, Disability and Health (ICF)*. Geneva, Switzerland: World Health Organization, pp. 7–20.

Worsley, R. et al. (2014). The association between vasomotor symptoms and depression during perimenopause: A systematic review. *Maturitas*, 77, 111–117.

Wright, N.C. et al. (2014). The recent prevalence of osteoporosis and low bone mass in the United States based on bone mineral density at the femoral neck or lumbar spine. *Journal of Bone and Mineral Research*, 29, 11, 2520–2526.

Zhang, X. et al. (2019). Association of sarcopenic obesity with the risk of all-cause mortality among adults over a broad range of different settings: A updated meta-analysis. *BMC Geriatrics*, 19, 183.

SUGGESTED READINGS

American College of Sports Medicine (2016). *ACSM's Exercise Management for Persons with Chronic Diseases and Disabilities* (4th ed.). Champaign, Ill.: Human Kinetics.

American College of Sports Medicine (2009). *ACSM's Resource for Clinical Exercise Physiology: Musculoskeletal, Neuromuscular, Neoplastic, Immunologic, and Hemotologic Conditions* (2nd ed.). Philadelphia: Wolters Kluwer/Lippincott Williams & Wilkins.

Anton, S.D. et al. (2015). Successful aging: Advancing the science of physical independence in older adults. *Ageing Research Reviews*, 24, 304–307.

Glossary

Absorption The uptake of nutrients across a tissue or membrane by the gastrointestinal tract.

Acceptable Macronutrient Distribution Range (AMDR) The range of intake for a particular energy source that is associated with reduced risk of chronic disease while providing intakes of essential nutrients.

Action The stage of the transtheoretical model of behavior change during which the individual is actively engaging in a behavior that was started less than six months ago.

Active listening Mode of listening in which the listener is concerned about the content, intent, and feelings of the message.

Activities of daily living (ADL) Activities normally performed for hygiene, bathing, household chores, walking, shopping, and similar activities.

Acute Descriptive of a condition that usually has a rapid onset and a relatively short and severe course; opposite of chronic.

Adequate Intake (AI) A recommended average daily nutrient intake level based on observed or experimentally determined approximations or estimates of mean nutrient intake by a group (or groups) of apparently healthy people. An AI is used when the Recommended Dietary Allowance cannot be determined.

Adherence The extent to which people follow their plans or treatment recommendations. Exercise adherence is the extent to which people follow an exercise program.

Adipose Fat cells stored in fatty tissues in the body.

Adiposity The state of being fat; fatness; obesity.

Aerobic capacity See Maximal oxygen uptake ($\dot{V}O_2$max).

Ageism The stereotyping, prejudice, and discrimination against people based on their age; believed to be the most socially normalized of any prejudice.

Ageusia Absence of the sense of taste.

Agility The ability to move quickly and easily; a skill-related component of physical fitness.

Agreement to participate Signed document that indicates that the client is aware of inherent risks and potential injuries that can occur from participation.

Allergen A usually harmless substance capable of triggering a response that starts in the immune system and results in an allergic reaction.

Alveoli Spherical extensions of the respiratory bronchioles and the primary sites of gas exchange between the lungs and the blood.

Alzheimer's disease An irreversible, progressive brain disorder that slowly destroys memory and thinking skills and, eventually, the ability to complete the simplest tasks. The most common cause of dementia among older adults.

Ambivalence A state of having mixed feelings about a change; arguing both for and against change simultaneously.

Amortization phase   The transition period between the eccentric and concentric actions during plyometrics; a crucial part of the stretch-shortening cycle that contributes to power development.

Anabolic   Muscle-building effects.

Anabolism   A state in which the body produces more protein than it breaks down; occurs in times of growth such as childhood, pregnancy, recovery from illness, and in response to muscular training when overloading the muscles promotes protein synthesis.

Anaerobic capacity   The maximal amount of adenosine triphosphate (ATP) resynthesized via non-mitochondrial pathways during short-duration maximal exercise.

Anaerobic gylcolysis   The metabolic pathway that uses glucose for energy production without requiring oxygen. Sometimes referred to as the lactic acid system or anaerobic glucose system, it produces lactic acid as a by-product.

Angina   See Angina pectoris.

Angina pectoris   A common symptom of coronary artery disease characterized by chest pain caused by an inadequate supply of oxygen and decreased blood flow to the heart muscle; an early sign of coronary artery disease. Symptoms may include pain or discomfort, heaviness, tightness, pressure or burning, numbness, aching, and tingling in the chest, back, neck, throat, jaw, or arms; also called angina.

Angiotensin II receptor antagonist   A class of drugs used to treat high blood pressure and other conditions by preventing angiotensin II from binding to angiotensin II receptors, thereby allowing blood vessels to dilate; also referred to as angiotensin-receptor blockers.

Angiotensin-converting enzyme (ACE) inhibitor   A class of drugs used to treat high blood pressure and other conditions by reducing the activity of angiotensin converting enzyme, which converts angiotensin I to angiotensin II.

Anorexia   An eating disorder characterized by a restriction of energy intake leading to a significant low body weight relative to normative values for sex, age, physical health, and developmental trajectory; intense fear of gaining weight or becoming fat; or persistent behavior that interferes with weight gain.

Anosmia   A complete loss of the sense of smell.

Anterior   Anatomical term meaning toward the front. Same as ventral; opposite of posterior.

Anterior cruciate ligament (ACL)   A primary stabilizing ligament of the knee that travels from the medial border of the lateral femoral condyle to its point of insertion anterolaterally to the medial tibial spine.

Anthropometry   The measurement of the size and proportions of the human body.

Antihistamine   A class of drugs that blocks histamine receptors involved in the allergic response.

Anxiety   A state of uneasiness and apprehension; occurs in some mental disorders.

Arrhythmia   A disturbance in the rate or rhythm of the heartbeat. Some can be symptoms of serious heart disease; may not be of medical significance until symptoms appear.

Artery   A blood vessel that carries oxygenated blood away from the heart to vital organs and the extremities.

Arthritis   Inflammation of a joint; a state characterized by the inflammation of joints.

Articular cartilage   Cartilage covering the ends of the bones inside diarthroidial joints; allows the ends of the bones to glide without friction.

Asthma A chronic inflammatory disorder of the airways that affects genetically susceptible individuals in response to various environmental triggers such as allergens, viral infection, exercise, cold, and stress.

Ataxia Failure of muscular coordination; irregularity of muscular action.

Atherosclerosis A specific form of arteriosclerosis characterized by the accumulation of fatty material on the inner walls of the arteries, causing them to harden, thicken, and lose elasticity.

Atrophy A reduction in muscle size (muscle wasting) due to inactivity or immobilization.

Attending A nonverbal communication skill that gives acknowledgement through posture, eye contact, and gestures. It entails being attentive through physical attention and putting the speaker at ease.

Auscultation Listening to the internal sounds of the body (such as the heartbeat), usually using a stethoscope.

Autoimmune disease Any of a group of disorders in which tissue injury is associated with the body's responses to its own constituents; they may be systemic (e.g., systemic lupus erythematosus) or organ-specific (e.g., autoimmune thyroiditis).

Automated external defibrillator (AED) A portable electronic device used to restore normal heart rhythms in victims of sudden cardiac arrest.

Autonomous regulation Regulation of behavior that occurs with self-endorsement or self-governance. Characterized by goals associated with personal interests and values instead of external pressure and feelings of being controlled. Also known as self-regulation and autonomous self-regulation

Autonomy The capacity of a rational individual to make an informed, un-coerced decision. Regulation by the self.

Balance The ability to maintain the body's position over its base of support within stability limits, both statically and dynamically; a health-related component of physical fitness.

Base of support (BOS) The areas of contact between the feet and their supporting surface and the area between the feet.

Basic activities of daily living Any daily activity performed for self-care, including personal hygiene, dressing and undressing, feeding, ambulating, continence, and toileting.

Beta blocker Medication that "blocks" or limits sympathetic nervous system stimulation. Acts to slow the heart rate and decrease maximal heart rate and is used for cardiovascular and other medical conditions.

Biological age A means of measuring age that focuses on biological, rather than chronological, processes; examines various biological processes and their effects on behavior.

Blood pressure (BP) The pressure exerted by the blood on the walls of the arteries; measured in millimeters of mercury (mmHg) with a sphygmomanometer.

Body composition The makeup of the body in terms of the relative percentage of fat-free mass and body fat; a health-related component of physical fitness.

Body fat A component of the body, the primary role of which is to store energy for later use.

Body-fat percentage The proportion of body composition representing the relative percentage of body fat. Calculated by dividing the fat mass by the total body mass, then multiplying by 100.

Body mass index (BMI) A relative measure of body height to body weight used to determine levels of health, from underweight to extreme obesity.

Bone mineral density (BMD) A measure of the amount of minerals (mainly calcium) contained in a certain volume of bone.

Bracing A mild contraction of the abdominal wall.

Bronchi The two large branches of the trachea leading into the lungs.

Bronchioles The smallest tubes that supply air to the alveoli (air sacs) of the lungs.

Bronchitis Acute or chronic inflammation of the bronchial tubes. See Chronic obstructive pulmonary disease (COPD).

Bronchoconstriction The constriction of the airways in the lungs caused by the tightening of surrounding smooth muscle, with consequent coughing, wheezing, and shortness of breath.

Bronchodilator Medication inhaled to dilate (enlarge) and relax the constricted bronchial smooth muscle.

Cachexia A loss of body weight (wasting) accompanied by muscle atrophy, weakness, and fatigue.

Calcaneal eversion Movement of the plantar surface of the calcaneus laterally away from the midline of the body.

Calcification A process in which calcium builds up in tissue, causing it to harden. This can be a normal (e.g., in bone tissue) or abnormal (e.g., in arteries) process.

Calcium channel blocker A class of blood pressure medications that relax and widen the blood vessels.

Carbohydrate The body's preferred energy source. Dietary sources include sugars (simple) and grains, rice, potatoes, and beans (complex). Carbohydrate is stored as glycogen in the muscles and liver and is transported in the blood as glucose. Each gram of carbohydrate contains four calories.

Cardiac output The amount of blood pumped by the heart per minute; usually expressed in liters of blood per minute. Cardiac output = Heart rate x Stroke volume.

Cardiopulmonary resuscitation (CPR) A procedure to support and maintain breathing and circulation for a person who has stopped breathing (respiratory arrest) and/or whose heart has stopped (cardiac arrest).

Cardiorespiratory fitness The ability to perform large muscle movement over a sustained period; related to the capacity of the heart-lung system to deliver oxygen for sustained energy production. Also called cardiorespiratory endurance or aerobic fitness.

Cardiovascular disease (CVD) A general term for any disease of the heart, blood vessels, or circulation.

Cardiovascular drift An increase in heart rate that occurs during prolonged, submaximal exercise without a change in workload to compensate for a decrease in stroke volume to maintain cardiac output.

Cartilage A smooth, semi-opaque material that absorbs shock and reduces friction between the bones of a joint.

Catabolism Metabolic pathways that break down molecules into smaller units and release energy.

Catecholamine Hormone (e.g., dopamine, epinephrine, and norepinephrine) released as part of the sympathetic response to exercise; acts both as neurotransmitter and hormone vital to the maintenance of homeostasis through the autonomic nervous system.

Center of gravity (COG)   The point around which all weight is evenly distributed; also called center of mass.

Center of mass (COM)   See Center of gravity (COG).

Central nervous system (CNS)   The brain and spinal cord.

Cerebrovascular disease   One of a group of brain dysfunctions related to disease of the blood vessels supplying the brain.

Cerebrovascular accident   Damage to the brain, often resulting in a loss of function, from impaired blood supply to part of the brain; more commonly known as a stroke.

Change talk   Any client speech that favors movement toward a particular change goal.

Cholesterol   A fatlike substance found in the blood and body tissues and in certain foods. Can accumulate in the arteries and lead to a narrowing of the vessels (atherosclerosis).

Chromosome   Rod-shaped or threadlike deoxyribonucleic acid (DNA)–containing structures of cellular organisms that contain genetic information.

Chronic   Descriptive of a condition that persists over a long period of time; opposite of acute.

Chronic bronchitis   Characterized by inflamed bronchiole tubes, increased mucus secretion, and a productive cough lasting several months to several years.

Chronic obstructive pulmonary disease (COPD)   A condition, such as asthma, bronchitis, or emphysema, in which there is chronic obstruction of air flow. See Asthma, Bronchitis, and Emphysema.

Chronological age   The length of time—in years or months since birth—a person has lived.

Cognitive   Pertaining to, or characterized by, that operation of the mind by which we become aware of objects of thought or perception; includes all aspects of perceiving, thinking, and remembering.

Cognitive restructuring   Intentionally changing the way one perceives or thinks about something.

Collagen   The main constituent of connective tissue, such as ligaments, tendons, and muscles.

Comparative negligence   A system used in legal defenses to distribute fault between an injured party and any defendant.

Compliance   The elastic resistance of a system or the ease with which an elastic structure can be stretched. The more compliant a structure is, the more elasticity it has. As a structure decreases in elasticity and compliance, it becomes stiffer.

Concentric   A type of isotonic muscle contraction in which the muscle develops tension and shortens when stimulated.

Congestive heart failure   Inability of the heart to pump blood at a sufficient rate to meet the metabolic demand or the ability to do so only when the cardiac filling pressures are abnormally high, frequently resulting in lung congestion.

Connective tissue   The tissue that binds together and supports various structures of the body. Ligaments and tendons are connective tissues.

Contemplation   The stage of the transtheoretical model of behavior change during which the individual is weighing the pros and cons of behavioral change.

Contributory negligence   A legal defense used in claims or suits when the plaintiff's negligence contributed to the act in dispute.

Coordination   The ability to process and execute appropriate actions or motor responses with proper sequence (timing) and magnitude to produce smooth, flowing movement; a skill-related component of physical fitness.

Coronary artery disease (CAD)   The major form of cardiovascular disease; results when the coronary arteries are narrowed or occluded, most commonly by atherosclerotic deposits of fibrous and fatty tissue; also called coronary heart disease.

Coronary heart disease (CHD)   See Coronary artery disease (CAD).

Costochondral   Relating to the costal cartilages (i.e., of the ribs).

Costovertebral   Relating to the ribs and the bodies of the thoracic vertebrae with which they articulate.

Cyanosis   A bluish discoloration, especially of the skin and mucous membranes, due to reduced hemoglobin in the blood.

Cytokines   Hormone-like low-molecular-weight proteins, secreted by many different cell types, which regulate the intensity and duration of immune responses and are involved in cell-to-cell communication.

Decisional balance   One of the four components of the transtheoretical model of behavior change. A choice-focused technique that can be used when coaching with neutrality, devoting equal exploration to the pros and cons of change or a specific plan.

Degenerative joint disease   A non-infectious, progressive disorder of the weight-bearing joints. The majority of degenerative joint disease is the result of mechanical instabilities or aging-related changes within the joint.

Dehydration   The process of losing body water; when severe can cause serious, life-threatening consequences.

Delayed-onset muscle soreness (DOMS)   Soreness that occurs 24 to 48 hours after strenuous exercise, the exact cause of which is unknown.

Dementia   A deteriorative mental state characterized by absence of, or reduction in, intellectual faculties; may be caused by disease or trauma.

Demyelinization   The destruction or removal of the myelin sheath of a nerve or nerves.

Deoxyribonucleic acid (DNA)   A large, double-stranded, helical molecule that is the carrier of genetic information.

Depression   1. The action of lowering a muscle or bone or movement in an inferior or downward direction. 2. A condition of general emotional dejection and withdrawal; sadness greater and more prolonged than that warranted by any objective reason.

Diabetes   A disease of carbohydrate metabolism in which an absolute or relative deficiency of insulin results in an inability to metabolize carbohydrates normally.

Diaphragmatic breathing   A deep, relaxing breathing technique that helps chronic obstructive pulmonary disease (COPD) patients improve their breathing capacity.

Diastolic blood pressure (DBP)   The pressure in the arteries during the relaxation phase (diastole) of the cardiac cycle; indicative of total peripheral resistance.

Dietary Approaches to Stop Hypertension (DASH) eating plan   An eating plan designed to reduce blood pressure; also serves as an overall healthy way of eating that can be adopted by nearly anyone; may also lower risk of coronary heart disease.

Digestion   The process of breaking down food into small enough units for absorption.

Disability   The inability to perform certain essential movements, such as dressing, walking, bathing, and climbing stairs.

Distal   Farthest from the midline of the body, or from the point of origin of a muscle.

Diuretic   Medication that produces an increase in urine volume and sodium excretion.

Diverticular disease   The general name for a common condition that causes small bulges (diverticula) or sacs to form in the wall of the large intestine (colon). Includes diverticulosis, diverticular bleeding, and diverticulitis.

Dopamine   A neurotransmitter that helps regulate movement and control the brain's reward and pleasure centers.

Dorsiflexion   Movement of the foot up toward the shin.

Dynamic balance   The ability to maintain balance while moving; requires an individual to lose, manipulate, and regain control of their center of mass over a changing base of support, such as when walking, marching, skipping, and running.

Dynapenia   The loss of muscle strength not caused by neurological or muscular disease that typically is associated with older age.

Dyslipidemia   A condition characterized by abnormal blood lipid profiles; may include elevated cholesterol, triglyceride, or low-density lipoprotein (LDL) levels and/or low high-density lipoprotein (HDL) levels.

Dysosmia   A distortion in the sense of smell such that one either experiences a smell incongruent with the actual smell (typically a pleasant smell is perceived as an unpleasant smell) or experiences a smell that does not exist.

Dyspnea   Difficult or labored breathing.

Dystrophy   Any disorder arising from defective or faulty nutrition, especially the muscular dystrophies.

Eccentric   A type of isotonic muscle action in which the muscle lengthens against a resistance when it is stimulated; sometimes called "negative work" or "negative reps."

Edema   Swelling resulting from an excessive accumulation of fluid in the tissues of the body.

Elasticity   The ability of tissue to regain its original shape and size after being deformed.

Electrocardiogram (ECG or EKG)   A recording of the electrical activity of the heart.

Electrolyte   A mineral that exists as a charged ion in the body and that is extremely important for normal cellular function.

Elicit-provide-elicit   An approach to providing information in which the exercise professional first asks permission to do so. When permission is granted, the professional follows with an open-ended question to understand what the client knows already (elicit). The professional follows with a small amount of highly relevant information (provide) and then checks back with the client to assess understanding and the response to the information (elicit).

Emotional arousal   A state of heightened physiological activity, emotions, and emotional behavior.

Empathetic responding   Responding based on the understanding of a person's experience from their perspective; it should acknowledge and increase the awareness of their experience and therefore make them more open to learning.

Empathy   The extent to which a professional communicates an accurate understanding of the client's perspectives and experiences; most commonly manifested as reflection.

Emphysema   An obstructive pulmonary disease characterized by the gradual destruction of lung alveoli and the surrounding connective tissue, in addition to airway inflammation, leading to reduced ability to effectively inhale and exhale.

Empty calories   Calories that provide very little nutritional value; should be limited in the diet; calories from solid fats and or added sugars.

Enzyme   A protein that speeds up a specific chemical reaction.

Epinephrine   A hormone released as part of the sympathetic response to exercise; also called adrenaline.

Estrogen   Generic term for estrus-producing steroid compounds produced primarily in the ovaries; the female sex hormones.

Eversion   Rotation of the foot to direct the plantar surface outward; occurs in the frontal plane.

Exculpatory clause   A clause within a waiver that bars the potential plaintiff from recovery.

Exercise-induced bronchoconstriction (EIB)   Transient and reversible airway narrowing triggered by vigorous exercise; also called exercise-induced asthma (EIA).

Exercise prescription   The development of individualized exercise programs based on exercise frequency, intensity, duration, and type.

Extension   The act of straightening or extending a joint, usually applied to the muscular movement of a limb.

External regulation   A form of controlled motivation in which an individual engages in an activity solely from external pressure to avoid punishment or gain rewards.

Extrinsic motivation   Motivation that comes from external (outside of the self) rewards, such as material or social rewards.

Fascia   Strong connective tissue that performs a number of functions, including enveloping and isolating the muscles of the body and providing structural support and protection (plural: fasciae).

Fast-twitch muscle fiber   One of several types of muscle fibers found in skeletal muscle tissue; also called type II fibers and characterized as having a low oxidative capacity but a high gylcolytic capacity; recruited for rapid, powerful movements such as jumping, throwing, and sprinting.

Fat   An essential nutrient that provides energy, energy storage, insulation, and contour to the body. Each gram of fat contains nine calories.

Fat mass   The actual amount of essential and non-essential fat in the body.

Fat-free mass   That part of the body composition that represents everything but fat—blood, bones, connective tissue, organs, and muscle; also called lean body mass.

Feedback   An internal response within a learner; during information processing, it is the correctness or incorrectness of a response that is stored in memory to be used for future reference. Also, verbal or nonverbal information about current behavior that can be used to improve future performance.

Femoral anteversion   A congenital condition in which the femur is rotated inward (medially).

First ventilatory threshold (VT1)   Intensity of aerobic exercise at which ventilation starts to increase in a nonlinear fashion in response to an accumulation of metabolic by-products in the blood.

Flexibility   The range of motion available at a joint or the degree of tissue extensibility available at a joint; a health-related component of physical fitness.

Flexion   The act of moving a joint so that the two bones forming it are brought closer together.

Food insecurity   A disruption of eating patterns or food intake because of lack of money and other resources.

Free-radical oxidation   A mechanism of cellular aging in which a highly unstable molecule of oxygen (i.e., a free-radical) with an uneven number of electrons in its outer shell attempts to link up with other molecules, thereby causing a series of destructive chain reactions; possible outcomes include reduced elasticity in the skin and declines in flexibility and range of motion.

Frontal plane   A longitudinal section that runs at a right angle to the sagittal plane, dividing the body into anterior and posterior portions.

Functional age   A measure of aging using various indications beyond chronological age; these indices include biological age, social age, and psychological age.

Functional capacity   The maximum physical performance represented by maximal oxygen consumption.

Functional limitation   A restriction in certain physical or mental tasks that can be the result of an impairment.

Gait   The manner or style of walking.

Gastroesophageal reflux disease   A chronic condition in which the lower esophageal sphincter allows gastric acids to reflux into the esophagus, causing heartburn, acid indigestion, and possible injury to the esophageal lining.

Gerontologist   A specialist in the scientific study of the clinical, biological, historical, and sociological problems of aging.

Gerontology   The study of aging.

Glomerular filtration rate   The volume of fluid filtered from the renal (kidney) glomerular capillaries into the Bowman's capsule per unit time; a measure of kidney function.

Glucose   A simple sugar; the form in which all carbohydrates are used as the body's principal energy source.

Gross negligence   A form of negligence that is worse than normal negligence. Generally, a waiver clause cannot prevent a suit for gross negligence or for wanton or recklessness or intentional misconduct in any state or jurisdiction.

Group waiver   Waiver that includes lines for multiple signatures.

Growth hormone   A hormone secreted by the pituitary gland that facilitates protein synthesis, fat metabolism, and overall growth in the body.

Hayflick limit   Finite number of times that a cell is able to reproduce. Suggests that cellular aging is, at least to some degree, preprogrammed.

Health belief model   A model to explain that people's emotions and ideas about illness, prevention, and treatment may influence health-related behaviors and decisions about changing (or not changing).

Health Insurance Portability and Accountability Act (HIPAA)   Enacted by the U.S. Congress in 1996, HIPAA requires the U.S. Department of Health and Human Services (HHS) to establish national standards for electronic health care information to facilitate efficient and secure exchange of private health data. The Standards for Privacy of Individually Identifiable Health Information ("Privacy Rule"), issued by the HHS, addresses the use and disclosure of individuals' health information—called "protected health information"—by providing federal protections and giving patients an array of rights with respect to personal health information while permitting the disclosure of information needed for patient care and other important purposes.

Healthy Mediterranean-Style Eating Pattern   One of three USDA Food Patterns featured in the *Dietary Guidelines for Americans*; modified from the Healthy

U.S.-Style Eating Pattern to more closely reflect eating patterns that have been associated with positive health outcomes in studies of Mediterranean-style diets.

Healthy U.S.-Style Eating Pattern   One of three USDA Food Patterns featured in the *Dietary Guidelines for Americans*; based on the types and proportions of foods Americans typically consume, but in nutrient-dense forms and appropriate amounts.

Healthy Vegetarian Eating Pattern   One of three USDA Food Patterns featured in the *Dietary Guidelines for Americans*; modified from the Healthy U.S.-Style Eating Pattern to more closely reflect eating patterns reported by self-identified vegetarians.

Heart rate (HR)   The number of heartbeats per minute.

Heart-rate reserve (HRR)   The reserve capacity of the heart; the difference between maximal heart rate and resting heart rate. It reflects the heart's ability to increase the rate of beating and cardiac output above resting level to maximal intensity.

Hemorrhagic stroke   Disruption of blood flow to the brain caused by the presence of a blood clot or hematoma.

High-density lipoprotein (HDL)   A lipoprotein that carries excess cholesterol from the arteries to the liver. High HDL levels are associated with a decreased risk for coronary heart disease.

High-intensity interval training (HIIT)   An exercise strategy alternating periods of short, intense anaerobic exercise with less-intense recovery periods.

Homeostasis   An internal state of physiological balance.

Homocysteine   A normal by-product of metabolism that can promote development of heart disease.

Hormone   A chemical substance produced and released by an endocrine gland and transported through the blood to a target organ.

Hydrostatic weighing   Weighing a person fully submerged in water. The difference between the person's mass in air and in water is used to calculate body density, which can be used to estimate the proportion of fat in the body.

Hypercholesterolemia   An excess of cholesterol in the blood.

Hyperglycemia   An abnormally high content of glucose (sugar) in the blood.

Hyperkyphosis   A kyphosis angle that exceeds the normal range, which may be a consequence of normal aging from decreased muscle strength and degenerative changes of the spine or other factors such as vertebral fractures.

Hyperlipidemia   An excess of lipids in the blood that could be primary, as in disorders of lipid metabolism, or secondary, as in uncontrolled diabetes.

Hypernatremia   A deficit of water relative to sodium, causing an electrolyte imbalance and a rise in serum sodium concentration. Can result from inadequate water intake, water loss, or sodium overload.

Hypertension   High blood pressure, or the elevation of resting blood pressure to 130/80 mmHg or greater.

Hypertonic   1. Having extreme muscular tension. 2. Having a solute concentration that is greater than the concentration of human blood.

Hypertrophy   An increase in the cross-sectional size of a muscle in response to progressive muscular training.

Hypogeusia   A diminished sense of taste.

Hypoglycemia   A deficiency of glucose in the blood commonly caused by too much insulin, too little glucose, or too much exercise where glycogen stores become depleted. Most commonly found in those with insulin-dependent diabetes and characterized by symptoms such as fatigue, dizziness, confusion, headache, nausea, or anxiety.

Hyponatremia   Abnormally low levels of sodium ions circulating in the blood; severe hyponatremia can lead to brain swelling and death.

Hypotension   Abnormally low blood pressure.

Impairment   A decrease in strength or function; can be anatomical or structural in nature.

Inflammation   A protective tissue response to injury or destruction of tissues, which serves to destroy, dilute, or wall off both the injurious agent and the injured tissues; classic signs include pain, heat, redness, swelling, and loss of function.

Inflammatory bowel syndrome   An umbrella term used to describe disorders causing chronic inflammation of the digestive tract. Includes Crohn's disease and ulcerative colitis and is a relapsing and remitting condition characterized by chronic inflammation at numerous sites in the gastrointestinal tract leading to abdominal pain and diarrhea.

Informed consent   A written statement signed by a client prior to testing that informs them of testing purposes, processes, and all potential risks and discomforts.

Inherent risk   Risks that can occur through normal participation in the stated activity. Inherent risks can only be avoided by declining to participate.

Instrumental activities of daily living (IADL)   Activities not necessary for fundamental functioning, but that allow an individual to live independently in a community and require more complex thinking and organizational skills; includes tasks such as housekeeping, managing money, communication, transportation, medications, and shopping. People usually begin asking for outside assistance when these tasks become difficult.

Insulin   A hormone released from the pancreas that allows cells to take up glucose.

Insulin resistance   An inability of muscle tissue to effectively use insulin, where the action of insulin is "resisted" by insulin-sensitive tissues.

Insulin sensitivity   The degree of sensitivity of a receptor site on a tissue cell for insulin, which functions to allow glucose to enter the cell.

Integrated regulation   The most autonomous form of extrinsic motivation. Occurs when a behavior and goals have become integrated into a person's self-concept. People who have internalized motivation for exercise benefits are said to have integrated regulation.

Intermittent claudication   Muscle pain (e.g., ache, cramp, numbness, or sense of fatigue), classically in the calf muscle, which occurs during exercise, such as walking, and is relieved by a short period of rest.

Intrinsic motivation   Motivation that comes from internal states, such as enjoyment or personal satisfaction. The enactment of a behavior because it is consistent with personal goals and values.

Inversion   Rotation of the foot to direct the plantar surface inward; occurs in the frontal plane.

Ischemic stroke   A sudden disruption of cerebral circulation in which blood supply to the brain is either interrupted or diminished.

Isometric   A type of muscular contraction in which the muscle is stimulated to generate tension but little or no joint movement occurs.

Kegel exercises Controlled isometric contraction and relaxation of the muscles that help control the flow of urine to strengthen and gain control of the pelvic floor muscles.

Kinetic chain The concept that joints and segments have an effect on one another during movement.

Korotkoff sounds Five different sounds created by the pulsing of the blood through the brachial artery; proper distinction of the sounds is necessary to determine blood pressure.

Kyphosis Posterior curvature of the spine, typically seen in the thoracic region.

Lactose intolerance A condition that results from a deficiency in the enzyme lactase, which is required to digest lactose; symptoms include cramps, bloating, diarrhea, and flatulence.

Lapse An expected slip or mistake that is usually a discreet event and is a normal part of the behavior-change process.

Lateral Away from the midline of the body, or the outside.

Lean body mass The components of the body (apart from fat), including muscles, bones, nervous tissue, skin, blood, and organs.

Ligament A strong, fibrous tissue that connects one bone to another.

Line of gravity (LOG) A theoretical vertical line passing through the center of gravity, dissecting the body into two hemispheres.

Lipid The name for fats used in the body and bloodstream.

Lipoprotein An assembly of a lipid and protein that serves as a transport vehicle for fatty acids and cholesterol in the blood and lymph.

Lordosis Excessive anterior curvature of the spine that typically occurs at the low back (may also occur at the neck).

Low-density lipoprotein (LDL) A lipoprotein that transports cholesterol and triglycerides from the liver and small intestine to cells and tissues; high levels may cause atherosclerosis.

Maintenance The stage of the transtheoretical model of behavior change during which the individual is incorporating the new behavior into their lifestyle and has been doing so for more than six months.

Malnutrition Refers to deficiencies, excesses, or imbalances in a person's intake of energy and/or nutrients; addresses three broad groups of conditions including (1) undernutrition (wasting or low weight-for-height, stunting or low height-for-age, and underweight or low weight-for-age); (2) Micronutrient-related malnutrition (a lack of or excess of important vitamins and minerals); and (3) Overweight, obesity, and diet-related noncommunicable disease (e.g., heart disease, diabetes and some cancers).

Maximal heart rate (MHR) The highest heart rate a person can attain.

Maximal oxygen uptake ($\dot{V}O_2max$) The maximum capacity for the body to take in, transport, and use oxygen during maximal exertion; a common indicator of physical fitness. Also called aerobic capacity.

Maximal voluntary contraction (MVC) The maximum effort of a muscle or muscle group during a muscular contraction.

Menopause Literally means the "end of monthly cycles"; the end of monthly menstrual periods, which marks the conclusion of a woman's reproductive capabilities.

Metabolic disease Any disease that affects normal metabolism, the process of converting food to energy at a cellular level.

Metabolic equivalent (MET) A simplified system for classifying physical activities where one MET is equal to the resting oxygen consumption, which is approximately 3.5 milliliters of oxygen per kilogram of body weight per minute (3.5 mL/kg/min).

Metabolic syndrome A cluster of factors associated with increased risk for coronary heart disease and diabetes—abdominal obesity indicated by a waist circumference ≥40 inches (102 cm) in men and ≥35 inches (88 cm) in women; levels of triglyceride ≥150 mg/dL (1.7 mmol/L); high-density lipoprotein levels <40 and 50 mg/dL (1.0 and 1.3 mmol/L) in men and women, respectively; blood pressure levels ≥130/85 mmHg; and fasting blood glucose levels ≥110 mg/dL (6.1 mmol/L).

Micronutrient A nutrient that is needed in small quantities for normal growth and development.

Minute ventilation ($\dot{V}_E$) A measure of the amount of air that passes through the lungs in one minute; calculated as the tidal volume multiplied by the ventilatory rate.

Mitochondria The "power plant" of the cells where aerobic metabolism occurs.

Mitosis A type of cell division; the process by which the body makes new cells for growth, development, and repair.

Mobility The degree to which an articulation is allowed to move before being restricted by surrounding tissues or structures.

Morbidity The disease rate; the ratio of sick to well persons in a community.

Mortality The death rate; the ratio of deaths that take place to expected deaths.

Motivation The psychological drive that gives purpose and direction to behavior.

Motivational interviewing (MI) A person-centered conversation style that encourages clients to honestly examine beliefs and behaviors, and that motivates clients to make a decision to change a particular behavior.

Muscular endurance The ability of a muscle or muscle group to exert force against a resistance over a sustained period of time; a health-related component of physical fitness.

Muscular fitness Having appropriate levels of both muscular strength and muscular endurance.

Muscular strength The maximal force a muscle or muscle group can exert during contraction; a health-related component of physical fitness.

Myocardial infarction An episode in which some of the heart's blood supply is severely cut off or restricted, causing the heart muscle to suffer and die from lack of oxygen. Commonly known as a heart attack.

Myocardial ischemia The result of an imbalance between myocardial oxygen supply and demand, most often caused by atherosclerotic plaques that narrow and sometimes completely block the blood supply to the heart.

Myocardium Muscle of the heart.

Negligence Failure of a person to perform as a reasonable and prudent professional would perform under similar circumstances.

Neoplastic Pertaining to any new and abnormal growth, specifically when the growth is uncontrolled and progressive.

Neuroendocrine system Relating to, or involving, the interaction between the nervous system and the hormones of the endocrine glands.

Neuropathy Any disease affecting a peripheral nerve. It may manifest as loss of nerve function, burning pain, or numbness and tingling.

Neuroplasticity   Growth and reorganization of neural networks in the brain as a result of new situations or changes in the environment.

Neurotransmitter   A chemical substance such as acetylcholine or dopamine that transmits nerve impulses across synapses.

Non-high-density lipoprotein (non-HDL)   Cholesterol other than high-density lipoprotein (HDL) circulating in the blood.

Norepinephrine   A hormone released as part of the sympathetic response to exercise; prepares the body for a fight or flight response.

Normotensive   Having normal blood pressure.

Nutrient   A component of food needed by the body. There are six classes of nutrients: water, minerals, vitamins, fats, carbohydrates, and proteins.

Nutrient density   Nutrient content of foods, expressed per reference amount, typically 100 kcal, 100 g, or per serving; nutrient to calorie ratio.

Obesity   An excessive accumulation of body fat. Usually defined as more than 20% above ideal weight, or over 25% body fat for men and over 32% body fat for women; also can be defined as a body mass index of ≥30 kg/m^2 or a waist girth of >40 inches (102 cm) in men and >35 inches (89 cm) in women.

Olfaction   The sense of smell.

Omega-3 fatty acid   An essential fatty acid that promotes a healthy immune system and helps protect against heart disease and other diseases; found in egg yolk and cold water fish and shellfish like tuna, salmon, mackerel, cod, crab, shrimp, and oyster. Also known as linolenic acid.

Omega-6 fatty acid   An essential fatty acid found in flaxseed, canola, and soybean oils and green leaves. Also known as linoleic acid.

One-repetition maximum (1-RM)   The amount of resistance that can be moved through the range of motion one time before the muscle is temporarily fatigued.

Onset of blood lactate accumulation (OBLA)   The point in time during high-intensity exercise at which the production of lactic acid exceeds the body's capacity to eliminate it; after this point, oxygen is insufficient at meeting the body's demands for energy. Also referred to as the second ventilatory threshold (VT2).

Open-ended question   A question that offers the client broad latitude and choice in how to respond.

Orthopnea   Form of dyspnea in which the person can breathe comfortably only when standing or sitting erect; associated with asthma, emphysema, and angina.

Ossification   The formation of bone.

Osteoarthritis   A degenerative disease; characterized by pain and stiffness in the joints. Most common form of arthritis.

Osteoarthrosis   Similar to osteoarthritis, but without the joint inflammation; a non-inflammatory disease of the joint in which the cartilage in the joint breaks down. This degenerative disease occurs as a result of injury, aging, and long-term wear and tear of cartilage in the joints.

Osteomalacia   Softening of the bone.

Osteopenia   A disorder in which bone density is below average, classified as 1.5 to 2.5 standard deviations below peak bone density.

Osteophytes   Bone spurs; the result of deterioration of the articular cartilage, causing a tremendous amount of pain.

Osteoporosis   A disorder, primarily affecting postmenopausal women, in which bone mineral density decreases and susceptibility to fractures increases.

Overtraining   Constant intense training that does not provide adequate time for recovery; symptoms include increased resting heart rate, impaired physical performance, reduced enthusiasm and desire for training, increased incidence of injuries and illness, altered appetite, disturbed sleep patterns, and irritability.

Overtraining syndrome   A condition brought on by overtraining; symptoms include increased resting heart rate, impaired physical performance, reduced enthusiasm and desire for training, increased incidence of injuries and illness, altered appetite, disturbed sleep patterns, and irritability.

Overweight   A term to describe an excessive amount of weight for a given height, using height-to-weight ratios.

Palpation   The use of hands and/or fingers to detect anatomical structures or an arterial pulse (e.g., carotid pulse).

Palpitation   A rapid and irregular heartbeat.

Papillae   Small nipple-like projections, such as a protuberance on the skin, at the root of a hair, taste buds on the tongue, or at the base of a developing tooth.

Paresthesia   An abnormal sensation such as numbness, prickling, or tingling.

Parkinson's disease (PD)   A degenerative disorder of the central nervous system that often impairs the sufferer's motor skills and speech; characterized by muscle rigidity, tremor, a slowing of physical movement and, in extreme cases, a loss of physical movement.

Paroxysmal nocturnal dyspnea   Attacks of severe shortness of breath and coughing that generally occur at night.

Pathology   Anatomic or functional manifestations of a disease.

Percent daily value (PDV)   How much a nutrient in a single serving of a packaged food or dietary supplement contributes to a person's daily diet; can be used to determine how a food fits into a daily meal plan, not just one meal or snack, for a person eating 2,000 calories per day.

Percutaneous transluminal coronary angioplasty   A procedure that uses a small balloon at the tip of a heart catheter to push open plaques; usually followed by the insertion of a stent.

Performance goal   A goal that represents change in a measurable variable, such as increases in strength scores, reductions in resting heart rate, or weight loss. Also called a product goal.

Perfusion   The passage of fluid through a tissue, such as the transport of blood through vessels from the heart to internal organs and other tissues.

Perimenopause   The transitional period of time before menstruation actually stops; the time nearing menopause.

Periodization   The systematic application of overload through the pre-planned variation of program components to optimize gains in strength (or any specific component of fitness), while preventing overuse, staleness, overtraining, and plateaus.

Peripheral artery disease (PAD)   Any disease caused by the obstruction of large peripheral arteries, which can result from atherosclerosis, inflammatory processes leading to stenosis, an embolism, or thrombus formation. Also called peripheral arterial disease.

Peripheral nervous system (PNS)   The parts of the nervous system that are outside the brain and spinal cord (central nervous system).

Peripheral neuropathy   Damage to nerves of the peripheral nervous system, which may be caused either by diseases of the nerve or from the side effects of systemic illness.

Peripheral vascular disease   A painful and often debilitating condition characterized by muscular pain caused by ischemia to the working muscles. The ischemic pain is usually due to atherosclerotic blockages or arterial spasms, referred to as claudication. Also called peripheral vascular occlusive disease (PVOD).

Physical Activity Readiness Questionnaire for Everyone (PAR-Q+)   A brief, self-administered medical questionnaire recognized as a safe pre-exercise screening measure for low-to-moderate (but not vigorous) exercise training.

Physically active   Meeting the recommended levels of regular physical activity.

Physically inactive   Not getting any moderate- or vigorous-intensity physical activity beyond basic movement from daily life activities.

Physiological age   See Biological age.

Planes of motion   The conceptual planes in which the body moves; called the sagittal, frontal, and transverse planes; often used as a way to describe anatomical movement.

Plantar flexion   Distal movement of the plantar surface of the foot; opposite of dorsiflexion.

Plaque   A combination of fat, cholesterol, calcium, and other substances found in blood that over time hardens and narrows arteries.

Plyometrics   High-intensity movements, such as jumping, involving high-force loading of body weight during the landing phase of the movement that take advantage of the stretch-shortening cycle.

Polypharmacy   The use of multiple medications by a patient, generally older adults; more specifically, it is often defined as the use of five or more regular medications.

Positive energy balance   A situation when the storage of energy exceeds the amount expended. This state may be achieved by either consuming too many calories or by not expending enough through physical activity.

Postexercise hypotension   Acute postexercise reduction in both systolic and diastolic blood pressure.

Posture   The arrangement of the body and its limbs.

Power   The capacity to move with a combination of speed and force; a skill-related component of physical fitness.

Precontemplation   The stage of the transtheoretical model of behavior change during which the individual is not intending to change within the next six months.

Preparation   The stage of the transtheoretical model of behavior change during which the individual is getting ready to make a change.

Presbyopia   A term meaning "old eye"; a gradual loss of the ability to see things clearly up close that occurs with age.

Presbyosmia   Age-related diminished sense of smell.

Previously physically inactive   Describes an individual who previously was not meeting the recommendations for regular physical activity.

Process goal   A goal a person achieves by doing something, such as completing an exercise session or attending a talk on stress management.

Product goal   See Performance goal.

Progesterone   Female sex hormone produced by the ovaries, adrenal cortex, and placenta that affects many aspects of female physiology, including menstrual cycles and pregnancy.

Pronation   Internal rotation of the forearm causing the radius to cross diagonally over the ulna and the palm to face posteriorly.

Proprioception   Sensation and awareness of knowing where one's body or body part is in space.

Protected health information   Health data created, received, stored, or transmitted by the Health Insurance Portability and Accountability Act (HIPAA)–covered entities and their business associates in relation to the provision of healthcare, healthcare operations, and payment for healthcare services. Protected health information includes individually identifiable health information, including demographic data, medical histories, test results, insurance information, and other information used to identify clients or provide healthcare services or healthcare coverage. 'Protected' means the information is protected under the HIPAA Privacy Rule.

Protein   A compound composed of a combination 20 amino acids that is the major structural component of all body tissue; one of the macronutrients found in a variety of animal and plant sources and helps to clot blood; balance bodily fluids; contract and build muscles; transport oxygen, vitamins, minerals, and fats around the body; and fight infections. Each gram of protein contains four calories.

Proximal   Nearest to the midline of the body or point of origin of a muscle.

Psychological age   A measurement of aging based on an individual's abilities of mental and cognitive functioning, including self-esteem, self-efficacy, learning, memory, and perception. How old one acts, feels, and behaves.

Pursed-lip breathing   A breathing technique that increases the amount of air taken in through the damaged tissues of the lungs (e.g., in COPD patients) and reduces the incidence of dyspnea.

Quickness   The quality of moving fast.

Range of motion (ROM)   The number of degrees that an articulation will allow one of its segments to move.

Rapport   A relationship marked by mutual understanding and trust.

Rating of perceived exertion (RPE)   A scale, originally developed by noted Swedish psychologist Gunnar Borg, that provides a standard means for evaluating a participant's perception of exercise effort. The original scale ranged from 6 to 20; a revised category ratio scale ranges from 0 to 10.

Readiness to change   A reference to how likely someone is to make a behavioral change based on their current stage of change (precontemplation, contemplation, preparation, action, or maintenance) according to the transtheoretical model of behavior change.

Recommended Dietary Allowance (RDA)   The levels of intake of essential nutrients that, on the basis of scientific knowledge, are judged by the Food and Nutrition Board to be adequate to meet the known needs of practically all healthy persons.

Reflecting   A feature of active listening in which the health coach or exercise professional makes a best guess at the underlying meaning of what a client has said.

Registered dietitian (RD)   A food and nutrition expert who has met the following criteria: completed a minimum of a bachelor's degree at a U.S. or regionally accredited university, or college and coursework accredited by the Accreditation Council for Education in Nutrition and Dietetics (ACEND); completed an ACEND-accredited supervised practice program;

passed a national examination; and completed continuing professional education requirements to maintain registration. Also called a registered dietitian nutritionist.

Relapse   In behavioral change, the return of an original problem after many lapses (i.e., slips or mistakes) have occurred.

Relapse-prevention model   A cognitive-behavioral approach to addressing behavioral change, with the goal of identifying and preventing high-risk situations.

Relative age   The extent to which an individual is aging faster or slower than an average person of the same age.

Renal plasma flow   The volume of plasma that flows through the kidney over a specified period of time.

Respiratory compensation threshold   See Second ventilatory threshold (VT2).

Respondeat superior   A legal doctrine wherein the actions of an employee can subject the employer to liability; Latin for "Let the master answer."

Resting energy expenditure   The amount of energy expended at rest; represents 60 to 75% of the body's total energy expenditure.

Resting heart rate (RHR)   The number of heartbeats per minute when the body is at complete rest; usually counted first thing in the morning before any physical activity.

Retinopathy   Any non-inflammatory disease of the retina.

Rheumatoid arthritis   An autoimmune disease that causes inflammation of connective tissues and joints.

Sagittal plane   The longitudinal plane that divides the body into right and left portions.

Sarcopenia   Decreased muscle mass; often used to refer specifically to an age-related decline in muscle mass or lean-body tissue that may result in diminished muscle strength and functional performance.

Sarcopenic obesity   The presence of obesity in combination with sarcopenia.

Satiety   A feeling of fullness.

Saturated fat   A fatty acid that contains no double bonds between carbon atoms; typically solid at room temperature and very stable.

Scoliosis   Excessive lateral curvature of the spine.

Scope of practice   The range and limit of responsibilities normally associated with a specific job or profession.

Second ventilatory threshold (VT2)   A metabolic marker that represents the point at which high-intensity exercise can no longer be sustained due to an accumulation of lactate.

Sedentary   Describing any waking behavior characterized by a low level of energy expenditure [less than or equal to 1.5 metabolic equivalents (METs)] while sitting, reclining, or lying.

Self-efficacy   One's perception of their ability to change or to perform specific behaviors (e.g., exercise).

Self–myofascial release   The act of rolling one's own body on a round foam roll or other training tool, massaging away restrictions to normal soft-tissue extensibility.

Senescence   The process or condition of growing old.

Serotonin   A neurotransmitter; acts as a synaptic messenger in the brain and as an inhibitor of pain pathways; plays a role in mood and sleep.

Serving   A standardized amount of food used to quantify recommended amounts or represent quantities that people typically consume.

Sinoatrial node   A group of specialized myocardial cells, located in the wall of the right atrium, that control the heart's rate of contraction; the "pacemaker" of the heart.

Sinus tachycardia   A regular cardiac rhythm in which the heart beats faster than normal and results in an increase in cardiac output; elevated heart rate over 100 beats per minute. Commonly occurs as a compensatory response to exercise or stress but becomes concerning when it occurs at rest.

Slow-twitch muscle fiber   A muscle fiber type designed for use of aerobic glycolysis and fatty acid oxidation, recruited for low-intensity, longer-duration activities such as walking and swimming. Also called type I muscle fiber.

SMART goal   A properly designed goal; SMART stands for specific, measurable, attainable, relevant, and time-bound.

Social age   Considers aging in terms of what is and is not socially acceptable behavior for a person of a particular age group.

Social support   The perceived comfort, caring, esteem, or help an individual receives from other people.

Somatosensory system   The physiological system relating to the perception of sensory stimuli from the skin and internal organs.

Specificity   Exercise training principle explaining that specific exercise demands made on the body produce specific responses by the body; also called exercise specificity.

Speed   Rate of movement; a skill-related component of physical fitness.

Sprain   A traumatic joint twist that results in stretching or tearing of the stabilizing connective tissues; mainly involves ligaments or joint capsules, and causes discoloration, swelling, and pain.

Stability   Characteristic of the body's joints or posture that represents resistance to change of position.

Standard of care   Appropriateness of a health coach or exercise professional's actions in light of current professional standards and based on the age, condition, and knowledge of the client or participant.

Static balance   The ability to maintain the body's center of mass within its base of support.

Static stretching   Holding a nonmoving (static) position to immobilize a joint in a position that places the desired muscles and connective tissues passively at their greatest possible length.

Statute of limitations   A formal regulation limiting the period within which a specific legal action may be taken.

Strain   A stretch, tear, or rip in the muscle or adjacent tissue such as the fascia or tendon.

Stress urinary incontinence (SUI)   Pressure (or stress) on the bladder resulting from physical movement or activity, such as coughing, sneezing, running, or heavy lifting. Not related to psychological stress.

Stroke   A sudden and often severe ischemic attack due to blockage of an artery into the brain.

Stroke volume (SV)   The amount of blood pumped from the left ventricle of the heart with each beat.

Successful aging   A four-component concept that considers absence of disease or well-managed disease, minimal to no depressive symptoms, good physical and cognitive function, and active life engagement.

Supination   External rotation of the forearm (radioulnar joint) that causes the palm to face anteriorly.

Sympathetic nervous system A branch of the autonomic nervous system responsible for mobilizing the body's energy and resources during times of stress and arousal (i.e., the fight or flight response). Opposes the physiological effects of the parasympathetic nervous system (e.g., reduces digestive secretions, speeds the heart, contracts blood vessels).

Sympathomimetic A characteristic of medications that mimic the effects of the sympathetic nervous system.

Syncope A transient state of unconsciousness during which a person collapses to the floor as a result of lack of oxygen to the brain; commonly known as fainting.

Synovial fluid A thick fluid produced by the synovial membrane that nourishes articular cartilages and lubricates joint surfaces.

Synovial membrane One of two layers making up the articular capsule that encloses synovial joints. This membrane is well supplied with capillaries and produces a thick fluid called synovial fluid that nourishes articular cartilages and lubricates joint surfaces.

Synovium The connective-tissue membrane that lines the cavity of a synovial joint and produces the synovial fluid; also called synovial membrane.

Systolic blood pressure (SBP) The pressure exerted by the blood on the vessel walls during ventricular contraction.

Tachycardia A heart rate over 100 beats per minute, typically as a result of a heart rhythm disorder.

Talk test A method for measuring exercise intensity using observation of respiration effort and the ability to talk while exercising.

Target heart rate Number of heartbeats per minute that indicates an appropriate exercise intensity levels for each individual; also called training heart rate. Usually expressed as a percentage of maximum heart rate.

T-cell Type of leukocyte (white blood cell) that is an essential part of the immune system.

Telemetry The use of instruments to record electrical signals from within the body, such as a heartbeat.

Telomere Specialized deoxyribonucleic acid (DNA) that sits at the end of a chromosome to prevent damage. Each time a cell divides, the telomere becomes shorter, limiting how many times a cell can divide before losing some of the important DNA on the chromosome.

Tendinitis Inflammation of a tendon.

Tendon A band of fibrous tissue forming the termination of a muscle and attaching the muscle to a bone.

Testosterone In males, the steroid hormone produced in the testes; involved in growth and development of reproductive tissues, sperm, and secondary male sex characteristics.

Tidal volume The volume of air inspired per breath.

Torsion The rotation or twisting of a joint by the exertion of a lateral force tending to turn it about a longitudinal axis.

Total peripheral resistance (TPR) The resistance to the passage of blood through the small blood vessels, especially arterioles.

Trans fat An unsaturated fatty acid that is converted into a saturated fat to increase the shelf life of some products.

Transient ischemic attack (TIA) A transient stroke that lasts only a few minutes; occurs when the blood supply to part of the brain is briefly interrupted. TIA symptoms, which usually occur suddenly, are similar to those of stroke but do not last as long.

Transtheoretical model of behavior change (TTM)   A theory of behavior that examines one's readiness to change and identifies five stages: precontemplation, contemplation, preparation, action, and maintenance. Also called the stages-of-change model.

Transverse plane   Anatomical term for the imaginary line that divides the body, or any of its parts, into upper (superior) and lower (inferior) parts. Also called the horizontal plane.

Triglyceride   Three fatty acids joined to a glycerol (carbon and hydrogen structure) backbone; how fat is stored in the body.

Type 1 diabetes   Form of diabetes caused by the destruction of the insulin-producing beta cells in the pancreas, which leads to little or no insulin production; generally develops in childhood and requires regular insulin injections; formerly known as insulin-dependent diabetes mellitus (IDDM) and childhood-onset diabetes.

Type 2 diabetes   Most common form of diabetes; typically develops in adulthood and is characterized by a reduced sensitivity of the insulin target cells to available insulin; usually associated with obesity; formerly known as non-insulin-dependent diabetes mellitus (NIDDM) and adult-onset diabetes.

Type I muscle fiber   See Slow-twitch muscle fiber.

Type II muscle fiber   See Fast-twitch muscle fiber.

Valsalva effect   Increased intrabdominal and intrathoracic pressure due to Valsalva maneuver.

Valsalva maneuver   Forced expiration against a closed glottis to compress the contents of the thoracic and abdominal cavity causing an increased intrabdominal and intrathoracic pressure.

Vasoconstriction   Narrowing of the opening of blood vessels (notably the smaller arterioles) caused by contraction of the smooth muscle lining the vessels.

Vasodilation   Increase in diameter of the blood vessels, especially dilation of arterioles leading to increased blood flow to a part of the body.

Vasomotor symptoms (VMS)   Hot flashes and night sweats associated with perimenopause and menopause.

Vasovagal response   A response that occurs from pressure placed on the vagus nerve, which slows the heart rate and can cause fainting.

Vegan   A vegetarian who also does not consume any animal products, including dairy products such as milk and cheese, eggs, and may exclude honey.

Vegetarian   A person who does not eat meat, fish, poultry, or products containing these foods.

Ventilatory threshold   Point of transition between predominantly aerobic energy production to anaerobic energy production; involves recruitment of fast-twitch muscle fibers and is identified via gas exchange during exercise testing.

Ventricular fibrillation (VF)   An irregular heartbeat characterized by uncoordinated contractions of the ventricle.

Vestibular system   Part of the central nervous system that coordinates reflexes of the eyes, neck, and body to maintain equilibrium in accordance with posture and movement of the head.

Vicarious liability   Legal term meaning that employers are responsible for the workplace conduct of their employees.

Visceral   Pertaining to the internal organs.

Viscosity   Refers to the thickness of a fluid, or a fluid's resistance to flow.

Visual system   The series of structures by which visual sensations are received from the environment and conveyed as signals to the central nervous system.

$\dot{V}O_2$max   See Maximal oxygen uptake ($\dot{V}O_2$max).

Waist circumference   Abdominal girth measured at the level of the umbilicus; values >40 inches (102 cm) in men and >35 inches (89 cm) in women are strong indicators of abdominal obesity and associated with an increased health risk.

Waiver   Voluntary abandonment of a right to file suit; not always legally binding.

Index

American Council on Exercise

G

gait

aging on, 65

assessments, 213–227. See also balance and gait assessments; specific assessments

evaluation, Tinetti, 226, 226t

gastrointestinal system function, on nutrition, 92–93

genetic theories, of aging, 69

Global Action Plan on Physical Activity 2018–2030: More Active People for a Healthier World (WHO), 71–73

Global Recommendations on Physical Activity for Health (WHO), 71

glomerular filtration rate, 96

gluteal muscles

dominant, squat, 243–244, 244f

self–myofascial release for, 274, 274f

glute bridge, 266t, 267f

goals (exercise)

action stage, 40–41, 42b–44b

assessment data and feasibility, 53

commitment and time frame, 54

evaluating original and setting new, 42b–44b

Muscular Training, programming, 261

performance, 51

physical activity, 51

pre-exercise interview, 121

process, 37b

product, 51

short-term, 53

revising, 40–41

SMART, 52–53

goal setting, 50–57

behavioral contract, 54, 54b

behavior vs. outcome focus, 53

commitment, time frame, 54

effective, 55b–57b

empowerment, 22

key considerations, 50–51

short-term goals, 40–41, 53

SMART goals, 52–53

grains

refined, food label, 112f, 113

whole

added, food label, 112f, 113

healthy eating patterns, 109

gross negligence, 142

growth hormone, 96

gum disease, 97

H

hamstrings

seated stretch, 303b, 303f

self–myofascial release for, 274, 274f

static stretching for, 274, 274f

hay baler, 290, 291b, 291f

Hayflick, Leonard, 68, 69

Hayflick limit, 69

health and fitness, 4–6

health belief model, 21–22, 21f

health benefits, 71, 72t. See also specific types

health benefits, physical activity, 71, 72t, 173–174

health challenges, 332–387

cardiovascular and cerebral disorders, 335–348, 335t

coronary artery disease, 335–340

Korotkoff sounds, 200, 202

kyphosis, 203, 264f

   muscle imbalances, 264t, 266b

   stability/mobility warm-up, 266t,
      267f–268f

L

labels, nutrition, reading, 111–114, 112f

lapse

   vs. relapse, 47

   temporary, 25

lateral lunge, 298b, 298f

latissimus dorsi, self–myofascial release for,
      266t, 268f

lat pull-down, 302b, 302f, 313f

lean body mass, 193

leg press, 309f

leukotriene modifiers, for asthma, 350

levalbuterol, for asthma, 350

liberation

   self-liberation, 26t

   social, 26t

lifestyle and health-history questionnaire,
      144, 145f–148f

ligaments, 77

line of gravity (LOG), 275

lipids, blood. See also cholesterol; specific
      types

   body fat on, 76

   physical activity on, 75–76

5-lipoxygenase inhibitor, for asthma,
      350

listening

   active, 7–8

   without interruption, 9

Load/Speed Training, 172–173, 173t

Load/Speed Training, programming, 296–320

   athletic performance, 314b–319b,
         315f–319f

      agility drills, 318f–319f

      ankle hops/hop progressions, 317f

      box jump progression, 318f

      cone/hurdle hops, 317f

      countermovement jump, 315f

      definitions and applications,
            314b–316b

      double-leg butt kicks, 317f

      split jump, 317f

      stride jump, 316f

   cool-down, 303b–304b, 303f–304f

   delayed-onset muscle soreness, 314

   jumping and hopping techniques, 320

   muscular strength improvement, 296

   muscular strength improvement, exercise
         guidelines, 305–307

      frequency, 305

      intensity, 305

      repetitions, 305–306

      sets, 306–307

      type, 307

   strength, examples, 308b–313b,
         308f–313f

      bend-and-lift, deadlift, 308f

      bend-and-lift, leg press, 309f

      bend-and-lift, squat, 308f

      pulling, lat pull-down, 313f

      pulling, mid row, 312f

      pulling, pull-up, 313f

      pushing, bench press, 310f

      pushing, incline press, 311f

      pushing, shoulder press, 311f

      pushing, triceps kickback, 312f

N

with bend-and lift and rotational movement, squat with 1-arm overhead spiral, 299b, 299f

incline press, 311f

shoulder press, 301b, 301f, 311f

triceps kickback, 301b, 301f, 312f

Q

quadriceps muscle

dominance, squat, 243

self–myofascial release for, 274, 274f

questionnaires

for exercise professionals, 124, 127f

fall-risk, 149–150, 149t

lifestyle and health-history, 144, 145f–148f

Physical Activity Readiness Questionnaire for Everyone, 130, 131t–134t

questions

direct, closed, 123

open-ended, 123

R

radial artery, pulse rate, 196, 196f

range of motion (ROM)

center of gravity control through, 172

muscular imbalance on, 204

programming, for mobility, 273–274, 274f

range-of-motion training

hip mobility/ROM, seated hamstrings stretch, 303b, 303f

seated 90-90° stretch, 304b, 304f

rapport, building positive, 7

rating of perceived exertion (RPE), 199

assessment, 199, 199f

Base Training, 168, 325, 325f

with beta blockers, 338b

with calcium channel blockers, 338b

Fitness Training, 168, 326–327

maximal heart rate, 199

Performance Training, 328

three-zone intensity model, 320–321, 322t

readiness to change, 27

Recommended Dietary Allowance (RDA), macronutrient, 103t, 104–105

record keeping, 151–153

correspondence, 152, 153f

exercise record, 151

HIPAA permission form, for medical doctor/personal trainer, 152, 153f

incident report, 151–152

medical history, 151

reevaluation, self-, 26t

regulation

autonomous, 39

external, 39

integrated, 39

reinforcement, management, 26t

relapse, 20

vs. lapse, 47

relapse prevention

model, 24–25

skills, 46–47

relationship

client–exercise professional, 11

helping, 26t

relative age, 63

release, medical, 150, 150f

reminders, exercise, 39

renal plasma flow, 96

American Council on Exercise